MORE 4U!

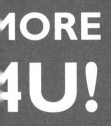

theclinics.com

This Clinics series is available online.

re's what
u get:

- Full text of EVERY issue from 2002 to NOW
- Figures, tables, drawings, references and more
- Searchable: find what you need fast

  Search | All Clinics ▼ | for | | GO |

- Linked to MEDLINE and Elsevier journals
- E-alerts

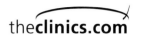

PEDIATRIC CLINICS

OF NORTH AMERICA

Diabetes Mellitus in Children

GUEST EDITOR
Mark A. Sperling, MD

December 2005 • Volume 52 • Number 6

SAUNDERS

An Imprint of Elsevier, Inc.
PHILADELPHIA   LONDON   TORONTO   MONTREAL   SYDNEY   TOKYO

W.B. SAUNDERS COMPANY
A Division of Elsevier Inc.

1600 John F. Kennedy Boulevard • Suite 1800 • Philadelphia, Pennsylvania 19103

http://www.theclinics.com

THE PEDIATRIC CLINICS OF NORTH AMERICA	Volume 52, Number 6
December 2005	ISSN 0031-3955
Editor: Carin Davis	ISBN 1-4160-2753-X

The ideas and opinions expressed in *The Pediatric Clinics of North America* do not necessarily reflect those of the Publisher. The Publisher does not assume any responsibility for any injury and/or damage to persons or property arising out of or related to any use of the material contained in this periodical. The reader is advised to check the appropriate medical literature and the product information currently provided by the manufacturer of each drug to be administered to verify the dosage, the method and duration of administration, or contraindications. It is the responsibility of the treating physician or other health care professional, relying on independent experience and knowledge of the patient, to determine drug dosages and the best treatment for the patient. Mention of any product in this issue should not be construed as endorsement by the contributors, editors, or the Publisher of the product or manufacturers' claims.

The Pediatric Clinics of North America (ISSN 0031-3955) is published bi-monthly by W.B. Saunders Company, Corporate and Editorial offices: 1600 JFK Boulevard, Suite 1800, Philadelphia, PA 19103-2822. Accounting and Circulation offices: 6277 Sea Harbor Drive, Orlando, FL 32887-4800. Periodicals postage paid at Orlando, FL 32862, and additional mailing offices. Subscription prices are $125.00 per year (US individuals), $260.00 per year (US institutions), $170.00 per year (Canadian individuals), $340.00 per year (Canadian institutions), $190.00 per year (international individuals), $340.00 per year (international institutions), $65.00 per year (US students), $100.00 per year (Canadian students), and $100.00 per year (foreign students). To receive student/resident rate, orders must be accompanied by name of affiliated institution, date of term, and the signature of program/residency coordinator on institution letterhead. Orders will be billed at individual rate until proof of status is received. Foreign air speed delivery is included in all Clinics subscription prices. All prices are subject to change without notice. POSTMASTER: Send address changes to *The Pediatric Clinics of North America*, W.B. Saunders Company, Periodicals Fulfillment, Orlando, FL 32887-4800. **Customer Service: 1-800-654-2452 (US). From outside of the US, call 1-407-345-4000.** E-mail: hhspcs@harcourt.com.

The Pediatric Clinics of North America is also published in Spanish by McGraw-Hill Inter-americana Editores S.A., Mexico City, Mexico; in Portuguese by Reichmann and Affonso Editores, Rua Comandante Coelho 1085, CEP 21250, Rio de Janeiro, Brazil; and in Greek by Althayia SA, Athens, Greece.

The Pediatric Clinics of North America is covered in *Index Medicus, Excerpta Medica, Current Contents, Current Contents/Clinical Medicine, Science Citation Index, ASCA, ISI/BIOMED*, and *BIOSIS*.

Printed in the United States of America.

GUEST EDITOR

MARK A. SPERLING, MD, Professor of Pediatrics, University of Pittsburgh School of
Medicine, Division of Endocrinology, Diabetes, and Metabolism, Department of
Pediatrics, Children's Hospital of Pittsburgh, Pittsburgh, Pennsylvania

CONTRIBUTORS

HOLLY ANTAL, PhD, Post-Doctoral Fellow in Psychology, Division of Psychology and
Psychiatry, Nemours Children's Clinic, Jacksonville, Florida

SILVA ARSLANIAN, MD, Division of Pediatric Endocrinology, Metabolism, and Diabetes
Mellitus, Children's Hospital of Pittsburgh, Pittsburgh, Pennsylvania

MARK A. ATKINSON, PhD, Sebastian Family Eminent Scholar, Director, The Center for
Immunology and Transplantation, University of Florida, Gainesville, Florida

FIDA BACHA, MD, Division of Pediatric Endocrinology, Metabolism, and Diabetes
Mellitus, Children's Hospital of Pittsburgh, Pittsburgh, Pennsylvania

DOROTHY BECKER, MBBCh, FCP, Professor, Department of Pediatrics, Director,
Division of Endocrinology, Children's Hospital of Pittsburgh, University of
Pittsburgh, Pittsburgh, Pennsylvania

LISA M. BUCKLOH, PhD, Clinical Research Psychologist, Division of Psychology and
Psychiatry, Nemours Children's Clinic, Jacksonville, Florida

ANNA CASU, MD, Post-Doctural Fellow, Division of Immunogenetics, Department of
Pediatrics, Rangos Research Center, Children's Hospital of Pittsburgh, University of
Pittsburgh School of Medicine, Pittsburgh, Pennsylvania

DENIS DANEMAN, MB, BCH, FRCPC, Professor of Pediatrics and Chief, Division of
Endocrinology, Department of Pediatrics, The Hospital for Sick Children and
University of Toronto, Toronto, Ontario, Canada

KIM C. DONAGHUE, MBBS, PhD, FRACP, Associate Professor, University of Sydney;
Head of Diabetes Services, Institute of Endocrinology and Diabetes, The Children's
Hospital at Westmead, Sydney, Australia

NICOLE GLASER, MD, Associate Professor, Department of Pediatrics, University of
California Davis, School of Medicine, Sacramento, California

SARAH J. GLASTRAS, MBBS (Hons), BSc Psychol (Hons), Institute of Endocrinology
and Diabetes, The Children's Hospital at Westmead, Sydney, Australia

NESLIHAN GUNGOR, MD, Division of Pediatric Endocrinology, Metabolism, and Diabetes Mellitus, Children's Hospital of Pittsburgh, Pittsburgh, Pennsylvania

NURSEN GURTUNCA, MD, FCP, Research Associate, Division of Endocrinology, Department of Pediatrics, University of Pittsburgh, Pittsburgh, Pennsylvania

MICHAEL J. HALLER, MD, Pediatric Endocrinology Fellow, University of Florida, Gainesville, Florida

TAMARA HANNON, MD, Division of Pediatric Endocrinology, Metabolism, and Diabetes Mellitus, Children's Hospital of Pittsburgh, Pittsburgh, Pennsylvania

DIEGO IZE-LUDLOW, MD, Pediatric Endocrinology Fellow, Division of Endocrinology, Diabetes, and Metabolism, University of Pittsburgh School of Medicine, Children's Hospital of Pittsburgh, Pittsburgh, Pennsylvania

ELKA JACOBSON-DICKMAN, MD, Fellow in Pediatric Endocrinology, Massachusetts General Hospital for Children and Harvard Medical School; Pediatric Endocrine Unit, Massachusetts General Hospital, Boston, Massachusetts

LYNNE LEVITSKY, MD, Associate Professor of Pediatrics, Massachusetts General Hospital for Children and Harvard Medical School; Chief, Pediatric Endocrine Unit, Massachusetts General Hospital, Boston, Massachusetts

INGRID LIBMAN, MD, PhD, Division of Pediatric Endocrinology, Metabolism, and Diabetes Mellitus, Children's Hospital of Pittsburgh, Pittsburgh, Pennsylvania

AMANDA SOBEL LOCHRIE, PhD, Clinical Research Psychologist, Division of Psychology and Psychiatry, Nemours Children's Clinic, Jacksonville, Florida

FAUZIA MOHSIN, MBBS, FCPS, Institute of Endocrinology and Diabetes, The Children's Hospital at Westmead, Sydney, Australia

MERANDA NAKHLA, MD, Clinical Fellow, Department of Pediatrics, Division of Pediatric Endocrinology, McGill University Health Center, Montréal, Québec, Canada

KUSIEL PERLMAN, MD, FRCPC, Associate Professor of Pediatrics, Division of Endocrinology, Department of Pediatrics, The Hospital for Sick Children and University of Toronto, Toronto, Ontario, Canada

MASSIMO PIETROPAOLO, MD, Associate Professor, Division of Immunogenetics, Department of Pediatrics, Rangos Research Center, Children's Hospital of Pittsburgh, University of Pittsburgh School of Medicine, Pittsburgh, Pennsylvania

CONSTANTIN POLYCHRONAKOS, MD, Professor, Department of Pediatrics, Division of Pediatric Endocrinology, McGill University Health Center, Montréal, Québec, Canada

MARIANNA RACHMIEL, MD, Senior Fellow, Division of Endocrinology, Department of Pediatrics, The Hospital for Sick Children and University of Toronto, Toronto, Ontario, Canada

CHRISTOPHER RYAN, PhD, Professor of Psychiatry, Psychology, Health and Community Systems; Director, University of Pittsburgh Institutional Review Board; Department of Psychiatry, University of Pittsburgh, Western Pennsylvania Psychiatric Institute and Clinic, Pittsburgh, Pennsylvania

DESMOND SCHATZ, MD, Professor and Associate Chairman of Pediatrics, Medical Director, Diabetes Center, University of Florida, Gainesville, Florida

KRISTIN A. SIKES, MSN, Yale Pediatric Diabetes Research Program, Yale School of Medicine, New Haven, Connecticut

MARK A. SPERLING, MD, Professor of Pediatrics, University of Pittsburgh School of Medicine, Division of Endocrinology, Diabetes, and Metabolism, Department of Pediatrics, Children's Hospital of Pittsburgh, Pittsburgh, Pennsylvania

AMY T. STEFFEN, BS, Yale Pediatric Diabetes Research Program, Yale School of Medicine, New Haven, Connecticut

WILLIAM V. TAMBORLANE, MD, Professor, Department of Pediatrics and General Clinical Research Center, Yale University School of Medicine, New Haven, Connecticut

MASSIMO TRUCCO, MD, Hillman Professor of Pediatric Immunology; Head, Division of Immunogenetics, Department of Pediatrics, Rangos Research Center, Children's Hospital of Pittsburgh, University of Pittsburgh School of Medicine, Pittsburgh, Pennsylvania

STUART A. WEINZIMER, MD, Associate Professor, Department of Pediatrics, Yale University School of Medicine, New Haven, Connecticut

TIM WYSOCKI, PhD, Director, Center for Pediatric Psychology Research, Nemours Children's Clinic, Jacksonville, Florida

CONTENTS

Diabetes is the extreme manifestation of a spectrum conditions in which the balance of insulin secretion and insulin action (or insulin resistance) has been altered. Loss of euglycemia is caused by relative insulin deficiency in the presence of insulin resistance, or by absolute insulin deficiency. There are related conditions in which an alteration of insulin resistance or β-cell dysfunction exists, but because of compensation glucose homeostasis has not been lost. The elucidation of the causes of insulin resistance and β-cell failure and the attention to the different degrees of insulin deficiency and insulin resistance allow for better diagnosis, treatment, and prevention of diabetes and its related conditions.

This article reviews our current understanding of the etiology, presentation, and management of type 1 diabetes. The discussion includes a review of the natural history of diabetes, the complex relationship between genetic and environmental risk for type 1 diabetes, and current methods for prediction of type 1 diabetes. The article also reviews the current management of children who have new-onset type 1 diabetes, age-appropriate management goals, and diabetes complications. Finally, the article discusses the future of diabetes screening programs and the progress toward the ultimate goal of curing type 1 diabetes.

patients and their parents. Although transient detrimental effects are clearly disturbing and may have severe results, there is surprisingly little evidence of long-term CNS damage, even after multiple hypoglycemic episodes, except in rare instances. Despite the latter evidence, we advocate that every treatment regimen be designed to prevent hypoglycemia without inducing unacceptable hyperglycemia and increasing the risk of micro- and macrovascular complications.

individuals before the clinical onset of the disease has provided a real opportunity for the identification of risk markers and the design of therapeutic intervention. With such a high degree of predictability using a combination of immunologic markers, strategies to prevent T1DM may become possible. A number of novel therapeutic strategies are under investigation in newly diagnosed T1DM patients and might ultimately be applied to prevent T1DM.

FORTHCOMING ISSUES

RECENT ISSUES

PEDIATRIC CLINICS OF NORTH AMERICA DECEMBER 2005

GOAL STATEMENT

The goal of *Pediatric Clinics of North America* is to keep practicing physicians and residents up to date with current clinical practice in pediatrics by providing timely articles reviewing the state-of-the-art in patient care.

ACCREDITATION

The *Pediatric Clinics of North America* is planned and implemented in accordance with the Essential Areas and Policies of the Accreditation Council for Continuing Medical Education (ACCME) through the joint sponsorship of the University of Virginia School of Medicine and Elsevier. The University of Virginia School of Medicine is accredited by the ACCME to provide continuing medical education for physicians.

The University of Virginia School of Medicine designates this educational activity for a maximum of 90 category 1 credits per year, 15 category 1 credits per issue, toward the AMA Physician's Recognition Award. Each physician should claim only those credits that he/she actually spent in the activity.

The American Medical Association has determined that physicians not licensed in the US who participate in this CME activity are eligible for AMA PRA category 1 credit.

Category 1 credit can be earned by reading the text material, taking the CME examination online at http://www.theclinics.com/home/cme, and completing the evaluation. After taking the test, you will be required to review any and all incorrect answers. Following completion of the test and evaluation, your credit will be awarded and you may print your certificate.

FACULTY DISCLOSURE/CONFLICT OF INTEREST

The University of Virginia School of Medicine, as an ACCME accredited provider, endorses and strives to comply with the Accreditation Council for Continuing Medical Education (ACCME) Standards of Commercial Support, Commonwealth of Virginia statutes, University of Virginia policies and procedures, and associated federal and private regulations and guidelines on the need for disclosure and monitoring of proprietary and financial interests that may affect the scientific integrity and balance of content delivered in continuing medical education activities under our auspices.

The University of Virginia School of Medicine requires that all CME activities accredited through this institution be developed independently and be scientifically rigorous, balanced and objective in the presentation/discussion of its content, theories and practices.

All authors/editors participating in an accredited CME activity are expected to disclose to the readers relevant financial relationships with commercial entities occurring within the past 12 months (such as grants or research support, employee, consultant, stock holder, member of speakers bureau, etc.). The University of Virginia School of Medicine will employ appropriate mechanisms to resolve potential conflicts of interest to maintain the standards of fair and balanced education to the reader. Questions about specific strategies can be directed to the Office of Continuing Medical Education, University of Virginia School of Medicine, Charlottesville, Virginia.

The authors/editors listed below have identified no financial or professional relationships for themselves or their spouse/partner: Holly Antal, PhD; Mark A. Atkinson, PhD; Fida Bacha, MD; Dorothy Becker, MBBCh; Lisa Buckloh, PhD; Anna Casu, MD; Carin Davis, Acquisitions Editor; Elka Jacobson-Dickman, MD; Kim C. Donaghue, MBBS, PhD, FRACP; Nicole Glaser, MD; Sarah J. Glastras, MBBS; Neslihan Gungor, MD; Nursen Gurtunca, MD; Michael J. Haller, MD; Tamara S. Hannon, MD; Diego Ize-Ludlow, MD; Ingrid Libman, MD, PhD; Amanda Lochrie, PhD; Fauzia Mohsin, MBBS; Meranda Nahkla, MD; Kusiel Perlman, MD; Massimo Pietropaolo, MD; Constantin Polychronakos, MD, FRCP; Marianna Rachmiel, MD; Christopher Ryan, PhD; Desmond A. Schatz, MD; Kristin A. Sikes, MSN, CPNP, APRN; Amy T. Steffen, BS; Massimo Trucco, MD; and Tim Wysocki, PhD, ABPP.

The authors listed below have identified the following financial or professional relationships for themselves or their spouse/partner:
Silva Arslanian, MD has grant/research support from Pfizer; and is a consultant for and receives grant/research support from Sanofi-Aventis.
Denis Daneman, MBBCh is a consultant and is on the speakers' bureau for NovoNordisk; and is an independent contractor for Eli Lilly.
Lynne Levitsky, MD has performed funded investigator initiated research with Genentech and Pfizer; and a funded clinical trial on IGF-1 with Tercica.
Mark A. Sperling, MD is a member of the speakers' bureau for Serono in the area of endocrinology.
William V. Tamborlane, MD is on the advisory board for MedTronic in the area of insulin pumps, and is on the advisory board for Novo Nordisk and Sanofi Aventis in the area of insulin analogs.
Stuart Weinzimer, MD is an independent contractor for Medtronics, Inc. in the field of diabetes technology, and an independent contractor for Novo Nordisk in the area of pediatric diabetes.

Disclosure of Discussion of Non-FDA Approved Uses for Pharmaceutical and/or Medical Devices: **The University of Virginia School of Medicine, as an ACCME provider, requires that all authors identify and disclose any "off label" uses for pharmaceutical and medical device products. The University of Virginia School of Medicine recommends that each physician fully review all the available data on new products or procedures prior to clinical use.**

TO ENROLL

To enroll in the *Pediatric Clinics of North America* Continuing Medical Education program, call customer service at **1-800-654-2452** or visit us online at www.theclinics.com/home/cme. The CME program is available to subscribers for an additional fee of $195.00.

PEDIATRIC CLINICS
OF NORTH AMERICA

Pediatr Clin N Am 52 (2005) xv–xvi

Preface

Diabetes Mellitus in Children

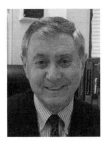

Mark A. Sperling, MD
Guest Editor

Diabetes mellitus is a complex disorder with profound consequences, both acute and long-term, for the health of the affected individual and for the cost of health care in society at large. The classical type 1 diabetes mellitus (T1DM)—also known as insulin-dependent diabetes mellitus (IDDM) and formerly called juvenile diabetes mellitus—is an autoimmune disease that is increasing in frequency worldwide, most rapidly in children under 5 years of age. Type 2 diabetes mellitus (T2DM), formerly considered a disease of those over the age of 40 years and a rarity in youth, now constitutes a sizable fraction of diabetes in older children and adolescents, with an incidence of 50% or more in some areas. The increase in T2DM clearly is related to the epidemic of obesity sweeping both the developed and developing world. The ability to predict T1DM is highly advanced, but preventing or delaying its clinical appearance is a problem that remains to be solved. By contrast, T2DM probably is preventable, though how and why obesity and lifestyle exert such a profound effect remains enigmatic.

However, much light has been shed on our understanding of the entities that constitute clinical diabetes mellitus and their management via newer insulins, newer devices for insulin delivery, newer oral agents, newer means to identify and treat complications, and newer directions for research to prevent and cure this disease.

The purpose of this issue of the *Pediatric Clinics of North America* is to bring these newer developments, so exciting to those of us working in the field, to the general reader working in the broad field of pediatrics. To do so, we have

0031-3955/05/$ see front matter © 2005 Elsevier Inc. All rights reserved.
doi:10.1016/j.pcl.2005.09.002   *pediatric.theclinics.com*

assembled a team of nationally recognized experts to cover 12 topics beginning with a conceptual framework for classification and concluding with a look to the future including cure by islet transplantation and stem cell therapy. In between are comprehensive and contemporary yet readable reviews of T1DM and T2DM; diabetic ketoacidosis and nonketotic hyperosomolar states; monogenic forms of diabetes, which, although rare, provide insight into the more common forms of diabetes mellitus; new insulins; pump therapy; oral agents; and the major clinical, psychosocial, and long-term complications of diabetes mellitus in children.

I am grateful to Elsevier for the opportunity to edit this issue and to my colleagues who acted as contributors. I can only hope that you, the reader, will enjoy and learn as much from them as I did and that this knowledge will be translated to the benefit of children who have diabetes mellitus.

Mark A. Sperling, MD
University of Pittsburgh School of Medicine
Division of Endocrinology, Diabetes, and Metabolism
Department of Pediatrics
Children's Hospital of Pittsburgh
3705 Fifth Avenue, DeSoto 4A-400
Pittsburgh, PA 15213, USA
E-mail address: masp@pitt.edu

ELSEVIER
SAUNDERS

PEDIATRIC CLINICS
OF NORTH AMERICA

Pediatr Clin N Am 52 (2005) 1533–1552

The Classification of Diabetes Mellitus: A Conceptual Framework

Diego Ize-Ludlow, MD, Mark A. Sperling, MD*

Division of Endocrinology, Diabetes, and Metabolism, University of Pittsburgh School of Medicine, Children's Hospital of Pittsburgh, 3705 Fifth Avenue, 4A-400, Pittsburgh, PA 15213–2583, USA

Classification, the systematic grouping of disease entities by etiology or other categories, is useful because it guides the thinking of physicians, informs their actions, and provides value to their patients. A classical example is anemia, in which hemoglobin of approximately 6 g/dL or less is associated with typical symptoms, such as pallor, fatigue, and shortness of breath irrespective of the cause. Although initial treatment may include transfusion, subsequent management is guided by the cause: essential factors for hemoglobin synthesis (iron, vitamin B_{12}, folic acid); correction of factors that promote excessive peripheral destruction of red blood cells (splenectomy, steroids for immune hemolysis, avoidance of drugs, such a sulfonamides in those with G6PD deficiency); and congenital or acquired defects in hemoglobin synthesis (hemoglobinopathy, bone marrow infiltration). Knowledge of the etiology of diabetes mellitus (DM) is not as advanced as that of anemia, but it has become increasingly apparent that the classification of DM as type 1, type 2, and "other" is inadequate. This article provides a rational conceptual framework for the classification of DM based on the rapidly evolving understanding of congenital or acquired defects in insulin secretion and congenital or acquired factors that affect insulin's ability to evoke its biologic effects (ie, insulin sensitivity or its mirror image, insulin resistance [IR]). DM results when the normal constant of the product of insulin concentration times the insulin action, a parabolic relationship (Fig. 1), is inadequate to prevent hyperglycemia and its clinical consequences of polyuria, polydipsia, and weight loss. When an increase in IR can be compensated by increased insulin secretion, DM does not result as long as this constant is maintained. By simul-

---

* Corresponding author.
E-mail address: masp+@pitt.edu (M.A. Sperling).

0031 3955/05/$ see front matter © 2005 Elsevier Inc. All rights reserved.
doi:10.1016/j.pcl.2005.07.001   *pediatric.theclinics.com*

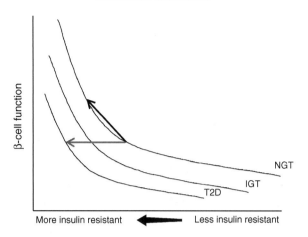

Fig. 1. The hyperbolic relationship of insulin resistance and β-cell function. In a subject with normal β-cell reserve an increase in insulin resistance results in increased insulin release and normal glucose tolerance (*black arrow*). In an individual where the capacity to increase insulin release is compromised, increased insulin resistance with no β-cell compensation results in progression from normal glucose tolerance to impaired glucose tolerance to diabetes (*gray arrow*). The product of insulin sensitivity (the reciprocal of insulin resistance) and acute insulin response (a measurement β-cell function) has been called "disposition index." This index remains constant in an individual with normal β-cell compensation in response to changes in insulin resistance. IGT, impaired glucose tolerance; NGT, normal glucose tolerance; T2D, type 2 diabetes.

taneously considering insulin secretion and insulin action in any given individual, it becomes possible to account for the natural history of DM in that subject: the reasons for its clinical appearance at that time, or its temporary resolution or exacerbation (eg, diabetic ketoacidosis in a patient with type 2 DM). Diabetes is the extreme phenotypical manifestation of the combination β-cell malfunction and IR. This syndrome can be the result of the severe failure of one of the components of the homeostatic system or of combinations of milder defects in each component (Fig. 2).

A clear clinical example of these relationships (see Figs. 1 and 2) is the classical presentation of type 2 diabetes. An obese individual with DM may return to normoglycemia through weight loss. The decrease in IR through weight loss allows the remaining β-cell function to achieve a new homeostatic balance, which could easily be lost with further increased IR (eg, by weight gain, pregnancy, illness), or by further impairment of the β-cell secretory function [1].

This concept is strongly supported by data obtained from knockout mice. The muscle insulin receptor knockout mice develop severe IR but compensatory hyperinsulinemia allows for regulation of the blood glucose in the normal range [2]. By contrast, β-cell defects with coexistent IR lead to diabetes, as is the case in the insulin receptor substrate-1/insulin receptor knockout [3]. Type 2 diabetes is most often a "two-hit" phenomenon, in which IR is accompanied by a β-cell defect preventing compensatory up-regulation of insulin secretion.

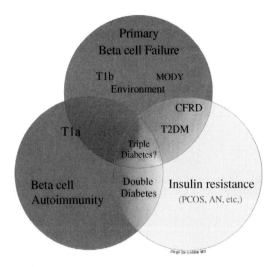

Fig. 2. The spectrum of β-cell failure and insulin resistance syndromes. β-cell failure can be genetic, as in MODY; acquired secondary to environment (drugs, virus, and so forth); or autoimmune. The combination of different degrees of these factors leads to the different manifestations of the β-cell failure and insulin resistance diseases. AN, acanthosis nigricans; CFRD, cystic fibrosis–related diabetes; MODY, maturity-onset diabetes of the young; PCOS, polycystic ovary syndrome; T1a, type 1a diabetes mellitus (autoimmune); T1b, type 1b diabetes (idiopathic); T2DM, type 2 diabetes mellitus.

In the following paragraphs, insulin secretion and insulin action are considered separately and then examples of their interaction in clinically relevant situations are provided. A rational framework for the classification of DM is provided, which informs and guides the reader in later articles in this issue describing various forms of DM.

Insulin secretion

Insulin secretion is at the core of all metabolic processes governing the disposition of the nutrients glucose, amino acids, and fats either for immediate energy use or for storage. Insulin secretion is tightly integrated with the cycle of feeding and fasting, and can be considered from the aspect of whole-body physiology and the biochemical-molecular events occurring in the β-cells of the pancreatic islet.

Physiology

During feeding, a complex interplay of neural, nutrient, hormonal, and chemical stimuli elicits insulin secretion (Fig. 3) [4–6]. The neural signals arise from visual and gustatory cues and augment insulin secretion largely by vagal parasympathetic pathways [4–7]. Vagal pathways may also modulate the brain's control of insulin secretion. The sympathetic arm of the autonomic nervous system

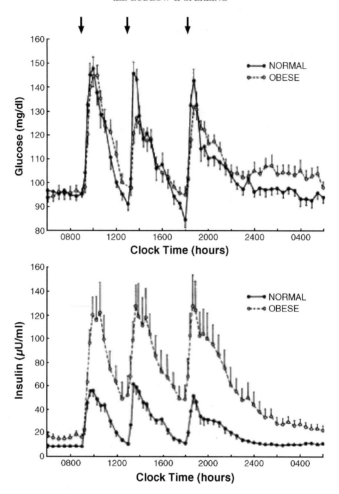

Fig. 3. Twenty-four–hour glucose and insulin profiles in normal and obese volunteers. Arrows represent meals. (*Adapted from* Polonsky KS, Given BD, Van Cauter E. Twenty-four-hour profiles and pulsatile patterns of insulin secretion in normal and obese subjects. J Clin Invest 1988;81:442–8; with permission.)

modulates insulin secretion by alpha and beta receptors. In general, stimulation of β-2 receptors increases insulin secretion, whereas α-adrenergic pathways, which predominate with epinephrine and norepinephrine, inhibit insulin secretion.

Nutrient signals involve all three classes with glucose predominating as the major stimulus; amino acids and fatty acids have individual hierarchies of stimulation but effectively amplify and augment glucose effects on insulin secretion. The islets, each encased in a cocoon-like structure and distributed throughout the exocrine pancreas, are ideally situated to sense nutrient composition, which must also signal exocrine cells to secrete their digestive enzymes. Exocrine and endocrine actions of the pancreas are linked and some data support

that β-cells may be derived from pancreatic ductular epithelium, further emphasizing their likely communication [8]. Within the islets, there is also communication between the various cell types; glucagon from the α-cells stimulates
insulin, and insulin suppresses glucagon, whereas somatostatin inhibits both insulin and glucagon.

The insulin response to glucose is age-dependent (Table 1), being highest
during the pubertal growth spurt and returning toward but not quite matching
prepubertal values by early adulthood. Increased growth hormone secretion
during puberty is likely responsible for increased insulin secretion by inducing
resistance to insulin action [9]. Placentally derived growth hormone–like hormones also are responsible for increased insulin secretion in the second half
of pregnancy. Inability to compensate for growth hormone–induced IR is a likely
key contributor to the increased incidence of clinically manifest DM in puberty
and for gestational diabetes in women [10]. Other hormones that antagonize
insulin action, such as glucocorticoids and combination estrogen-progesterone as
found in oral contraceptives, also result in increased insulin secretion. Ghrelin, a
gastrointestinal peptide that stimulates growth hormone secretion and appetite,
and leptin, a hormone produced by fat cells, which regulates satiety indirectly,
also modulate insulin secretion; ghrelin stimulates, whereas leptin lowers insulin
secretion [4–6,11,12].

For any given level of glycemia, orally ingested glucose elicits a greater
insulin response than when the same glycemic profile is achieved by glucose
infused intravenously. This has given rise to the concept of incretins, gut-derived
hormonal signals that amplify insulin response to ingested food [13]. The incretin
effect, which amplifies the insulin response to glucose by some 50% to 75%, is
mediated largely by two intestinal hormones, glucagon-like peptide-1 and
glucose-dependent insulinotropic polypeptide. The incretin effect is markedly
impaired in type 2 DM, mostly because of impaired glucagon-like peptide-1
secretion. Interest in restoring glucagon-like peptide 1 effects has resulted in the
development of a drug recently approved by the Food and Drug Administration,
exenatide, a peptide derived from lizards that activates the mammalian receptor
for glucagon-like peptide-1, resulting in increased insulin secretion, suppressed

Table 1
Glucose and insulin responses to oral glucose tolerance test in prepubertal and pubertal subjects

	Prepubertal		Pubertal	
Glucose dose	1.75 g/kg	55 g/m^2	1.75 g/kg	55 g/m^2
Subjects	(N = 9)	(N = 8)	(N = 10)	(N = 9)
Fasting glucose mg/dL	82 ± 3.1	75.6 ± 4.1	84.3 ± 3	83.2 ± 3.7
Peak glucose	151.6 ± 8.5	143.3 ± 7.5	152.2 ± 7.9	148.8 ± 11.5
Area glucose mg/dL × 4 h	421 ± 17	409.5 ± 16	432.7 ± 18	429.1 ± 30
Area insulin μU/mL × 4 h	118.5 ± 17.3[*]	115.4 ± 16.5[§]	299.1 ± 77.6[*]	365.4 ± 114.8[§]

Values represent mean ± SEM.
    [*, §] Like symbols compared, prepubertal versus pubertal ($P < 0.05$).
Adapted from Bloch CA, Clemons P, Sperling MA. Puberty decreases insulin sensitivity. J Pediatr
1987;110(3):481–7.

glucagon, and delayed gastric emptying [14,15]. The drug is approved for use in patients with type 2 diabetes. Studies in type 1 DM suggest that when given with insulin before meals, the drug can decrease exaggerated glycemic excursions by up to 90%, emphasizing its therapeutic potential for both children and adults with either type 1 or type 2 DM [14].

The effects of glucagon-like peptide-1 in suppressing glucagon secretion and delaying gastric emptying are also mimicked by amylin, a peptide hormone cosecreted with insulin from pancreatic β-ells [16]. In experimental studies in children with type 1 DM, synthetic amylin, given together with the recommended bolus dose in patients treated by an insulin pump, significantly reduced the immediate postprandial hyperglycemia and glucagon secretion [17]. This drug, due for release in 2005, may prove of benefit to reduce postprandial glucose excursions in children with type 1 DM.

The result of this physiologic interaction is that insulin secretion is tightly linked to the cycle of feeding and fasting. The early insulin response to ingested meals is the physiologic counterpart of the biphasic response to intravenous glucose, so important for signaling immediate and ongoing disposition of ingested nutrients [18].

Biochemical and molecular aspects of insulin secretion

Insulin is synthesized as a prohormone, proinsulin, with the amino terminus of the A chain linked to the carboxy terminus of the B chain by a connecting peptide called C peptide (Fig. 4). Enzymatic cleavage by carboxypeptidase at the

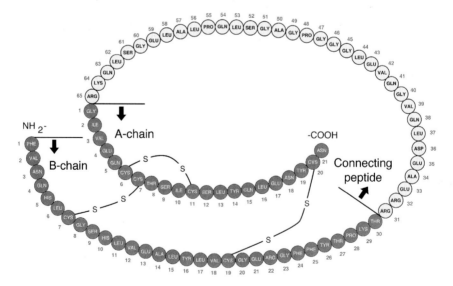

Fig. 4. Human proinsulin. Insulin is derived from the cleavage of the connecting peptide (C peptide) from the proinsulin molecule. C peptide is secreted in equimolar amounts with insulin and has a longer half-life.

CLASSIFICATION OF DIABETES MELLITUS

appropriate sites results in the two chains of insulin linked by disulfide bonds and C peptide; both are cosecreted along with amylin. Inappropriate cleavage at the NH_2 or COOH terminus results in an abnormal insulin with less biologic potency, thereby predisposing to DM [19]. Because C peptide is so different than insulin or proinsulin, measurement of C peptide is useful to distinguish endogenous insulin secretion (C peptide at least as high as insulin) from exogenously administered insulin, wherein insulin is high but C peptide is low because of suppression of endogenous insulin secretion. The two major uses of C peptide measurements are assessment of residual insulin secretion in new-onset DM treated with insulin, and distinction of factitious insulin administration from endogenous secretion in hypoglycemia [20].

The combination of insulin measurements in isolated islets, electrophysiologic studies by patch clamp techniques, and molecular approaches have revolutionized the understanding of insulin secretion in health and disease [21]. The β-cell transforms chemical signals from glucose metabolism to electrical signals that allow K^+ and Ca^{++} channels to open or close and result in release of insulin. These concepts are summarized in Fig. 5. In the resting state, the β-cell synthesizes and stores insulin as granules distributed close to the cell membrane or more centrally in the cytoplasm. The ATP-sensitive K^+ channel, K_{ATP}, is composed of four separate KIR 6.2 subunits that form a pore, which is surrounded by four sulfonylurea receptor (SUR1) subunits. Each K_{ATP} channel is an octamer; synthesis and assembly of these subunits is critical for insulin secretion. In the resting state, the ratio of ATP/ADP is such that the K_{ATP} remains open, permitting

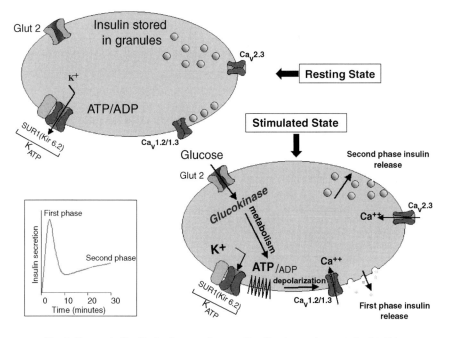

Fig. 5. Pancreatic β-cell stimulus-secretion coupling for glucose (see text for details).

efflux of the K^+ so that the cell membrane is hyperpolarized and a family of Ca^{++} channels remains closed. With glucose ingestion or infusion, glucose enters the β-cell by the non–insulin sensitive glucose transporter, GLUT 2, and is rapidly phosphorylated by glucokinase with subsequent metabolism to generate energy as ATP. The change in ATP/ADP closes the K_{ATP} as does sulfonylurea acting on its receptor SUR1. This causes a buildup of potassium within each cell ultimately resulting in depolarization of the cell membrane. In turn, depolarization opens the voltage-gated calcium channel $Ca_v1.2/1.3$, resulting in a rapid release of the immediate pool of available insulin and accounting for the first phase of insulin release that occurs within the first 3 to 5 minutes (see inset of Fig. 5). Ongoing metabolism of glucose mobilizes preformed or newly synthesized insulin from the interior of the cell by calcium entering a second distinct group of calcium channels, known as Ca_v 2.3 and located distal to the K_{ATP}. This results in the sustained second phase of insulin secretion. In this model, defects of insulin secretion can occur because of faulty formation of β-cells, faulty genetic control of factors that regulate insulin synthesis, defects in metabolic steps of glycolysis, or defects in the K_{ATP} channel secondary to mutations in the Kir 6.2 or SUR1 components and in the calcium channel family described previously. Examples of each of these mutations have been reported and although relatively rare, they may collectively contribute to impaired insulin secretion, which when coupled to increasing IR as occurs in obesity, results in type 2 DM, because β-cells cannot compensate for the increased IR [22]. Likewise, these defects may contribute to type 1 DM because less damage to β-cells is required by autoimmune destruction before failure is unmasked.

Glucotoxicity or lipotoxicity are concepts that imply exhaustion or functional interference, but not death, of β-cells and may also contribute to apparent β-cell failure. Remarkably, in most circumstances, early failure of insulin secretion is manifest by impairment of the first-phase response to intravenous glucose. The mechanisms for this are not fully understood. Failure of first-phase insulin response, however, can be used to predict those who may go on to develop clinical DM [23]. Measures of β-cell function in terms of insulin secretion are

Table 2
Measures of β-cell function

Measure	Reference
Fasting insulin or C peptide	[24,25]
Homeostatic model assessment: β-cell function	[24,25]
Insulin profile during oral glucose tolerance test	(see Table 1)
Hyperglycemic clamp	[24,25]
The insulinogenic index*	[24]
Mixed meal tolerance test	[78]
Insulin profile during intravenous glucagon tolerance test	[26]
Arginine stimulation	[27]

* The insulinogenic index is calculated as the ratio of increment in the plasma insulin level to that of plasma glucose level during the first 30 minutes after the ingestion of glucose (1.75 g/kg, maximum 75 g).

summarized in Table 2 [24–27]. For each of the listed tests, one must rely on the age-specific values considered normal for the specific laboratory.

Insulin resistance

Definition

Insulin resistance is defined by the decrease in the ability of insulin to induce glucose uptake by insulin-sensitive tissues and to suppress hepatic glucose production. Insulin sensitivity, the reciprocal of IR, is widely used, especially because it is the sensitivity to insulin that is assessed during the euglycemic hyperinsulinemic clamp, considered the gold standard measurement.

Measurement of insulin resistance

Currently, there is no consensus on a test of IR that can be applied to routine clinical practice. Until better assessment tools are available, indices of IR derived from fasting insulin and glucose values or from an oral glucose tolerance test can be used to assess the IR and β-cell function of an individual. This could be particularly useful in individuals at high risk of developing diabetes (eg, impaired glucose tolerance or high genetic risk) to tailor possible interventions and to aid in the treatment choices (Table 3) [24,25,28–31].

Fasting insulin

In the presence of a normal glucose level an elevated fasting insulin level suggests IR. The problem with this assumption is that the range of normal glucose levels makes this interpretation difficult. For this reason the insulin concentration in plasma can usually only be interpreted in the light of the prevailing glucose concentration, as it is done using the insulin sensitivity indices discussed next.

Insulin dose

In type 1 diabetes, where there is little or no endogenous insulin production, the dose required to obtain euglycemia is related to the degree of IR. Doses above 1.5 U/kg/d are strongly suggestive of IR. The multiplicity of factors affecting the insulin doses and the reliability of patients reported doses limit the accuracy of this estimation.

Euglycemic hyperinsulinemic clamp

The euglycemic hyperinsulinemic clamp is currently considered the gold standard measurement of IR. It is based on the assessment of insulin sensitivity

Table 3
Measurements of insulin resistance

Test	Labor intensity	Method	Uses	Interpretation of results	Validated in children
Euglycemic clamp	Blood glucose measurements every 3–10 min over 150–180 min	Constant rate IV insulin infusion and variable rate IV glucose infusion	Research; regarded as the gold standard	Insulin resistance is estimated from the ratio of mean glucose infusion to the mean insulin concentration over the last 20–30 min of the clamp	Yes [24]
HOMA or QUICKI	Three basal samples at 5-min intervals (one sample often used)	Overnight fast	Epidemiologic studies or longitudinally within an individual	Computer-derived nomogram or computerized table (HOMA) Mathematical equation (QUICKI)	Yes [25,29,30]
CIGMA	Three samples at 50, 55, and 60 min	IV glucose infusion (5 mg/kg/min for 60 min)	Epidemiologic studies or longitudinally within an individual	Computer-derived nomogram or computerized table	No
FSIVGTT-minimal model	Twenty-five samples over 3 h	IV glucose bolus +/– IV bolus of tolbutamide or insulin at 20 min	Research	Computer program	Yes [31]
OGTT derived insulin sensitivity indices	Six to 7 samples over 2 h	Oral glucose after overnight fast	Epidemiologic studies or longitudinally within an individual	Mathematical equation	Yes [28]

Abbreviations: CIGMA, continuous infusion of glucose with model assessment; FSIVGTT, frequently sampled intravenous glucose tolerance test; HOMA, homeostatic model assessment; IV, intravenous; OGTT, oral glucose tolerance test; QUICKI, quantitative insulin sensitivity check index.

(the reciprocal of IR). During this test a fixed amount of insulin is infused. A variable rate of glucose infusion is used to keep blood glucose level constant to avoid any effect of counterregulatory hormones on insulin sensitivity. The greater the sensitivity to insulin, the greater is the amount of glucose needed to maintain euglycemia. The amount of infused glucose once a steady state is reached is the main determinant of the test (M value [$mg \cdot min^{-1} \cdot kg$ body weight^{-1}]). Because of its precision in quantitating insulin sensitivity under physiologic conditions of insulinemia and glycemia, and because it can be combined with other methods (eg, tracer glucose infusion, indirect calorimetry), the euglycemic hyperinsulinemic clamp remains the preferred technique to evaluate the contribution of impaired insulin sensitivity to overall glucose homeostasis. Unfortunately, the invasive and complex nature of the test limits its use in epidemiologic studies or clinical practice.

Minimal models: frequently sampled intravenous glucose tolerance test and minimal modeling

Minimal models work by using individual patient data from intravenous glucose tolerance tests, and establishing the profile of both insulin and glucose. Because insulin causes glucose to fall and glucose causes insulin to rise, the feedback loop can be mathematically analyzed to estimate the β-cell function and IR [32].

The frequently sampled intravenous glucose tolerance test is less labor-intensive than the euglycemic hyperinsulinemic clamp: there is no need for the continuous adjustment of glucose infusion rates, so bedside glucose readings are not necessary. It is also, however, a time-consuming and expensive test.

Homeostatic model assessment

The homeostatic model assessment (HOMA) of β-cell function and IR is a method for assessing β-cell function and IR from basal glucose and insulin or C peptide concentrations. It is based on mathematical modeling of the interaction of β-cell function and IR in steady state.

HOMA1, the original model from Matthews and coworkers [33], contained a simple mathematical approximation of the original nonlinear solution to the iterative equations. These equations are simplified to as follows. For IR: HOMA1-IR = (FPI × FPG)/22.5. For β-cell function: HOMA1-%B = (20 × FPI)/(FPG − 3.5), where FPI is fasting plasma insulin concentration in milliunit per liter and FPG is fasting plasma glucose in millimole per liter.

The group that published these equations later developed a corrected nonlinear computer model (HOMA2) [34]. The computer model can be used to determine insulin sensitivity (%S) and β-cell function (%B) from paired fasting plasma glucose and insulin or C peptide concentrations across a range of 1 to 2200 pmol/L for insulin and 1 to 25 mmol/L for glucose. Because the model was calculated in a steady state situation it should not be used when glucose levels are in the hypoglycemic range or other non–steady-state situations. Also, the model is based on the relationship of IR and β-cell function, so that both estimations should be reported.

It is recommended to use this model when HOMA is compared with other models (HOMA2 model is available from www.OCDEM.ox.ac.uk). The group who designed the model has recently published a review on its use [35].

Quantitative insulin sensitivity check index

The quantitative insulin sensitivity check index [36] is similar to the simple equation form of the HOMA model in all comparative respects, except that QUICKI uses a log transform of the insulin x glucose product. It has the same disadvantage and limitations as the use of HOMA: QUICKI = 1/log(FPI) + log(FPG) = 1/([log(FPI × FPG]), where FPG (milligrams per deciliter) is the fasting glucose concentration and FPI (microunit per milliliter) is the fasting insulin concentration.

In the revised QUICKI, to improve the performance of this estimation Perseghin and coworkers [37] included fasting free fatty acids in the calculation. Incorporation of the fasting FFA concentration (FFA, measured in millimole per liter) into QUICKI leads to a revised QUICKI, which is calculated a follows: revised QUICKI = 1/log(FPI) + log(FPG) + log (FFA). The revised equation showed an improvement in its association with insulin sensitivity in healthy, nonobese individuals. This modified index has not been validated in children.

Continuous infusion of glucose with model assessment

Continuous infusion of glucose with model assessment is a steady-state mathematical model, which assesses the glucose and insulin responses to a low-dose glucose infusion. It has not been widely benchmarked, however, and used by only a few groups [38].

Indexes of insulin sensitivity from the oral glucose tolerance test

Although the oral glucose tolerance test is not designed to asses IR, indices of IR have been developed [39–44]. Two of these indices have been validated in children [28].

Clearly, most of these tools are used for research purposes. The HOMA and QUICKI, however, could be quantified from a single fasting glucose and insulin determination and may find application in clinical practice.

The interaction of insulin resistance and β-cell function

Having presented the major aspects of insulin secretion and IR, some examples of DM and its related disorders according to their main determinant are now discussed: predominantly insulin deficiency, predominantly IR, or resulting from relative insulin deficiency in the context of IR.

Diabetes with predominantly insulin deficiency

Type 1 diabetes

Type 1 diabetes is the form of the disease caused primarily by β-cell destruction. This condition is characterized by severe insulin deficiency and dependence on exogenous insulin to prevent ketosis and to preserve life; it was called insulin-dependent DM. The natural history of this disease indicates that there are preketotic, non–insulin-dependent phases both before and after the initial diagnosis. Although the onset is predominantly in childhood, the disease may occur at any age.

It is possible that nonautoimmune and autoimmune destruction of β-cells could coexist, but the current classification considers two subtypes. In type 1a there is evidence suggesting an autoimmune origin of β-cell destruction, mostly determined by the presence of circulating antibodies against islet cells; insulin antibodies in the absence of exposure to exogenous insulin; or antibodies to glutamic acid decarboxylase, and/or islet cell-associated phosphatase. This autoimmune entity also is associated with certain HLAs. Patients with type 1a are also more likely to have other concomitant autoimmune disorders, such as autoimmune thyroiditis, Addison's disease, and celiac disease.

The type 1b form of diabetes is characterized by low insulin and C peptide levels similar to those in type 1a, although there is no evidence of an autoimmune etiology of the β-cell destruction. As in autoimmune diabetes, patients are prone to ketoacidosis. This idiopathic diabetes reflects the still limited knowledge of the etiology of many forms of diabetes.

Maturity-onset diabetes of the young

Maturity-onset diabetes of the young comprises a heterogeneous group of disorders of monogenic defects in β-cell function. It is believed that a more appropriate term for this group is monogenic diabetes of the young. The maturity-onset diabetes of the young syndromes are characterized by dominant inheritance with at least two and preferably three consecutive generations, and onset before age 25 to 30 years. The first maturity-onset diabetes of the young gene was found in 1992 [45], and since then six forms of maturity-onset diabetes of the young syndromes have been described (see also the article by Nakhla and Polychronakos elsewhere in this issue).

Mitochondrial diabetes

Mitochondrial diabetes, also called maternally inherited diabetes and deafness, is characterized by a progressive decline in β-cell function. Cases of mitochondrial diabetes are often misdiagnosed as type 1 or type 2 diabetes depending on degree and age of progression of the insulinopenia. The diagnosis should be suspected when there is a marked history of diabetes associated with bilateral deafness in most carriers that follows a maternal inheritance. The most common mutation associated with this type of diabetes is the A3243G mutation in the mitochondrial DNA-encoded tRNA. The molecular mechanism by which the A3243G mutation affects insulin secretion may involve an attenuation of cytosolic ADP-ATP levels causing the resetting of the glucose sensor in the pancreatic β-cell [46]. The A3243G mutation is present in heteroplasmic form (the patient carries a mixture of normal and mutant mitochondria) and there is a trend toward a lower age of onset at high heteroplasmy values [47].

Hearing impairment generally precedes the onset of clinically manifest diabetes by several years and changes in pigmentation of the retina are also present in many carriers of the A3243G mutation [46]. Patients with mitochondrial diabetes show a pronounced age-dependent deterioration of pancreatic function with a mean age of presentation of 38 years [46]. The same mitochondrial variant is found in the MELAS syndrome (mitochondrial myopathy, encephalopathy, lactic acidosis, and stroke-like syndrome), although diabetes in not part of this syndrome [48].

Diabetes and other syndromes with predominantly insulin resistance

A number of mutations of the insulin receptor resulting in diabetes have been identified. Although these are rare causes of diabetes they should be considered in a patient with marked features of IR and exceptionally high insulin levels. These mutations lead to at least three clinical syndromes, all of them characterized by findings secondary to IR (Table 4) [49].

Lipoatrophic diabetes

Lipoatrophic diabetes presents with paucity of fat, IR, and hypertriglyceridemia. There are several forms, including face-sparing partial lipoatrophy (the Dunnigan syndrome or the Koberling-Dunnigan syndrome), an autosomal-dominant form caused by mutations in the lamin A/C gene, and congenital generalized lipoatrophy (the Seip-Berardinelli syndrome), an autosomal-recessive form [50].

Metabolic syndrome

The metabolic syndrome, also called the IR syndrome, has become the major health problem of this time. This clinical phenotype is characterized by abdomi-

Table 4
Insulin receptor mutation syndromes

Syndrome	Clinical characteristics
Type A insulin resistance	Insulin resistance, acanthosis nigricans, and hyperandrogenism
Leprechaunism	Multiple abnormalities, including intrauterine growth retardation, fasting hypoglycemia, and death within the first 1 to 2 years of life
Rabson-Mendenhall syndrome	Short stature, protuberant abdomen, and abnormalities of teeth and nails

nal obesity, dyslipidemia, elevated blood pressure, IR, and a proinflammatory state and is one of the major risk factors for cardiovascular disease [51,52]. Although some single-gene defects affecting satiety or energy homeostasis have been shown to produce this syndrome, in most cases it is the consequence of the interaction of multiple genes with lifestyle factors of excessive carbohydrate and fat consumption and lack of exercise. IR as an integral part of the syndrome is likely both the cause and consequence of many of the metabolic alterations seen in this syndrome. It is not surprising that the metabolic syndrome is a risk factor for type 2 diabetes, because adding β-cell failure to the prevailing IR leads to loss of glucose homeostasis.

Polycystic ovary syndrome

Polycystic ovarian syndrome is a reproductive disorder characterized by hyperandrogenism and chronic anovulation not caused by specific diseases of the ovaries, adrenals, and pituitary. It is one of the most common hormonal disorders in women, with a prevalence estimated between 5% and 10% [53–55].

Women with the polycystic ovary syndrome are more insulin resistant than are controls [56]. In these women, insulin acts synergistically with luteinizing hormone to increase the androgen production by ovarian theca cells. Insulin also inhibits hepatic synthesis of sex hormone–binding globulin, the main carrier protein for testosterone, and increases the proportion of testosterone that circulates in the unbound, biologically available, or free, state.

The sole presence of IR does not lead to diabetes and 30% to 40% of women with the polycystic ovary syndrome have impaired glucose tolerance, and as many as 10% have type 2 diabetes by their fourth decade [57,58]. This implies that most women with polycystic ovarian syndrome are able to compensate for their degree of IR and those whose β-cell function is abnormal or deteriorates progress to diabetes.

Diabetes resulting from combined insulin deficiency and insulin resistance

Type 2 diabetes mellitus

Type 2 DM is the most common form of diabetes in adults, and its prevalence in children is increasing. It is characterized by IR and defective insulin secretion, either of which can be the predominant feature. Patients with type 2 DM usually have IR and relative rather than absolute insulin deficiency. Pediatric patients with type 2 DM are likely to be overweight or obese and present with glycosuria without ketonuria, absent or mild polyuria and polydipsia, and little or no weight loss. Up to 33% have ketonuria at diagnosis, and 5% to 25% of patients who are subsequently classified as having type 2 diabetes have ketoacidosis at presentation. Children with type 2 diabetes usually have the metabolic syndrome, have a family history of type 2 diabetes, and are more likely to be of non-European ancestry (African, Hispanic, Asian, and American Indian descent) [59]. Type 2 DM patients are most likely antibody negative, although in adults a syndrome of clinical type 2 diabetes with positive autoantibodies has been described as latent autoimmune diabetes [60]. Acanthosis nigricans and polycystic ovarian syndrome, disorders associated with IR and obesity, are common in youth with type 2 diabetes.

Currently, children with type 2 diabetes are usually diagnosed over the age of 10 years and are in middle to late puberty. With increased obesity and IR in the population, more and younger individuals with poor β-cell function develop diabetes.

Longitudinal studies examining the progression from normal glucose tolerance to impaired glucose tolerance in Pima Indians have demonstrated that the transition from normal glucose tolerance to impaired glucose tolerance was associated with an increase in body weight, a modest increase in IR, and a significantly greater decline in insulin secretion when measured by the first-phase insulin response to intravenous glucose [61].

Cystic fibrosis–related diabetes

About 5% to 10% of patients with cystic fibrosis have diabetes based on fasting glucose levels, but the prevalence of glucose homeostasis abnormalities has been described in up to 34% [62,63]. The clinical course of these patients is characterized by a slow progression from normal glucose tolerance to impaired glucose tolerance and ultimately fasting hyperglycemia [62,63], with no tendency to ketosis. Patients frequently become glucose intolerant at times of illness. This is presumably caused by limited insulin secretion, which cannot compensate for the stress-induced resistance to insulin action. One such "stress" is the use of glucocorticoid bursts to dampen pulmonary inflammation. Poor β-cell function seems to be the major contributor to cystic fibrosis–related diabetes. In comparison with controls, normal glucose-tolerant cystic fibrosis patients have higher glucose levels at 30, 60, and 90 minutes associated with a delayed rise in insulin levels [64–67] and a decreased first-phase insulin release [68]. It is possible that the alteration in β-cell function may be caused by altered function of the cystic fibrosis transmembrane conductance regulator because it is expressed in pancreatic islets [69]. Although there are conflicting reports on the involvement of IR in cystic fibrosis–related diabetes [70–77], the trend of worsening in glucose tolerance with ageing and exacerbations of pulmonary disease is suggestive of an episodic worsening of IR. Increased inflammatory milieu or medications (ie, steroids) are likely to explain a significant part of the increase in IR.

Cystic fibrosis–related diabetes is a good example of the balance of insulin secretion and IR. Most patients have enough β-cell function to maintain normoglycemia, and this balance is lost in periods of increased IR.

Summary

Diabetes is the extreme manifestation of a spectrum of conditions in which the balance of insulin secretion and insulin action (or IR) has been altered. Loss of euglycemia is caused by relative insulin deficiency in the presence of IR, or by absolute insulin deficiency. There are related conditions in which an alteration of IR or β-cell dysfunction exists, but because of compensation (increased insulin secretion or increased insulin sensitivity) glucose homeostasis has not been lost. Patients with these conditions are at increased risk of developing diabetes if the compensatory mechanisms fail. There are multiple causes of IR and of β-cell failure. The elucidation of these causes and the attention to the different degrees of insulin deficiency and IR allow for better diagnosis, treatment, and prevention of diabetes and its related conditions.

References

[1] Bergman RN, Ader M, Huecking K, et al. Accurate assessment of beta-cell function: the hyperbolic correction. Diabetes 2002;51(Suppl 1):S212–20.

[2] Bruning JC, Michael MD, Winnay JN, et al. A muscle-specific insulin receptor knockout exhibits features of the metabolic syndrome of NIDDM without altering glucose tolerance. Mol Cell 1998;2:559–69.

[3] Bruning JC, Winnay J, Bonner-Weir S, et al. Development of a novel polygenic model of NIDDM in mice heterozygous for IR and IRS-1 null alleles. Cell 1997;88:561–72.

[4] Badman MK, Flier JS. The gut and energy balance: visceral allies in the obesity wars. Science 2005;307:1909–14.

[5] Porte Jr D, Baskin DG, Schwartz MW. Insulin signaling in the central nervous system: a critical role in metabolic homeostasis and disease from *C. elegans* to humans. Diabetes 2005;54: 1264–76.

[6] Schwartz MW, Porte Jr D. Diabetes, obesity, and the brain. Science 2005;307:375–9.

[7] Rossi J, Santamaki P, Airaksinen MS, et al. Parasympathetic innervation and function of endocrine pancreas requires the glial cell line-derived factor family receptor alpha2 (GFRalpha2). Diabetes 2005;54:1324–30.

[8] Kemp DM, Thomas MK, Habener JF. Developmental aspects of the endocrine pancreas. Rev Endocr Metab Disord 2003;4:5–17.

[9] Amiel SA, Caprio S, Sherwin RS, et al. Insulin resistance of puberty: a defect restricted to peripheral glucose metabolism. J Clin Endocrinol Metab 1991;72:277–82.

[10] Buchanan TA, Xiang AH. Gestational diabetes mellitus. J Clin Invest 2005;115:485–91.

[11] Kojima M, Kangawa K. Ghrelin: structure and function. Physiol Rev 2005;85:495–522.

[12] Williams DL, Cummings DE. Regulation of ghrelin in physiologic and pathophysiologic states. J Nutr 2005;135:1320–5.

[13] Vilsboll T, Holst JJ. Incretins, insulin secretion and type 2 diabetes mellitus. Diabetologia 2004;47:357–66.

[14] Dupre J. Glycaemic effects of incretins in type 1 diabetes mellitus: a concise review, with emphasis on studies in humans. Regul Pept 2005;128:149–57.

[15] Dupre J, Behme MT, McDonald TJ. Exendin-4 normalized postcibal glycemic excursions in type 1 diabetes. J Clin Endocrinol Metab 2004;89:3469–73.

[16] Lutz TA. Pancreatic amylin as a centrally acting satiating hormone. Curr Drug Targets 2005;6: 181–9.

[17] Heptulla RA, Rodriguez LM, Bomgaars L, et al. The role of amylin and glucagon in the dampening of glycemic excursions in children with type 1 diabetes. Diabetes 2005;54:1100–7.

[18] Caumo A, Luzi L. First-phase insulin secretion: does it exist in real life? Considerations on shape and function. Am J Physiol Endocrinol Metab 2004;287:E371–85.

[19] Gabbay KH. The insulinopathies. N Engl J Med 1980;302:165–7.

[20] Sperling MA. Insulin biosynthesis and C-peptide: practical applications from basic research. Am J Dis Child 1980;134:1119–21.

[21] Hussain K, Cosgrove KE. From congenital hyperinsulinism to diabetes mellitus: the role of pancreatic β-cell Katp channels. Pediatr Diabetes 2005;1:1–11.

[22] Porter JR, Barrett TG. Monogenic syndromes of abnormal glucose homeostasis: clinical review and relevance to the understanding of pathology of insulin resistance and beta cell failure. J Med Genet 2005:16.

[23] Diabetes Prevention Trial-Type 1 Diabetes Study Group. Effects of insulin in relatives of patients with type 1 diabetes mellitus. N Engl J Med 2002;346:1685–91.

[24] Uwaifo GI, Fallon EM, Chin J, et al. Indices of insulin action, disposal, and secretion derived from fasting samples and clamps in normal glucose-tolerant black and white children. Diabetes Care 2002;25:2081–7.

[25] Gungor N, Saad R, Janosky J, et al. Validation of surrogate estimates of insulin sensitivity and insulin secretion in children and adolescents. J Pediatr 2004;144:47–55.

[26] Scheen AJ, Castillo MJ, Lefebvre PJ. Assessment of residual insulin secretion in diabetic patients using the intravenous glucagon stimulatory test: methodological aspects and clinical applications. Diabetes Metab 1996;22:397–406.

[27] Greenbaum C, Seidel K, Pihoker C. The case for intravenous arginine stimulation in lieu of mixed-meal tolerance tests as outcome measure for intervention studies in recent-onset type 1 diabetes. Diabetes Care 2004;27:1202–4.

[28] Yeckel CW, Weiss R, Dziura J, et al. Validation of insulin sensitivity indices from oral glucose tolerance test parameters in obese children and adolescents. J Clin Endocrinol Metab 2004; 89:1096–101.

[29] Keskin M, Kurtoglu S, Kendirci M, et al. Homeostasis model assessment is more reliable than the fasting glucose/insulin ratio and quantitative insulin sensitivity check index for assessing insulin resistance among obese children and adolescents. Pediatrics 2005;115:e500–3.

[30] Conwell LS, Trost SG, Brown WJ, et al. Indexes of insulin resistance and secretion in obese children and adolescents: a validation study. Diabetes Care 2004;27:314–9.

[31] Cutfield WS, Bergman RN, Menon RK, et al. The modified minimal model: application to measurement of insulin sensitivity in children. J Clin Endocrinol Metab 1990;70:1644–50.

[32] Bergman RN, Phillips LS, Cobelli C. Physiologic evaluation of factors controlling glucose tolerance in man: measurement of insulin sensitivity and beta-cell glucose sensitivity from the response to intravenous glucose. J Clin Invest 1981;68:1456–67.

[33] Matthews DR, Hosker JP, Rudenski AS, et al. Homeostasis model assessment: insulin resistance and beta-cell function from fasting plasma glucose and insulin concentrations in man. Diabetologia 1985;28:412–9.

[34] Levy JC, Matthews DR, Hermans MP. Correct homeostasis model assessment (HOMA) evaluation uses the computer program. Diabetes Care 1998;21:2191–2.

[35] Wallace TM, Levy JC, Matthews DR. Use and abuse of HOMA modeling. Diabetes Care 2004;27:1487–95.

[36] Katz A, Nambi SS, Mather K, et al. Quantitative insulin sensitivity check index: a simple, accurate method for assessing insulin sensitivity in humans. J Clin Endocrinol Metab 2000;85: 2402–10.

[37] Perseghin G, Caumo A, Caloni M, et al. Incorporation of the fasting plasma FFA concentration into QUICKI improves its association with insulin sensitivity in nonobese individuals. J Clin Endocrinol Metab 2001;86:4776–81.

[38] Wallace TM, Matthews DR. The assessment of insulin resistance in man. Diabet Med 2002;19: 527–34.

[39] Soonthornpun S, Setasuban W, Thamprasit A, et al. Novel insulin sensitivity index derived from oral glucose tolerance test. J Clin Endocrinol Metab 2003;88:1019–23.

[40] Matsuda M, DeFronzo RA. Insulin sensitivity indices obtained from oral glucose tolerance testing: comparison with the euglycemic insulin clamp. Diabetes Care 1999;22:1462–70.

[41] Belfiore F, Iannello S, Volpicelli G. Insulin sensitivity indices calculated from basal and OGTT-induced insulin, glucose, and FFA levels. Mol Genet Metab 1998;63:134–41.

[42] Cederholm J, Wibell L. Insulin release and peripheral sensitivity at the oral glucose tolerance test. Diabetes Res Clin Pract 1990;10:167–75.

[43] Gutt M, Davis CL, Spitzer SB, et al. Validation of the insulin sensitivity index (ISI(0,120)): comparison with other measures. Diabetes Res Clin Pract 2000;47:177–84.
[44] Stumvoll M, Mitrakou A, Pimenta W, et al. Use of the oral glucose tolerance test to assess insulin release and insulin sensitivity. Diabetes Care 2000;23:295–301.
[45] Hattersley AT, Turner RC, Permutt MA, et al. Linkage of type 2 diabetes to the glucokinase gene. Lancet 1992;339:1307–10.
[46] Maassen JA, 't Hart LM, Van Essen E, et al. Mitochondrial diabetes: molecular mechanisms and clinical presentation. Diabetes 2004;53(Suppl 1):S103–9.
[47] Ohkubo K, Yamano A, Nagashima M, et al. Mitochondrial gene mutations in the tRNA(Leu(UUR)) region and diabetes: prevalence and clinical phenotypes in Japan. Clin Chem 2001;47:1641–8.
[48] Moraes CT, Ricci E, Bonilla E, et al. The mitochondrial tRNA(Leu(UUR)) mutation in mitochondrial encephalomyopathy, lactic acidosis, and strokelike episodes (MELAS): genetic, biochemical, and morphological correlations in skeletal muscle. Am J Hum Genet 1992;50:934–49.
[49] Hegele RA. Monogenic forms of insulin resistance: apertures that expose the common metabolic syndrome. Trends Endocrinol Metab 2003;14:371–7.
[50] Oral EA. Lipoatrophic diabetes and other related syndromes. Rev Endocr Metab Disord 2003;4:61–77.
[51] Grundy SM, Brewer Jr HB, Cleeman JI, et al. Definition of metabolic syndrome: report of the National Heart, Lung, and Blood Institute/American Heart Association conference on scientific issues related to definition. Arterioscler Thromb Vasc Biol 2004;24:e13–8.
[52] Ten S, Maclaren N. Insulin resistance syndrome in children. J Clin Endocrinol Metab 2004;89:2526–39.
[53] Diamanti-Kandarakis E, Kouli CR, Bergiele AT, et al. A survey of the polycystic ovary syndrome in the Greek island of Lesbos: hormonal and metabolic profile. J Clin Endocrinol Metab 1999;84:4006–11.
[54] Knochenhauer ES, Key TJ, Kahsar-Miller M, et al. Prevalence of the polycystic ovary syndrome in unselected black and white women of the southeastern United States: a prospective study. J Clin Endocrinol Metab 1998;83:3078–82.
[55] Asuncion M, Calvo RM, San Millan JL, et al. A prospective study of the prevalence of the polycystic ovary syndrome in unselected caucasian women from Spain. J Clin Endocrinol Metab 2000;85:2434–8.
[56] Dunaif A, Segal KR, Futterweit W, et al. Profound peripheral insulin resistance, independent of obesity, in polycystic ovary syndrome. Diabetes 1989;38:1165–74.
[57] Ehrmann DA, Barnes RB, Rosenfield RL, et al. Prevalence of impaired glucose tolerance and diabetes in women with polycystic ovary syndrome. Diabetes Care 1999;22:141–6.
[58] Legro RS, Kunselman AR, Dodson WC, et al. Prevalence and predictors of risk for type 2 diabetes mellitus and impaired glucose tolerance in polycystic ovary syndrome: a prospective, controlled study in 254 affected women. J Clin Endocrinol Metab 1999;84:165–9.
[59] American Diabetes Association. Type 2 diabetes in children and adolescents. Diabetes Care 2000;23:381–9.
[60] Landin-Olsson M. Latent autoimmune diabetes in adults. Ann N Y Acad Sci 2002;958:112–6.
[61] Weyer C, Tataranni PA, Bogardus C, et al. Insulin resistance and insulin secretory dysfunction are independent predictors of worsening of glucose tolerance during each stage of type 2 diabetes development. Diabetes Care 2001;24:89–94.
[62] Lanng S, Hansen A, Thorsteinsson B, et al. Glucose tolerance in patients with cystic fibrosis: five year prospective study. BMJ 1995;311:655–9.
[63] Mackie AD, Thornton SJ, Edenborough FP. Cystic fibrosis-related diabetes. Diabet Med 2003;20:425–36.
[64] Holl RW, Wolf A, Thon A, et al. Insulin resistance with altered secretory kinetics and reduced proinsulin in cystic fibrosis patients. J Pediatr Gastroenterol Nutr 1997;25:188–93.
[65] Dobson L, Sheldon CD, Hattersley AT. Conventional measures underestimate glycaemia in cystic fibrosis patients. Diabet Med 2004;21:691–6.

[66] Yung B, Noormohamed FH, Kemp M, et al. Cystic fibrosis-related diabetes: the role of peripheral insulin resistance and beta-cell dysfunction. Diabet Med 2002;19:221–6.
[67] Holl RW, Heinze E, Wolf A, et al. Reduced pancreatic insulin release and reduced peripheral insulin sensitivity contribute to hyperglycaemia in cystic fibrosis. Eur J Pediatr 1995;154:356–61.
[68] De Schepper J, Hachimi-Idrissi S, Smitz J, et al. First-phase insulin release in adult cystic fibrosis patients: correlation with clinical and biological parameters. Horm Res 1992;38:260–3.
[69] Polychronakos C. Early onset diabetes mellitus: tip or iceberg? Pediatr Diabetes 2004;5:171–3.
[70] Austin A, Kalhan SC, Orenstein D, et al. Roles of insulin resistance and beta-cell dysfunction in the pathogenesis of glucose intolerance in cystic fibrosis. J Clin Endocrinol Metab 1994;79:80–5.
[71] Moran A, Pyzdrowski KL, Weinreb J, et al. Insulin sensitivity in cystic fibrosis. Diabetes 1994;43:1020–6.
[72] Lombardo F, De Luca F, Rosano M, et al. Natural history of glucose tolerance, beta-cell function and peripheral insulin sensitivity in cystic fibrosis patients with fasting euglycemia. Eur J Endocrinol 2003;149:53–9.
[73] Cucinotta D, De Luca F, Gigante A, et al. No changes of insulin sensitivity in cystic fibrosis patients with different degrees of glucose tolerance: an epidemiological and longitudinal study. Eur J Endocrinol 1994;130:253–8.
[74] Lanng S, Thorsteinsson B, Roder ME, et al. Insulin sensitivity and insulin clearance in cystic fibrosis patients with normal and diabetic glucose tolerance. Clin Endocrinol (Oxf) 1994;41:217–23.
[75] Hardin DS, Leblanc A, Marshall G, et al. Mechanisms of insulin resistance in cystic fibrosis. Am J Physiol Endocrinol Metab 2001;281:E1022–8.
[76] Hardin DS, LeBlanc A, Para L, et al. Hepatic insulin resistance and defects in substrate utilization in cystic fibrosis. Diabetes 1999;48:1082–7.
[77] Tofe S, Moreno JC, Maiz L, et al. Insulin-secretion abnormalities and clinical deterioration related to impaired glucose tolerance in cystic fibrosis. Eur J Endocrinol 2005;152:241–7.
[78] Ergun-Longmire B, Marker J, Zeidler A, et al. Oral insulin therapy to prevent progression of immune-mediated (type 1) diabetes. Ann NY Acad Sci 2004;1029:260–77.

PEDIATRIC CLINICS

OF NORTH AMERICA

Pediatr Clin N Am 52 (2005) 1553–1578

Type 1 Diabetes Mellitus: Etiology, Presentation, and Management

Michael J. Haller, MD[a], Mark A. Atkinson, PhD[b], Desmond Schatz, MD[c],*

[a]Division of Pediatric Endocrinology, University of Florida College of Medicine, PO Box 100296, Gainesville, FL 32610, USA
[b]The Center for Immunology and Transplantation, University of Florida College of Medicine, Room R3-128, ARB, Gainesville, FL 32610–0275, USA
[c]Diabetes Center, University of Florida College of Medicine, PO Box 100296, Gainesville, FL 32610, USA

Type 1 diabetes mellitus (T1D) is a heterogeneous disorder characterized by autoimmune-mediated destruction of pancreatic beta cells that culminates in absolute insulin deficiency. T1D is most commonly diagnosed in children and adolescents, usually presents with symptomatic hyperglycemia, and imparts the immediate need for exogenous insulin replacement. Approximately one fourth of patients with T1D are diagnosed as adults and often are labeled as having latent autoimmune disease of adults, however. Approximately 5% to 10% of adults diagnosed with type 2 diabetes actually may have T1D. Terms such as "juvenile diabetes" and "insulin-dependent diabetes" have been replaced because they no longer adequately reflect our understanding of the natural history and pathophysiology of T1D. This article provides an in-depth review regarding our current understanding of the epidemiology, etiology, presentation, and management of T1D as it relates to childhood and adolescence.

Epidemiology: incidence and prevalence

T1D is one of the most common chronic diseases of childhood. Even with the recent epidemic of type 2 diabetes, T1D accounts for approximately two thirds of

---

* Corresponding author.
  E-mail address: schatda@peds.ufl.edu (D. Schatz).

all cases of diabetes in children [1]. In the United States, more than 150,000 children younger than 18 years old have T1D [2]. The prevalence of T1D in US children is 1.7 to 2.5 cases per 1000 individuals, and the incidence is between 15 and 17 per 100,000/year [3]. In the United States, 10,000 to 15,000 new cases of T1D are diagnosed each year.

It seems that two peaks of T1D presentation occur in childhood: one between 5 and 7 years of age and the other at puberty. The incidence of T1D varies with seasonal changes and geography. Incidence rates are higher in autumn and winter and are lower in the summer. Some studies have suggested that the incidence of this disease is related positively to distance north of the equator; however, obvious exceptions do occur [4]. The incidence and prevalence of T1D varies dramatically around the world, with more than a 400-fold variation in incidence among reporting countries [5]. T1D is uncommon in China, India, and Venezuela, where the incidence is only 0.1 per 100,000. The disease is far more common in Sardinia and Finland, with the incidence approaching 50 cases per 100,000 individuals per year. Rates of more than 20 cases per 100,000 are observed in Sweden, Norway, Portugal, Great Britain, Canada, and New Zealand [5]. Wide variations have been observed between neighboring areas in Europe and North America. Estonia, separated from Finland by less than 75 miles, has a T1D incidence less than one third that of Finland. Puerto Rico has an incidence similar to the mainland United States (17 cases per 100,000), whereas neighboring Cuba has an incidence of less than 3 cases per 100,000 [5].

The incidence of T1D is increasing throughout the world, with marked changes especially being observed in young children from countries with historically high incidence rates (eg, children younger than 5–7 years of age in Norway). Sweden and Norway have reported a 3.3% annual increase in T1D rates, and Finland has observed a 2.4% annual rise in incidence [3]. Increases in T1D incidence rates cannot be explained by mere changes in socioeconomic status. Although many autoimmune diseases disproportionately affect women, T1D seems to affect men and women equally. Some reports indicate a modest excess in T1D cases in male patients younger than 20 years, however [6,7]. Taken collectively, differences in disease prevalence and changes in incidence rates suggest that a combination of multiple genetic and environmental factors contribute to T1D risk [5].

Economics of health care

As of 2002, the total costs attributable to diabetes care in the United States were estimated at $132 billion, whereas the direct costs of diabetes care were estimated at $91.8 billion [8]. Patients with diabetes were responsible for 1 in every $5.40 spent on health care in the United States, and individuals with diabetes had medical expenditures 2.4 times higher than patients without diabetes [8]. Although a disproportionate amount of these resources can be accounted for by adults with diabetes-related complications and patients requiring inpatient treatment, children faced with a lifetime of frequent glucose monitoring and insulin injections still have health care costs twice as high as children who do not have diabetes [9]. As a result, arguments have suggested that the economic strategy of the US health care system involve investment in intensive diabetes management to reduce the enormous future costs of long-term diabetes-related complications. Although the Diabetes Control and Complications Trial demonstrated that intensive therapy reduces the risk of complications, such an approach has not proved feasible for many patients with the disease [10]. As a result, some clinicians question the practical implementation of intensive therapy because mandating multiple daily insulin injections, frequent blood glucose monitoring, and altered nutritional and exercise practices substantially affects patients' and families' lifestyles.

Etiology

Natural history of prediabetes

Over the past 30 years, the ability to predict the development of T1D has improved dramatically with the combined use of genetic, autoantibody, and metabolic markers. The most often cited model of the natural history of T1D suggests that genetically susceptible individuals with a fixed number of beta cells are exposed to a putative environmental trigger that induces beta cell autoimmunity [11]. The development of islet reactive autoantibodies is a marker of ongoing autoimmune disease, but it is predominantly activated autoreactive T cells that destroy beta cells, which results in a progressive and predicable loss in insulin secretory function. Because clinical T1D typically does not present until approximately 80% to 90% of the beta cells have been destroyed, there is a marked gap between the onset of autoimmunity and the onset of diabetes (Fig. 1).

Recently, some aspects of the classic model have been challenged. For example, data suggest that pancreatic beta cells have considerable regenerative properties [12]. The degree of beta cell destruction required for symptomatic onset is also questioned, with recent studies suggesting that 40% to 50% of beta cells are viable at the onset of hyperglycemia. This finding may explain why, despite persistent autoimmunity, insulin secretory function may remain stable for long periods of time in persons with T1D. Only when autoimmunity overwhelms the regenerative capabilities of the beta cells does insulin secretory function decline (denoted by loss of first phase insulin secretion measured during intravenous glucose tolerance testing). Loss of first phase insulin response is followed by a period of glucose intolerance and a period of clinically "silent" diabetes.

An improved understanding of the natural history of prediabetes remains critical for directing future studies aimed at the prevention of T1D. Improved markers of disease risk, further identification of environmental agents that influence the disease, and continued identification of genes that influence disease

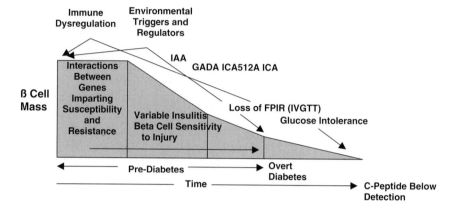

Fig. 1. Model of the pathogenesis and natural history of T1D. The modern model expands and updates the traditional model by inclusion of information gained through an improved understanding of the roles for genetics, immunology, and environment in the natural history of T1D. FPIR, first phase insulin response; GAD, glutamic acid decarboxylase autoantibodies; IAA, insulin autoantibodies; ICA, islet cell autoantibodies; ICA 512, autoantibodies against the islet tyrosine phosphatase; IVGTT, intravenous glucose tolerance test. (*Adapted from* Atkinson MA, Eisenbarth GS. Type 1 diabetes: new perspectives on disease pathogenesis and treatment. Lancet 2001;358(9277):225; with permission.)

susceptibility are all examples of information needed to impact efforts toward the goal of disease prevention.

Genetics

Despite being strongly influenced by genetic factors, T1D does not fit any mendelian pattern of inheritance and is considered a complex, multifactorial disease. Early familial aggregation and twin studies supported the aforementioned importance for genetic and environmental risk factors in T1D. Individuals in the United States who have a first-degree relative with T1D have a 1 in 20 risk of developing T1D, whereas the general population has a 1 in 300 lifetime risk [13]. Monozygotic twins have a concordance rate of 30% to 50%, whereas dizygotic twins have a concordance rate of 6% to 10%. Eighty-five percent of cases of T1D occur in individuals with no family history of the disease. Differences in risk also depend on which parent has diabetes. Children of mothers who have T1D have only a 2% risk of developing T1D, whereas children of fathers who have T1D have a 7% risk (Box 1) [14]. To date, more than two dozen susceptibility loci have been associated with susceptibility to T1D (Table 1). In and of itself, no single gene is either necessary or sufficient to predict the development of T1D.

The first T1D susceptibility locus identified, the human leukocyte antigen (HLA) complex, provides the greatest contribution (40%–60%) to genetic susceptibility. There are three classes of HLA genes, with class II genes having the strongest association with T1D. Because class II HLA genes encode for molecules that participate in antigen presentation, the effect of major histocom-

---

Box 1. Genetic susceptibility to type 1 diabetes mellitus

General population: 0.3%

Relatives: 2–50%

  Twins
  • Monozygotic: 30%–50%
  • Dizygotic: 6%–10%
  Siblings: 5%
  Offspring
  • Of affected father: 7%
  • Of affected mother: 2%
  Parents: 3%

---

patibility complex allelic variability on T1D risk may, for example, be explained by differences in the presentation of islet cell antigens, either by promoting anti-self reactivity or by failing to impart regulated immune responses. Most patients who have T1D carry the HLA-DR3 or -DR4 class II antigens, with 30% being DR3/DR4 heterozygous. In white persons, the DR3/DR4 genotype confers the highest T1D risk, followed by DR4 and DR3 homozygosity, respectively [13]. Conversely, the class II allele, DQB1*0602, in linkage disequilibrium with DR2, is associated with protection from the development of T1D and is found in less than 1% of patients with T1D (Table 2).

Table 1
Type 1 diabetes mellitus susceptibility loci

Locus	Chromosome	Markers	Genes
IDDM 1	6p21.31-21.32	IDDMHLA, HLA	PSMB8, TAP2
IDDM 2	11p15.5	5′INS-VNTR, TH	INS
IDDM 3	15q26.2	D15S107	—
IDDM 4	11q12.1-13.2	FGF3, D11S1917, MDU1, ZFM1, RT6, ICE, CD3, LRP5	LRP5
IDDM 5	6q25.1	ESR, a046Xa9, MnSOD	—
IDDM 6	18q12.2-21.1	D18S487, D18S64, JK	BCL2, TNFRSF11A
IDDM 7	2q32.1	D2S152, D251391, GAD1	—
IDDM 8	6q26-27	D6S281, D6S264, D6S446	—
IDDM 9	3q22.3-26.2	D3S1303	CP, IL12A
IDDM 10	10p11.1-12.1	D10S193, D10S208, GAD2	CXCL12, GAD2
IDDM 11	14q31.3-32.12	D14S67	—
IDDM 12	2q33.2-33.3	CTLA-4, CD28	CTLA-4, CD28
IDDM 13	2q35	D2S137, D2S164, IGFBP2, IGFBP5	—
IDDM 15	6q21	IDDMFYN, D6S283, D6S434, D6S1580	—
IDDM 17	10q25.1-25.3	D10S554, D10S592	CASP7
IDDM 18	5q31.3	IDDMIL12B, IL12B	IL12B

Table 2
Absolute risk for type 1 diabetes mellitus according to DR/DQ genotypes

DR/DQ	Risk	First-degree relative	Population
DR 3/4, DQ 0201/0302	Very high	1/4–5	1/15
DR 4/4, DQ 0300/0302	High	1/6	1/20
DR 3/3, DQ 0201/0201	High	1/10	1/45
DR4/x, DQ 0302/x (x≠0602)	Moderate	1/15	1/60
X/X	Low	1/125	1/600
DR0403 or DQ0602	Protected	1/15,000	1/15,000

As indicated, non-HLA genes are also associated with T1D. For example, the IDDM2 locus has been mapped to a variable number of tandem repeats located upstream of the insulin gene. Disease association studies in case control and family cohorts show that the number of tandem repeats is associated with T1D risk, with shorter repeats conferring higher risk and longer repeats conferring lower risk. Another non-HLA gene associated with T1D is CTLA-4 (cytotoxic T lymphocyte associated-4) [15]. First identified in a family study of T1D, this gene encodes a molecule that plays an important role in the regulation of T-cell function and immune responses. Other specific genes finding some degree of recent support include PTPN22 and SUMO4, each of which is believed to provide influence to immune responsiveness [16,17]. As our understanding of the function of susceptibility and resistant genes grows, we will continue to gain new insights into the relationship between genetic risk and the autoimmunity that culminates in T1D.

Autoimmunity and autoantibodies

As indicated, T1D is an autoimmune disease that culminates in destruction of the pancreatic beta cells, characterized histologically by insulitis and associated islet cell damage. The autoimmunity in T1D is specific to the insulin-producing beta cells. The specific mechanisms responsible for inducing the autoimmunity in T1D have yet to be elucidated, however. Many different theories have been promulgated to explain this induction, including molecular mimicry (sharing of antigenic properties) (ie, amino acid sequences between beta cells and possible environmental agents leading to the generation of an immune response), alteration of self-antigens, defective major histocompatibility complex expression, breakdown in central tolerance (ie, failure to establish immunity to self-antigens in early life), deleterious trafficking of dendritic cells from beta cells to pancreatic lymph nodes, and defects in peripheral tolerance (ie, aberrant T-cell activation). The role for the cellular immune response in T1D has been remarkably controversial. Because nearly all studies performed to date have involved characterization away from the site of injury (ie, performed on cells from peripheral blood and not the pancreatic islets), we have elected to avoid their review in this article but reference other articles dedicated to such descriptions [18–20].

Regardless of the proposed causes of the autoimmunity, biopsy is the only true means of directly demonstrating beta cell injury. Because in most settings pancreatic biopsies have not been considered ethically feasible (because of reasons of safety), autoimmunity in T1D typically has been identified by the presence of circulating autoantibodies to islet cell antigens, which in addition to their presence at the time of diagnosis often can be detected long before the disease becomes clinically evident. Islet cell autoantibodies (ICAs), autoantibodies to glutamic acid decarboxylase (GAD65A), insulin autoantibodies (IAAs), and autoantibodies directed at a transmembrane tyrosine phosphatase (ICA512A) are the most prevalent and best characterized, but the potential for other autoantibody/autoantigen combinations remains. It is critical to note that autoantibodies have no known etiologic role in diabetes and—simply put—are believed to represent the "smoke of the fire" in the pancreas and not the fire itself. Recent studies in animal models of T1D purporting a crucial role for B lymphocytes in disease development may allow for a previously unappreciated role for autoantibodies in presentation of self-antigens to the cytotoxic T cells responsible for beta cell destruction.

T1D-associated autoantibodies are present in 70% to 80% of patients newly diagnosed with the disease. In contrast, 0.5% of the general population and 3% to 4% of relatives of patients who have T1D are autoantibody positive [21]. Although autoantibodies are surrogate measures for beta cell autoimmunity, autoantibody titer and the absolute number of autoantibodies (eg, one, two) are independent predictors of T1D risk. Specifically, when present in combination, at higher titers, at a younger age, or with the high-risk HLA genes, autoantibodies allow for a more accurate prediction of T1D risk. ICA titers of >40 Juvenile Diabetes Foundation units carry a 60% to 70% risk of developing diabetes over 5 to 7 years [21]. When present at a young age, ICAs denote a much greater risk than when present in older subjects. When present in the first few years of life, the 10-year risk of developing diabetes is nearly 90%, whereas a 40-year-old individual who is ICA positive has a 30% 10-year risk. After 10 years of overt diabetes, less than 5% of patients have detectable ICA. Although IAAs may be the first autoantibodies to appear in the development of T1D, they are not by themselves strong predictors of developing T1D. When present in combination with other autoantibodies, however, the risk for T1D increases significantly. In the large, NIH-funded Diabetes Prevention Trial–Type 1, the 5-year risk of T1D was 20% to 25% for subjects with one autoantibody, 50% to 60% for subjects with two autoantibodies, nearly 70% for persons with three autoantibodies, and almost 80% for persons with four autoantibodies [22].

Another peculiar aspect of IAAs is that they must be measured within 1 week of the start of exogenous insulin therapy, because insulin antibodies in response to exogenously injected insulin also are detected and are indistinguishable from IAAs. GAD65A, like ICAs, are observed in 60% to 70% of patients who have new-onset T1D. Unlike ICA, GAD65A often persist for many years after diagnosis in patients with T1D and may be more useful in diagnosing latent autoimmune disease of adults than ICAs [23]. IA-2 has an extracellular, transmembrane, and cytoplasmic domain, and autoantibodies to several forms of IA-2 have been observed in persons who have T1D. Because more than one laboratory independently identified this molecule, it also has been referred to in the literature as the ICA512 autoantigen. The IA-2 antigen, like GAD, is expressed in many tissues, including brain, pituitary, and pancreas [24].

In summary, the identification and description of autoantibodies in T1D has allowed us to gain remarkable insight into the natural history of this disease. In combination with a growing understanding of genetic susceptibility, we are currently able to predict accurately which patients will develop T1D [25]. As efforts continue to help researchers understand the etioimmunopathogenesis of T1D, many questions still remain as to the role for cellular immunity and issues related to which specific environmental triggers induce or regulate the auto-immunity related to T1D.

Environment

T1D results from the interaction of genes, the environment, and the immune system. The presence of disparate geographic prevalence, rising worldwide in-cidence, and 50% discordance rate in identical twins provides evidence that environmental agents are operative [26]. Because the islet-specific autoantibodies frequently can be detected within the first few years of life [27–29], it seems that triggering environmental encounters may occur early in development. Because there is invariably a latent period between the appearance of T1D-associated autoantibodies and onset of disease, additional environmental factors—probably interacting with genetic factors—also seem to modulate the rate of development of the disease [30].

Early nutrition and infection have been the most frequently implicated early environmental influences [31]. There is, however, no direct evidence to date that either nutrition or infection plays a major role in causation, albeit one example is often cited as providing such evidence [32,33]. Prenatal rubella infection is associated with beta cell autoimmunity in up to 70% and diabetes in up to 40% of infected children [32,34–38]. Postnatal infection is not associated with increased risk, however. The introduction of universal rubella vaccination has virtually abolished this disease and the occurrence of this form of diabetes, which proves that in some cases T1D can be prevented by modification of environmental factors.

A relationship between beta cell autoimmunity and exposure to enteroviral infections in utero also has been proposed [33,39,40]. Studies from Finland and Sweden suggested that maternal enterovirus infection may increase the likelihood of subsequent T1D development in offspring [33,39]. Higher levels of antibodies to procapsid enterovirus antigens were found in the pregnant sera of mothers of children who developed diabetes. The presence of antibodies against entero-viruses in people with autoimmunity does not prove a causal relationship, however. It should be noted that the number of women exposed to enteroviral infection during pregnancy is decreasing and that infection in early childhood has become less common [41]. Islet-related autoantibodies also have been detected after mumps, measles, chickenpox, and rotavirus infections [42–44]. These considerations do not exclude arguments based on changing antigenicity of foods or viruses or timing of exposure to them. Persons with autoimmunity also may be more prone to enteroviral infection, may have a stronger humoral response to infection because of their particular HLA genotype, or may be in a nonspecific hyperimmune state marked by elevation of antibody levels to various exogenous antigens [31]. With this background, it is clear that well-planned prospective studies in larger populations are essential. The Environmental Determinants of Type 1 Diabetes in Youth study is one such example that was formed recently and at an international level will document exposure to various infectious and other environmental agents throughout pregnancy and early infancy.

In terms of noninfectious influences, the association between a potential protective effect of breastfeeding and early exposure to cow's milk on the incidence of autoimmunity and T1D remains controversial [45–50]. Gerstein's extensive meta-analysis demonstrated a weak but statistically significant association (odds ratio approximately 1.5) between T1D and a shortened period of breastfeeding and cow's milk exposure before 3 to 4 months of age [51]. In the biobreeding rat and nonobese diabetic mouse models of T1D, diet plays an important role in the development of the disease, yet which dietary components are important remains unclear. Among them is casein, a major protein fraction of cow's milk. Feeding semi-purified diets with simple sugars replacing complex carbohydrates and hydrolyzed casein as the protein source routinely retards the development of diabetes in rodents [52,53]. Another component is bovine serum albumin. Karjalainen and colleagues showed that antibodies to bovine serum albumin, which are immunologically distinct from human serum albumin, were present in 100% of Finnish children who have new-onset T1D but were absent in controls [48]. Structural similarities between bovine serum albumin and an islet protein (ICA_{69}) were proposed as an appealing pathogenic concept of molecular mimicry, by which the early introduction of cow's milk would allow absorption of the intact protein before gut maturation, thus immunizing an infant and directing an immune response to the islets through its ICA_{69} mimic [54]. There is strong evidence to counter each argument put forth to advance the cow's milk hypothesis, however [45]. No association between early exposure to cow's milk and beta cell autoimmunity in young siblings and offspring of patients who have diabetes has been shown in several other studies. Increased practice of breastfeeding in developed countries is inconsistent with a rising incidence of childhood diabetes [55]. We and others were unable to show any link between the presence of antibodies to bovine serum albumin and T1D [47,56]. Finally, ICA_{69} has been found in several other organs beside pancreatic cells, and cross-reactivity of these antibodies with bovine serum albumin has not been confirmed.

The ingestion of nutrient-containing elements of plants such as soy and wheat also seem to have an effect on the development of diabetes, at least as defined in studies of nonobese diabetic mice [57]. In humans, two recent studies—the Diabetes Autoimmunity Study in the Young and the German study of offspring of T1D parents—provided evidence that susceptibility to T1D is associated with the timing of exposure to cereal and gluten [58,59]. In the Diabetes Autoimmunity Study in the Young, initial exposure to cereal between birth and 3 months of age and after 7 months of age imparted risk of autoimmunity. In the German study of offspring of T1D parents, Zeigler and colleagues [59] demonstrated an increased risk for autoimmunity in infants initially exposed to gluten before 3 months of age and found no increased risk in infants initially exposed to gluten after 6 months of age. Although both studies provided interesting findings, their conclusions are in some ways contradictory and demonstrate the need for larger collaborative investigations to determine appropriately how early dietary exposures affect risk for autoimmunity.

The highest incidence of T1D worldwide occurs in Finland (currently approximately 50 cases per 100,000/year). Sun exposure in northern Finland is limited and low serum concentrations of vitamin D in Finland are common. Hypponen and colleagues [60] have suggested that ensuring adequate vitamin D supplementation for infants could help to reverse the increasing incidence of T1D. It has been proposed that vitamin D compounds may act as selective immunosuppressants, as illustrated by their ability to either prevent or markedly suppress development of autoimmune disease in animal models of T1D [61]. Vitamin D has been shown to stimulate transforming growth factor beta-1 and interleukin-4, which may suppress inflammatory T cell (Th1) activity [62].

Toxic doses of nitrosamine compounds also can cause diabetes because of the generation of free radicals [63,64]. The effect of dietary nitrate, nitrite, or nitrosamine exposure on human T1D risk is less clear [65,66]. Several perinatal risk factors for childhood diabetes are also associated with the development of T1D [67]. The effect of maternal-child blood group incompatibility is fairly strong (both ABO and Rh factor with ABO > Rh) and must be explored further. Other perinatal factors that confer increased risk include pre-eclampsia, neonatal respiratory distress, neonatal infections, caesarian section, birth weight, gestational age, birth order, and maternal age [68–72]. It is important to determine whether these factors really contribute and how they may act or be confounded by other unknown risk factors. Rodent studies also suggested that administration of diphtheria-tetanus-pertussis vaccine at 2 months of age increases the incidence of diabetes compared with the incidence in unvaccinated individuals or in individuals vaccinated at birth. In prospective studies, however, no association has been demonstrated between early childhood immunizations and beta cell autoimmunity [73,74].

Finally, researchers have argued that the rising incidence of T1D could be accounted for by protective factors in the environment that have been lost [75]. In support of this theory, the rise in the rates of asthma and allergy has been parallel to that of T1D. The hygiene hypothesis proposes that exposure to infective agents in early childhood is necessary for maturation of the neonatal immune response. In the absence of such exposure, the model predicts a failure of early immune regulation that may permit, depending on genetic susceptibility, the development of autoimmunity (Th1) or allergic (Th2) disease [76,77]. This is consistent with the fact that the nonobese diabetic mouse is less likely to develop diabetes in the presence of pinworms and other infections, yet specific evidence for the hygiene hypothesis in human T1D is minimal [76].

The list of suggested environmental triggers and regulators of disease in T1D remains considerable. Only through the continued effort of large, prospective, multicenter screening programs will we be able to determine which environmental and genetic factors are most responsible for the development of this disease.

Presentations: classic, silent, and diabetic ketoacidosis

The presentation of new-onset T1D is distributed among three typical patterns: classic new onset, silent diabetes, and diabetic ketoacidosis (DKA). Although most children present with classic new-onset diabetes, in many locations, DKA still accounts for 20% to 40% of all new diagnoses [78]. Silent diabetes, which is less commonly seen at diagnosis, is typically seen in children either involved in diabetes research studies or picked up by families in which one member already has the disease.

Children who have classic new-onset T1D typically present with polydipsia, polyuria, polyphagia, weight loss, and lethargy. Classic-onset T1D is differentiated from DKA because children who have classic onset have enough preserved beta cell function to avoid metabolic decompensation with resultant acidosis. The symptoms of classic diabetes are caused by prolonged hyperglycemia. Once blood glucose concentrations exceed the renal threshold for reabsorption (approximately 180mg/dL), glycosuria ensues with the resultant osmotic diuresis, dehydration, and thirst. Over time, increasingly poor glucose uptake by tissues, resultant chronic glycosuria, and breakdown of amino acids for gluconeogenic substrate with fat breakdown to supply fatty acids for ketogenesis all contribute to weight loss.

Classic T1D is usually diagnosed in the outpatient setting when a slightly ill-appearing child presents to the pediatrician for evaluation of weight loss and other nonspecific symptoms. A high index of suspicion for diabetes should be a concern for all physicians. The classic polyuria is not told to the physician, but recurrence of bedwetting, unusually wet diapers in a child who seems to be dehydrated, recurrent monilial infection in the diaper area, and persistent thirst should arouse suspicion. Glucosuria and hyperglycemia are easily confirmed in a physician's office by test strips and glucose meters. Children who have silent (ie, diagnosed early in the course of) T1D are typically diagnosed by families or physicians with a high index of suspicion. Often these children have other family members with T1D and their parents are more likely to have them undergo testing or have them screened in research studies. Children with a silent presentation often require little insulin because they have greater residual beta cell mass.

Most patients who have new-onset diabetes without DKA can receive initial management and education as outpatients in a tertiary care setting. In areas without a pediatric referral hospital, inpatient management may be needed to facilitate proper education and initiation of therapy. Outpatient management with early teaching of basic diabetes management tasks often gives the family a sense of being in control and reduces the initial emotional impact for the child and family.

The clinic setting is much more comfortable for education than the emotionally highly charged hospital environment. Outpatient management greatly reduces the initial cost of T1D management.

DKA is characterized by complete lack of insulin production such that glucose use is crippled and triglycerides must be broken down to provide the body with energy. The resulting byproducts of fatty acid metabolism—the ketones aceto-acetate and beta-hydroxybutyrate—further exacerbate the osmotic diuresis and cause acidosis. Dehydration and poor perfusion also may lead to lactic acidosis. The consequences of insulin deficiency are shown in Fig. 2.

Children who present with DKA require immediate hospitalization, insulin replacement, and rehydration. An initial arterial pH of < 7.3, serum bicarbonate concentration of < 15 mEq/L, and clinical signs of dehydration, vomiting, or mental status changes dictate hospitalization. Rapid deep respirations, known as Kussmaul breathing, often are present when significant acidosis occurs. Kuss-maul breathing results from the body's attempt to compensate for the metabolic acidosis by exhaling excess CO_2. Kussmaul respiration must be distinguished from reactive airways disease (asthma) or other causes of respiratory distress. Glucocorticoids and sympathomimetics given in the mistaken belief that the

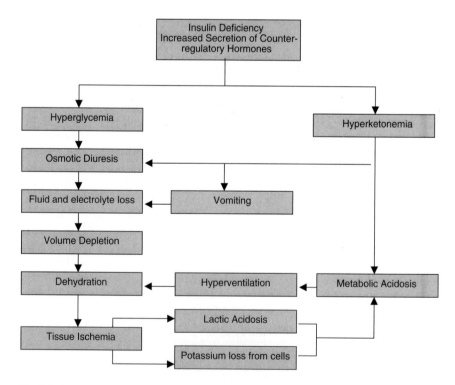

Fig. 2. Pathogenesis of DKA. This figure outlines the pathophysiology of insulin deficiency leading to hyperglycemia, hyperketonemia, dehydration, and acidosis.

deep, sighing respirations of acidosis are caused by airway obstruction are a common cause of exacerbating DKA.

The overall mortality rate from pediatric DKA in the United States is approximately 0.5%. More than 90% of the deaths associated with pediatric T1D are related to DKA and cerebral edema, which occurs almost exclusively in children and adolescents [79]. Approximately 1% of DKA episodes are complicated by cerebral edema with its extremely high morbidity and mortality.

Initial management of DKA includes fluid resuscitation, close monitoring of vital signs, securing intravenous access, and obtaining blood and urine specimens for laboratory analysis. Urine ketones, pH (arterial or venous), electrolytes, and blood glucose are usually the only laboratory tests needed to provide proper management. Based on the pathophysiology of DKA, successful management involves rehydration, appropriate replacement of electrolytes, and correction of the underlying defect, namely, insulin deficiency. (For an in-depth discussion of DKA management, please see the article by Glaser elsewhere in this issue.) Once acidosis has resolved, subcutaneous insulin regimens can be started.

Management

Overall the goals for management of T1D in children are as follows:

- Setting of realistic goals for each child and family. Factors to be considered include a patient's age, developmental status, family involvement and social situation, economic factors, and hypoglycemic history in persons with established disease
- Near normalization of blood glucose levels and HbA1c measurements or, where not possible, improvement on subsequent follow-up
- Prevention of DKA
- Avoidance of severe hypoglycemia
- Assuring as near normal quality of life as is possible within the constraints of the factors outlined in the first goal
- Maintaining normal growth, development, and maturation
- Providing readily available multidisciplinary support, including nutritional education and psychological support
- Maintaining close surveillance and prevention of microvascular and macrovascular complications (see article by Glastras and colleagues elsewhere in this issue)

Management in new-onset diabetes

For almost all children and their families, the diagnosis of diabetes is overwhelming. The initial management and education can be divided into two phases: (1) stabilization and the teaching of survival skills over the first few days and (2) ongoing diabetes management skills designed to teach a patient and family day-to-day management. All patients are seen on the day of diagnosis. If a patient is stable metabolically (ie, without DKA), has a stable social situation, and is older than 5 years, we manage the situation on an outpatient basis. Initially, the family is asked to return daily until education is completed and the family feels comfortable with their ability to manage the basics of their child's diabetes. After this intensive teaching, the family maintains close contact with the nurse and doctor on a daily basis until they seem able to cope with the situation.

Stabilization and teaching of survival skills

On the day the diagnosis is confirmed, families are given a simple overview of diabetes. Because there are often feelings of guilt, we reassure the family that there is no known cause of diabetes and that no food, activity, or anything they did contributed to its development. Survival skills are taught. All patients are started on insulin therapy. If stable, we typically start a patient on a total dose of insulin of 0.5 to 1 U/kg/d (see later discussion).

The next day the family returns for further education from the diabetes nurse. Information is provided on the pathophysiology of hyperglycemia and hypo-glycemia and the "do's" and "don'ts" of living with diabetes. This education usually takes 2 to 3 days. The family is taught about the insulin types, how to mix and inject the insulin, and how to rotate sites. They are also taught the importance and mechanics of monitoring blood glucose levels and checking the urine for ketones at times of illness and elevated blood glucose measurements (> 250 mg/dL). The child and family are taught to test the blood glucose initially before each mealtime, before bed, and once a week between 2AM and 4AM. Hypoglycemia recognition and treatment (including the use of glucagon) is taught, as is sick day management. A basic guideline is given for planning meals and snacks and what must be done if the blood glucose level is too high or low. Carbohydrate counting is not taught at this time. The importance of a healthy, balanced nutritional plan with various foods from all the basic food groups is emphasized.

Once the health care team is comfortable with a family's ability to manage the diabetes at home, the child is allowed to return to home and school. The family is instructed to call daily in the morning for the first week after diagnosis for insulin dose adjustment. The frequency of contact abates as the family becomes more confident with diabetes management abilities. It is imperative that the school be apprised of the child's diagnosis and written materials be provided on the essential skills necessary for the detection and management of hypoglycemia and hyperglycemia. Contact numbers are also provided in cases of an emergency.

Ongoing diabetes management

Within the next 4 to 6 weeks, two to three additional sessions are scheduled with a diabetes nurse and nutritionist and with a psychologist and social worker as necessary. Clearly, education relating to the pathophysiology of diabetes, the causes of hyperglycemia and hypoglycemia, target glucose levels, how different insulin preparations work, the importance of 2-hour postprandial blood glucose testing, the interaction of food, exercise, and insulin, and the impact of stress and illness is critical to good control. These concepts and the importance of good control are stressed repeatedly. Approximately 2 months after diagnosis, an in-depth review of the topics takes place, and short- and long-term treatment goals are mutually agreed upon by the family and multidisciplinary team. Potential barriers (eg, familial, psychosocial, and school) are identified and appropriate intervention instituted.

Subcutaneous insulin regimens: neutral protamine Hagedorn and rapid acting analogs

Although multiple insulin regimens exist, we prefer to start new-onset T1D patients on a simple combination of neutral protamine Hagedorn (NPH) insulin and a rapid-acting analog, such as aspart or lispro given two or three times daily (see the article by Daneman elsewhere in this issue on details of insulin types and mixtures available). Most children who have symptomatic T1D at diagnosis require a total insulin dose of approximately 1 U/kg/d at diagnosis. Pubertal children typically are more insulin resistant and often require 1 to 1.5 U/kg/d. When using NPH with short-acting insulin regimens, the total daily insulin dosage is typically divided into two thirds in the morning and one third in the evening. The morning dose is usually given as two thirds NPH and one third rapid-acting analog. The evening dose is usually given as one half NPH and one half rapid-acting analog. NPH insulin begins to work 2 hours after injection, peaks 5 to 7 hours after injection, and lasts 13 to 16 hours. Rapid-acting analogs, such as lispro or aspart, begin to work 15 minutes after injection, peak 1 to 3 hours after injection, and last 3 to 5 hours (Table 3) [80].

In addition to scheduled insulin doses, supplemental short-acting insulin should be given to bring elevated glucose values into the target range. Once patients and their families have developed a rudimentary understanding of diabetes management, we teach them to apply a correction factor to determine how much additional insulin is needed to correct elevated blood glucoses. The correction factor can be estimated by dividing 1600 by the total daily dose of insulin. The result gives an approximation of the glucose lowering effect of 1 U

Table 3
Insulin preparations

Type	Onset (h)	Peak (h)	Duration (h)
Short acting			
aspart/ lispro	0.25	1–3	3–5
regular	0.25 – 0.5	2–4	6–8
Intermediate			
NPH	2	5–7	13–16
Long acting			
glargine	1–2	No peak	24

of rapid acting insulin or the insulin sensitivity. For example, a child on 32 U of insulin per day would have an insulin sensitivity of 1600/32 or 50. We would then advise that the child receive an additional 1 U of rapid-acting insulin for every 50 mg/dL glucose above the defined target (typically >120 mg/dL over age 8 years).

Glargine and continuous subcutaneous insulin infusion

Basal-bolus insulin usage that employs glargine insulin and rapid-acting analogs and CSII has increased. Glargine and continuous subcutaneous insulin infusion (CSII) are most often offered to children who already have demonstrated the ability to manage their diabetes somewhat independently and to preschool-aged children who have committed parents. In families with previous diabetes knowledge, insulin glargine or CSII should be considered at diagnosis. Several studies have demonstrated the ability of CSII and insulin glargine to improve metabolic control and hypoglycemia frequency in young children and toddlers. Although CSII and glargine regimens require more frequent blood glucose testing and insulin administration than fixed doses, many children and parents accept the increased work required because of the lifestyle flexibility afforded by this schedule. Despite these advantages, overall glycemic control may not improve just because a child is switched to CSII or glargine. All regimens will fail unless a child and family are committed to performing the diabetes tasks necessary to succeed. Before changing therapy, we require children interested in using glargine or CSII to attend a carbohydrate counting and pump class, monitor their blood glucose a minimum of four to six times per day, call weekly with blood glucose results, and record carbohydrate intake and insulin boluses based on a prescribed insulin-to-carbohydrate ratio and correction factors.

Initial glargine doses are typically calculated by using 60% to 70% of the total intermediate-acting insulin previously given. For initial pump rates, most children use 70% to 80% of their previous total daily amount of subcutaneous insulin, with 60% of their previous intermediate-acting insulin dose given as a basal dose divided over 24 hours. Meal coverage is determined by using insulin-to-carbohydrate ratios. Ratios in children tend to be anywhere from 1:30 for young children to 1:5 for adolescents at the peak of insulin resistance. Supplemental insulin calculated as correction factors before beginning CSII or insulin glargine therapy should continue to be used (see the article by Weinzimer and colleagues elsewhere in this issue— on insulin pump therapy).

Potential adjuncts to insulin therapy

Despite the development of long- and rapid-acting insulin analogs, subcutaneous insulin administration is still unable to match normal insulin secretion perfectly. Additional therapies are needed to provide patients who have T1D with maximal glucose control. The potential role of glucagon-like peptide-1 analogs, which have shown promise as adjunct therapy for type 2 diabetes in augmenting insulin response, and amylin, a hormone that is normally co-secreted with insulin and may dampen glucagon secretion, are currently being explored as potential therapies in patients who have T1D [81,82].

Self blood glucose monitoring

Self blood glucose monitoring is the cornerstone of diabetes management. Intensive diabetes management mandates that patients perform frequent self blood glucose monitoring at least four to six times a day. Frequent self blood glucose monitoring empowers patients and their families and enhances the understanding of insulin, food, and exercise effects on blood glucose. It also affords multiple opportunities to provide additional insulin to correct hyperglycemia and improve control. Regardless of the insulin regimen being prescribed, frequency of self blood glucose monitoring correlates directly with improved glucose control [83]. Because the Diabetes Control and Complications Trial demonstrated the importance of maintaining tight glycemic control on minimizing microvascular disease, intensive diabetes management is the standard of care. The inconvenience, cost, and pain of self blood glucose monitoring may limit its use for some patients.

In addition to finger tip glucose monitoring, continuous glucose monitoring systems may allow for more intensive self blood glucose monitoring. Current continuous glucose monitoring systems use a subcutaneous catheter that transmits data on interstitial fluid glucose to a transmitter that is worn much like an insulin pump. After 3 days, the transmitter is downloaded and the data can be reviewed retrospectively. Real-time continuous glucose monitoring systems, which would provide readings on a digital screen every 5 minutes, are expected to be available in the near future [84].

Medical nutritional therapy

Perhaps the most important—yet often neglected—part of diabetes management is medical nutritional therapy. Although physicians often focus on insulin dosing and self blood glucose monitoring, optimal management requires proper recognition of the balance among insulin, exercise, and food. All families with a newly diagnosed child should receive consultation with a nutritionist, and most children and their families should be given a refresher course annually. Because the obesity epidemic has not spared the T1D population, increasing efforts must be made to encourage physical activity and limitation of excess caloric intake. Specifically, children should be encouraged to perform 30 to 60 minutes of exercise at least five times per week. Caloric intake should include approximately 50% to 55% of calories from carbohydrates, 15% to 20% from protein, and 30% from fat. The American Diabetes Association no longer recommends a specific diet and advises that individualized adjustments be made depending on activity and other metabolic demands.

With the increasing popularity of CSII and glargine insulin regimens, children who have diabetes must have an adequate understanding of how carbohydrates, protein, and fat affect blood glucose. Detailed carbohydrate counting instruction should be a cornerstone of diabetes education for all children who have diabetes, especially children who use CSII or glargine. When children are asked to report their prescribed carbohydrate ratio and correction factor, we should ask them directly to calculate a meal time insulin dose based on a typical meal and their current blood glucose. Using real world examples helps determine if a child or family needs more detailed nutritional education.

Sick day management

When children who have diabetes have an illness, the primary goal is to avoid ketoacidosis. Urine must be checked for ketones frequently. If ketones are present, additional regular insulin should be given and repeated every 4 hours if necessary. For moderate ketone levels, an additional 15% to 20% of the total daily insulin dose should be given; for large ketone levels, 25% to 30% of the total daily insulin dose should be given. When children have an illness that limits their oral intake or have low blood sugars, insulin adjustments can be difficult. For children on standard combinations of NPH and rapid-acting analogs who refuse to eat, small amounts of easily absorbable glucose may be necessary to avoid hypoglycemia. Doses of rapid-acting analogs also can be held until immediately after a child has eaten to determine if and how much of the dose should be given. Children who are not eating well and are on combination therapy with NPH and rapid-acting analogs may need a 25% to 30% reduction in their NPH dose to avoid hypoglycemia. On the other hand, children who use CSII or glargine may require a 10% to 15% increase in basal rates on sick days to avoid lipolysis.

Hypoglycemia

Fear of or actual hypoglycemia is one of the most important factors that limits the implementation of intensive diabetes management. Because even the best diabetes management provides exogenous insulin in a nonphysiologic manner, appropriate management of hypoglycemia must be discussed at initiation of insulin therapy and should be reviewed at each clinic visit. For the initial treatment of hypoglycemia in a responsive child, 15 g of rapid acting carbohydrate (eg, 4 oz juice, three glucose tablets) should be given, which should raise the blood glucose level 15 to 20 mg/dL after 10 minutes. Families also must be taught how to mix and administer glucagon (0.5–1 mg intramuscularly) in case a child is unconscious or seizing or does not respond to oral glucose.

Avoidance of severe hypoglycemia is critical in young children because of concerns over damaging active brain development. Children who are tightly controlled and experience a severe hypoglycemic event often have markedly higher HbA1c for several years. This occurs because parents of children who have experienced a severe hypoglycemic event often develop a significant fear of hypoglycemia and respond by withholding appropriate insulin or overfeeding. To avoid severe hypoglycemia, we advise patients to reduce insulin doses when they experience three or more blood glucose levels less than 60 mg/dL at the same time of day in 1 week, two or more blood glucose levels less than 50 mg/dL at the same time of day in 1 week, or any one blood glucose level less than 40 mg/dL. We also advise our patients that HbA1c goals must be adjusted for age. For further information, please see the article by Becker and Ryan elsewhere in this issue.

Age-specific goals

The risks of severe hypoglycemia must be balanced with the long-term risk of microvascular and macrovascular complications. In children, HbA1c goals must be age adjusted to minimize the frequency of serious hypoglycemia. Unlike adults, children who experience recurrent hypoglycemia at an early age (< 5 years) may be at increased risk for long-term neuropsychological impairment. Premeal glycemic goals for toddlers and preschoolers should be 100 to 180 mg/dL, overnight levels should be 110 to 200 mg/dL, and the HbA1c goal should be between 7.5% and 8.5%. School-aged children (6–12 years) should begin to tighten their control with premeal glucose levels of 90 to 180 mg/dL, overnight levels more than 100 mg/dL, and HbA1c ≤ 8%. In adolescents, the issues of adolescent rebellion and independence require a somewhat more individualized approach. Once a child is in the teenage years, premeal blood glucose levels should be 80 to 120 mg/dL and their lifetime goal should be to maintain HbA1c < 7%. This goal is difficult for most teens to achieve, however, and the American Diabetes Association has recommended an HbA1c goal of 7.5% for this age group, with an ideal HbA1c of ≤ 7% if achievable without hypoglycemia. It is imperative that each child have realistic individualized goals. Encouraging independence, avoiding major parent-child conflict, focusing on small successes, and trying to minimize the psychological impact of diabetes may require goals to be adjusted temporarily.

School issues

Most children spend most of their day in school. Schools must be equipped to deal with children who have diabetes. The overall goal for schools that have children who have diabetes should be to maintain excellent diabetes care while minimizing interruptions to the learning environment. Children must be allowed to check blood glucose levels, give supervised insulin injections, and treat hypoglycemia in close proximity to the classroom. It is preferable to have a school nurse familiar with diabetes management to oversee a child's diabetes management. Many schools do not have a nurse, however, or if they do, he or she may not be comfortable with diabetes management. When a school nurse is not available, specific training must be provided to a specified diabetes liaison.

Teachers also should be aware of the symptoms and treatment of hypoglycemia, and fast-acting carbohydrates (eg, juice or instant glucose) should be available in all classroom settings. A glucagon emergency kit should be kept in the nurse's station. A child's parent is responsible for providing all diabetes supplies.

In most schools, children must go to the school nurse's station to check blood sugars, give insulin, and treat hypoglycemia. In these situations, children should be accompanied by an aide or a classmate if there is a considerable distance between the classroom and the nurse's station. School nurses or the diabetes liaison also should be provided with specific protocols for treating hypoglycemia, checking for ketones, and giving insulin. The health care team is responsible for providing the school personnel with an individual diabetes management care plan.

Giving insulin at school can be a complex problem. When children are on a combination of NPH and rapid-acting analogs, insulin injections at school are not typically required. With the increasing number of children using CSII and glargine insulin, however, school nurses are often responsible for overseeing lunchtime insulin injections. Parents and physicians must be sure that nurses or diabetes liaisons are aware of a child's specific blood glucose goals and are appropriately trained either to give or oversee insulin injections. Frequent communication between school nurses and a child's diabetes care team is important to adjust insulin doses continuously and promote age-appropriate HbA1c goals.

Finally, physical fitness is important for maintaining cardiovascular health and improving metabolic control. Managing children who have diabetes during physical education can be a challenge. Coaches should be trained to allow children who have diabetes appropriate access to fluids and carbohydrates. If physical education is expected to last more than 30 minutes, a 10% to 20% reduction in the insulin dose or a juice box or small snack can be used to avoid hypoglycemia. Glucose testing also should be made available at the site and should be allowed any time a child feels hypoglycemic. The symptoms of physical exertion are often difficult to distinguish from those of hypoglycemia. Full participation in physical education should be expected. Creating an exercise program for children who have diabetes that provides for appropriate monitoring with expectation of full participation is important for teaching children that diabetes should not exclude them from any activities.

Complications

Complications of T1D include retinopathy, nephropathy, neuropathy, and cardiovascular disease. The Diabetes Control and Complications Trial demonstrated the importance of tight glucose control in minimizing these complications. Because most complications from T1D do not present until 10 to 15 years after diagnosis, however, children often underestimate the importance of glycemic control. Because glucose control is linked directly to complication rates, screening for diabetes complications should begin with a HbA1c at every clinic visit. Blood pressure also should be monitored closely and children who have hypertension (blood pressure higher than the ninety-fifth percentile) should be treated aggressively. To screen for neuropathy, a microfilament should be used to check finger and toe sensation at each clinic visit.

Once a child is 10 years old and has had diabetes for 5 years, urine microalbumin should be obtained annually to screen for nephropathy. If the urine albumin/creatinine ratio is more than 30 mg/g, a first morning sample should be obtained to rule out orthostatic proteinuria. If albuminuria persists on more than two to three confirmatory samples, angiotensin-converting enzyme inhibitor therapy should be initiated. Lipid profiles should be obtained on all children once glucose control has been established. If the low density lipoprotein (LDL) is < 100 mg/dL, screening should be repeated once every 5 years. If the LDL is elevated, screening should be repeated annually. Current guidelines recommend pharmacologic treatment for LDL > 160 mg/dL with a goal LDL of < 100 mg/dL. Statins are currently considered first-line therapy for hyperlipidemia [85]. Safety and efficacy have been established in children such that statin therapy can be initiated after 10 years of age [86]. Pharmacologic treatment should be considered in patients who have LDL between 130 and 160 mg/dL with additional cardiovascular risk factors. To screen for retinopathy, a dilated eye examination should be performed by an ophthalmologist annually once a child is 10 years old and has had diabetes for more than 3 years. (See the article by Glastras and colleagues elsewhere in this issue—on screening and management of complications in childhood diabetes.)

Prevention strategies

Screening

To prevent T1D effectively, we must have an effective intervention and effective means of identifying persons at risk for the disease. Although we still lack a proven and efficacious intervention, the application of autoantibody and genetic screening allows for precise identification of at-risk populations. The challenge remains to establish T1D screening programs that provide further insight into the pathogenesis of diabetes so that more effective prevention strategies can be developed.

Future

The design and implementation of well-organized and carefully designed randomized, controlled clinical trials within the past 10 years suggest that progress already has been made toward the disease's ultimate prevention. In the United States, the diabetes prevention trial for T1D was launched in 1994 with the goal of determining whether antigen-based therapies using parenteral or oral insulin would prevent or delay the onset of diabetes in at-risk relatives [87]. In the

European Nicotinamide Diabetes Intervention Trial, relatives of T1D probands were randomized to either nicotinamide or placebo [88]. One of the major impediments to effective intervention trials has been the paradox that accurate prediction improves over time, whereas the potential for effective intervention declines (Fig. 3). Although the diabetes prevention trial for T1D and the European Nicotinamide Diabetes Intervention Trial failed to alter the natural history of diabetes, both studies added significantly to our understanding of the natural history of diabetes.

The current prevention trials have generated collaborative interactions across and between continents. Initially piloted in Finland but currently with several collaborative sites in Europe and North America, the Trial to Reduce IDDM in the Genetically at Risk seeks to determine whether genetically at-risk infants who are not exposed to cow's milk for the first 6 months of life will be protected from the subsequent development of diabetes [89]. The most recent prevention/ intervention development is the creation of the multicenter cooperative group known as TrialNet. This collaborative network is similar to the childhood cancer

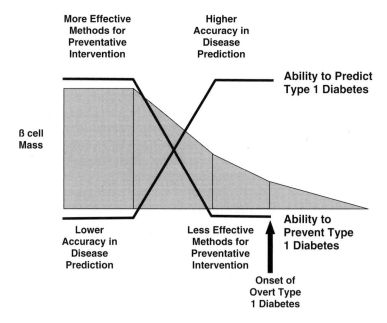

Fig. 3. The "treatment dilemma" for T1D. Many studies from animal models of T1D in combination with a much more limited series of investigations in human beings suggest that early intervention not only is more effective in terms of disease prevention but also often requires more benign forms of therapy. In contrast, the ability to identify an individual who will develop T1D (among an at-risk population) increases as the individual approaches onset of overt disease. FPIR, first phase insulin response; GAD, glutamic acid decarboxylase autoantibodies; IAA, insulin autoantibodies; ICA, islet cell autoantibodies; ICA 512, autoantibodies against the islet tyrosine phosphatase; IVGTT, intravenous glucose tolerance test. (*Adapted from* Atkinson MA, Eisenbarth GS. Type 1 diabetes: new perspectives on disease pathogenesis and treatment. Lancet 358(9277):222; with permission.)

cooperative groups and enables the undertaking of multiple pilot studies that involve primary and secondary prevention strategies in different population groups at different stages of the disease process. These studies not only will ascertain the efficacy of intervention but also should lead to greater insight into the pathogenesis of the disease.

References

[1] Fagot-Campagna A, Pettitt DJ, Engelgau MM, et al. Type 2 diabetes among North American children and adolescents: an epidemiologic review and a public health perspective. J Pediatr 2000;136(5):664–72.

[2] Centers for Disease Control and Prevention. Diabetes projects. Available at: http://www.cdc. gov/diabetes/projects/cda2.htm. Accessed August 15, 2005.

[3] Karvonen M, Viik-Kajander M, Moltchanova E, et al. Incidence of childhood type 1 diabetes worldwide: Diabetes Mondiale (DiaMond) Project Group. Diabetes Care 2000;23(10): 1516–26.

[4] Rosenbauer J, Herzig P, von Kries R, et al. Temporal, seasonal, and geographical incidence patterns of type I diabetes mellitus in children under 5 years of age in Germany. Diabetologia 1999;42(9):1055–9.

[5] LaPorte REMM, Chang Y-F. Prevalence and incidence of insulin-dependent diabetes. Bethesda (MD): National Institutes of Health; 1995.

[6] Krischer JP, Cuthbertson DD, Greenbaum C. Male sex increases the risk of autoimmunity but not type 1 diabetes. Diabetes Care 2004;27(8):1985–90.

[7] Weets I, Van Autreve J, Van der Auwera BJ, et al. Male-to-female excess in diabetes diagnosed in early adulthood is not specific for the immune-mediated form nor is it HLA-DQ restricted: possible relation to increased body mass index. Diabetologia 2001;44(1):40–7.

[8] Hogan P, Dall T, Nikolov P. Economic costs of diabetes in the US in 2002. Diabetes Care 2003;26(3):917–32.

[9] Icks A, Rosenbauer J, Haastert B, et al. Direct costs of pediatric diabetes care in Germany and their predictors. Exp Clin Endocrinol Diabetes 2004;112(6):302–9.

[10] Tamborlane WV, Ahern J. Implications and results of the Diabetes Control and Complications Trial. Pediatr Clin North Am 1997;44(2):285–300.

[11] Eisenbarth GS. Type I diabetes mellitus: a chronic autoimmune disease. N Engl J Med 1986; 314(21):1360–8.

[12] Rosenberg L. In vivo cell transformation: neogenesis of beta cells from pancreatic ductal cells. Cell Transplant 1995;4(4):371–83.

[13] Redondo MJ, Fain PR, Eisenbarth GS. Genetics of type 1A diabetes. Recent Prog Horm Res 2001;56:69–89.

[14] Hamalainen AM, Knip M. Autoimmunity and familial risk of type 1 diabetes. Curr Diab Rep 2002;2(4):347–53.

[15] Anjos SM, Tessier MC, Polychronakos C. Association of the cytotoxic T lymphocyte-associated antigen 4 gene with type 1 diabetes: evidence for independent effects of two polymorphisms on the same haplotype block. J Clin Endocrinol Metab 2004;89(12):6257–65.

[16] Guo D, Li M, Zhang Y, et al. A functional variant of SUMO4, a new I kappa B alpha modifier, is associated with type 1 diabetes. Nat Genet 2004;36(8):837–41.

[17] Zheng W, She JX. Genetic association between a lymphoid tyrosine phosphatase (PTPN22) and type 1 diabetes. Diabetes 2005;54(3):906–8.

[18] Yoon JW, Jun HS. Cellular and molecular pathogenic mechanisms of insulin-dependent diabetes mellitus. Ann N Y Acad Sci 2001;928:200–11.

[19] Roep BO. The role of T-cells in the pathogenesis of Type 1 diabetes: from cause to cure. Diabetologia 2003;46(3):305–21.

[20] Durinovic-Bello I. Autoimmune diabetes: the role of T cells, MHC molecules and autoantigens. Autoimmunity 1998;27(3):159–77.

[21] Schatz D, Krischer J, Horne G, et al. Islet cell antibodies predict insulin-dependent diabetes in United States school age children as powerfully as in unaffected relatives. J Clin Invest 1994;93(6):2403–7.

[22] Winter WE, Harris N, Schatz D. Immunological markers in the diagnosis and prediction of autoimmune type 1a diabetes. Clin Diabetes 2002;20(4):183–91.

[23] Lohmann T, Kellner K, Verlohren HJ, et al. Titre and combination of ICA and autoantibodies to glutamic acid decarboxylase discriminate two clinically distinct types of latent autoimmune diabetes in adults (LADA). Diabetologia 2001;44(8):1005–10.

[24] Solimena M, Dirkx Jr R, Hermel J, et al. ICA 512, an autoantigen of type I diabetes, is an intrinsic membrane protein of neurosecretory granules. EMBO J 1996;15(9):2102–14.

[25] Atkinson MA. Thirty years of investigating the autoimmune basis for type 1 diabetes: why can't we prevent or reverse this disease? Diabetes 2005;54(5):1253–63.

[26] Olmos P, A'Hern R, Heaton DA, et al. The significance of the concordance rate for type 1 (insulin-dependent) diabetes in identical twins. Diabetologia 1988;31(10):747–50.

[27] Ziegler AG, Hummel M, Schenker M, et al. Autoantibody appearance and risk for development of childhood diabetes in offspring of parents with type 1 diabetes: the 2-year analysis of the German BABYDIAB Study. Diabetes 1999;48(3):460–8.

[28] Rewers M, Bugawan TL, Norris JM, et al. Newborn screening for HLA markers associated with IDDM: diabetes autoimmunity study in the young (DAISY). Diabetologia 1996;39(7):807–12.

[29] Akerblom HK, Knip M, Simell O. From pathomechanisms to prediction, prevention and improved care of insulin-dependent diabetes mellitus in children. Ann Med 1997;29(5):383–5.

[30] Leslie RD, Elliott RB. Early environmental events as a cause of IDDM: evidence and implications. Diabetes 1994;43(7):843–50.

[31] Graves PM, Norris JM, Pallansch MA, et al. The role of enteroviral infections in the development of IDDM: limitations of current approaches. Diabetes 1997;46(2):161–8.

[32] Menser MA, Forrest JM, Bransby RD. Rubella infection and diabetes mellitus. Lancet 1978; 1(8055):57–60.

[33] Dahlquist GG, Ivarsson S, Lindberg B, et al. Maternal enteroviral infection during pregnancy as a risk factor for childhood IDDM: a population-based case-control study. Diabetes 1995;44(4): 408–13.

[34] Ginsberg-Fellner F, Witt ME, Yagihashi S, et al. Congenital rubella syndrome as a model for type 1 (insulin-dependent) diabetes mellitus: increased prevalence of islet cell surface antibodies. Diabetologia 1984;27(Suppl):87–9.

[35] Bodansky HJ, Grant PJ, Dean BM, et al. Islet-cell antibodies and insulin autoantibodies in association with common viral infections. Lancet 1986;2(8520):1351–3.

[36] Blom L, Nystrom L, Dahlquist G. The Swedish childhood diabetes study: vaccinations and infections as risk determinants for diabetes in childhood. Diabetologia 1991;34(3):176–81.

[37] Clarke WL, Shaver KA, Bright GM, et al. Autoimmunity in congenital rubella syndrome. J Pediatr 1984;104(3):370–3.

[38] Karounos DG, Wolinsky JS, Thomas JW. Monoclonal antibody to rubella virus capsid protein recognizes a beta-cell antigen. J Immunol 1993;150(7):3080–5.

[39] Hyoty H, Hiltunen M, Knip M, et al. A prospective study of the role of coxsackie B and other enterovirus infections in the pathogenesis of IDDM: Childhood Diabetes in Finland (DiMe) Study Group. Diabetes 1995;44(6):652–7.

[40] Clements GB, Galbraith DN, Taylor KW. Coxsackie B virus infection and onset of childhood diabetes. Lancet 1995;346(8969):221–3.

[41] Viskari HR, Koskela P, Lonnrot M, et al. Can enterovirus infections explain the increasing incidence of type 1 diabetes? Diabetes Care 2000;23(3):414–6.

[42] Helmke K, Otten A, Willems WR, et al. Islet cell antibodies and the development of diabetes mellitus in relation to mumps infection and mumps vaccination. Diabetologia 1986;29(1):30–3.

[43] Champsaur HF, Bottazzo GF, Bertrams J, et al. Virologic, immunologic, and genetic factors in insulin-dependent diabetes mellitus. J Pediatr 1982;100(1):15–20.

[44] Honeyman MC, Coulson BS, Stone NL, et al. Association between rotavirus infection and pancreatic islet autoimmunity in children at risk of developing type 1 diabetes. Diabetes 2000; 49(8):1319–24.

[45] Schatz DA, Maclaren NK. Cow's milk and insulin-dependent diabetes mellitus: innocent until proven guilty. JAMA 1996;276(8):647–8.

[46] Norris JM, Beaty B, Klingensmith G, et al. Lack of association between early exposure to cow's milk protein and beta-cell autoimmunity. Diabetes Autoimmunity Study in the Young (DAISY). JAMA 1996;276(8):609–14.

[47] Atkinson MA, Bowman MA, Kao KJ, et al. Lack of immune responsiveness to bovine serum albumin in insulin-dependent diabetes. N Engl J Med 1993;329(25):1853–8.

[48] Karjalainen J, Martin JM, Knip M, et al. A bovine albumin peptide as a possible trigger of insulin-dependent diabetes mellitus. N Engl J Med 1992;327(5):302–7.

[49] Martin JM, Trink B, Daneman D, et al. Milk proteins in the etiology of insulin-dependent diabetes mellitus (IDDM). Ann Med 1991;23(4):447–52.

[50] Borch-Johnsen K, Joner G, Mandrup-Poulsen T, et al. Relation between breast-feeding and incidence rates of insulin-dependent diabetes mellitus: a hypothesis. Lancet 1984;2(8411):1083–6.

[51] Gerstein HC. Cow's milk exposure and type I diabetes mellitus: a critical overview of the clinical literature. Diabetes Care 1994;17(1):13–9.

[52] Elliott RB, Martin JM. Dietary protein: a trigger of insulin-dependent diabetes in the BB rat? Diabetologia 1984;26(4):297–9.

[53] Coleman DL, Kuzava JE, Leiter EH. Effect of diet on incidence of diabetes in nonobese diabetic mice. Diabetes 1990;39(4):432–6.

[54] Pietropaolo M, Castano L, Babu S, et al. Islet cell autoantigen 69 kD (ICA69): molecular cloning and characterization of a novel diabetes-associated autoantigen. J Clin Invest 1993; 92(1):359–71.

[55] Wright AL. The rise of breastfeeding in the United States. Pediatr Clin North Am 2001;48(1):1–12.

[56] Ivarsson SA, Mansson MU, Jakobsson IL. IgG antibodies to bovine serum albumin are not increased in children with IDDM. Diabetes 1995;44(11):1349–50.

[57] Scott FW, Marliss EB. Conference summary: diet as an environmental factor in development of insulin-dependent diabetes mellitus. Can J Physiol Pharmacol 1991;69(3):311–9.

[58] Norris JM, Barriga K, Klingensmith G, et al. Timing of initial cereal exposure in infancy and risk of islet autoimmunity. JAMA 2003;290(13):1713–20.

[59] Ziegler AG, Schmid S, Huber D, et al. Early infant feeding and risk of developing type 1 diabetes-associated autoantibodies. JAMA 2003;290(13):1721–8.

[60] Hypponen E, Laara E, Reunanen A, et al. Intake of vitamin D and risk of type 1 diabetes: a birth-cohort study. Lancet 2001;358(9292):1500–3.

[61] Saggese G, Federico G, Balestri M, et al. Calcitriol inhibits the PHA-induced production of IL-2 and IFN-gamma and the proliferation of human peripheral blood leukocytes while enhancing the surface expression of HLA class II molecules. J Endocrinol Invest 1989;12(5):329–35.

[62] Mathieu C, Casteels K, Waer M, et al. Prevention of diabetes recurrence after syngeneic islet transplantation in NOD mice by analogues of 1,25(OH)2D3 in combination with cyclosporin A: mechanism of action involves an immune shift from Th1 to Th2. Transplant Proc 1998; 30(2):541.

[63] Pont A, Rubino JM, Bishop D, et al. Diabetes mellitus and neuropathy following Vacor ingestion in man. Arch Intern Med 1979;139(2):185–7.

[64] Schein PS, Alberti KG, Williamson DH. Effects of streptozotocin on carbohydrate and lipid metabolism in the rat. Endocrinology 1971;89(3):827–34.

[65] Kostraba JN, Gay EC, Rewers M, et al. Nitrate levels in community drinking waters and risk of IDDM: an ecological analysis. Diabetes Care 1992;15(11):1505–8.

[66] Dahlquist GG, Blom LG, Persson LA, et al. Dietary factors and the risk of developing insulin dependent diabetes in childhood. BMJ 1990;300(6735):1302–6.

[67] Dahlquist GG, Patterson C, Soltesz G. Perinatal risk factors for childhood type 1 diabetes in Europe: the EURODIAB Substudy 2 Study Group. Diabetes Care 1999;22(10):1698–702.

[68] McKinney PA, Parslow R, Gurney K, et al. Antenatal risk factors for childhood diabetes

mellitus: a case-control study of medical record data in Yorkshire, UK. Diabetologia 1997;40(8): 933–9.

[69] Patterson CC, Carson DJ, Hadden DR, et al. A case-control investigation of perinatal risk factors for childhood IDDM in Northern Ireland and Scotland. Diabetes Care 1994;17(5):376–81.

[70] Flood TM, Brink SJ, Gleason RE. Increased incidence of type I diabetes in children of older mothers. Diabetes Care 1982;5(6):571–3.

[71] Blom L, Dahlquist G, Nystrom L, et al. The Swedish childhood diabetes study: social and perinatal determinants for diabetes in childhood. Diabetologia 1989;32(1):7–13.

[72] Dahlquist G, Kallen B. Maternal-child blood group incompatibility and other perinatal events increase the risk for early-onset type 1 (insulin-dependent) diabetes mellitus. Diabetologia 1992; 35(7):671–5.

[73] Hummel M, Ziegler AG. Vaccines and the appearance of islet cell antibodies in offspring of diabetic parents: results from the BABY-DIAB Study. Diabetes Care 1996;19(12):1456–7.

[74] Classen JB. The timing of immunization affects the development of diabetes in rodents. Autoimmunity 1996;24(3):137–45.

[75] Todd JA. A protective role of the environment in the development of type 1 diabetes? Diabet Med 1991;8(10):906–10.

[76] Singh B. Stimulation of the developing immune system can prevent autoimmunity. J Autoimmun 2000;14(1):15–22.

[77] Black P. Why is the prevalence of allergy and autoimmunity increasing? Trends Immunol 2001; 22(7):354–5.

[78] Mallare JT, Cordice CC, Ryan BA, et al. Identifying risk factors for the development of diabetic ketoacidosis in new onset type 1 diabetes mellitus. Clin Pediatr (Phila) 2003;42(7):591–7.

[79] Dunger DB, Sperling MA, Acerini CL, et al. ESPE/LWPES consensus statement on diabetic ketoacidosis in children and adolescents. Arch Dis Child 2004;89(2):188–94.

[80] Murray L, editor. Physicians' Desk Reference. 59th edition. Montvale (NJ): Thompson; 2005.

[81] Dupre J, Behme MT, McDonald TJ. Exendin-4 normalized postcibal glycemic excursions in type 1 diabetes. J Clin Endocrinol Metab 2004;89(7):3469–73.

[82] Heptulla RA, Rodriguez LM, Bomgaars L, et al. The role of amylin and glucagon in the dampening of glycemic excursions in children with type 1 diabetes. Diabetes 2005;54(4):1100–7.

[83] Haller MJ, Stalvey MS, Silverstein JH. Predictors of control of diabetes: monitoring may be the key. J Pediatr 2004;144(5):660–1.

[84] Gross TM, Bode BW, Einhorn D, et al. Performance evaluation of the MiniMed continuous glucose monitoring system during patient home use. Diabetes Technol Ther 2000;2(1):49–56.

[85] Silverstein J, Klingensmith G, Copeland K, et al. Care of children and adolescents with type 1 diabetes: a statement of the American Diabetes Association. Diabetes Care 2005;28(1):186–212.

[86] McCrindle BW, Helden E, Cullen-Dean G, et al. A randomized crossover trial of combination pharmacologic therapy in children with familial hyperlipidemia. Pediatr Res 2002;51(6): 715–21.

[87] Type 1 Diabetes Study Group. Diabetes prevention trial: effects of insulin in relatives of patients with type 1 diabetes mellitus. N Engl J Med 2002;346(22):1685–91.

[88] Gale EA, Bingley PJ, Emmett CL, et al. European icotinamide Diabetes Intervention Trial (ENDIT): a randomised controlled trial of intervention before the onset of type 1 diabetes. Lancet 2004;363(9413):925–31.

[89] Julius MC, Schatz DA, Silverstein JH. The prevention of type I diabetes mellitus. Pediatr Ann 1999;28(9):585–8.

PEDIATRIC CLINICS
OF NORTH AMERICA

Pediatr Clin N Am 52 (2005) 1579–1609

Type 2 Diabetes Mellitus in Youth: The Complete Picture to Date

Neslihan Gungor, MD, Tamara Hannon, MD,
Ingrid Libman, MD, PhD, Fida Bacha, MD,
Silva Arslanian, MD*

*Division of Pediatric Endocrinology, Metabolism, and Diabetes Mellitus,
Children's Hospital of Pittsburgh, 3705 Fifth Avenue, Pittsburgh, PA 15213, USA*

Type 2 diabetes mellitus (T2DM) historically was considered a disease of adults, with autoimmune type 1 diabetes mellitus (T1DM) accounting for almost all cases of pediatric diabetes. T2DM was recognized as a disease of the pediatric age group by the late 1970s. It has turned into a significant public health problem, with escalating numbers of new cases referred to as an "epidemic" by the American Diabetes Association (ADA) [1,2]. The problem is not limited to North America; it also has been reported in children from Europe [3–10], Asia [11–15], Africa [16], and Australia [17].

T2DM is a heterogeneous condition in which the clinical manifestation of hyperglycemia is a reflection of the impaired balance between insulin sensitivity and insulin secretion [18,19]. Clinical experience and research in youth T2DM are in an early stage because of the relative novelty of the condition in pediatrics. This article discusses the amassed information in T2DM of youth to date with respect to the epidemiology, pathophysiology, risk factors, clinical presentation, screening, and management strategies.

This work was supported by the United States Public Health Service grant RO1 HD27503 (SA), K24 HD01357 (SA), the Pittsburgh Foundation (NG), MO1-RR00084 General Clinical Research Center, the University of Pittsburgh Obesity and Nutrition Research Center (NG), the Thrasher Research Fund, the Cochrane-Weber Endowed Fund, the Bristol Myers Squibb Company, Eli Lilly and Company, and the Renziehausen Trust Fund.

* Corresponding author.
E-mail address: Silva.Arslanian@chp.edu (S. Arslanian).

Epidemiology

By the turn of the century it was reported that some children presented with a mild and slowly progressive type of the disease unlike T1DM [20]. It was not until 1979, however, that recognition of T2DM in children and adolescents emerged, as described by a series of six obese Pima Indian children with strong parental history of T2DM [21]. Since then, T2DM has been reported in children from all over the world.

Currently, almost all information on the epidemiology of youth T2DM in the literature is compiled from case reports of tertiary diabetes clinics. Except in the native populations of the United States, Canada, Japan, and Taiwan, there are no population-based studies of childhood T2DM (Table 1) [22–28]. Based on population-based registries that monitor the epidemiology of T1DM, rates of T1DM are typically lower in African-American children than in white children. Data from the Allegheny County Registry from Pennsylvania showed for the first time a higher incidence of diabetes for African Americans (17.6/100,000) than for whites (16.5/100,000), which was explained by a threefold higher diabetes incidence in 15- to 19-year-old African Americans (30.7/100,000) com-

Table 1

Selected estimates of the magnitude of type 2 diabetes mellitus in children and adolescents in population-based studies

Study	Years	Race/ethnicity	Age (y)	No. of cases	Estimates
Population-based studies					**Prevalence per 1000**
Australia	1994	Aborigines	7–18		13.1
Arizona (USA)	1992–1996	Pima Indians	10–14	15	22.3
Arizona	1992–1996	Pima Indians	15–19	27	50.9
Manitoba (Canada)	1996–1997	First Nations	4–19	8	11.1
Manitoba	1996–1997	First Nations	10–19	7	36.0 (girls) 0 (boys)
Montana and Wyoming (USA)	1997–2001	American Indians	0–19	88	29.3
Population-based studies					**Incidence per 100,000**
New Mexico (USA)	1991–1992	Navajo Indians	12–19	2	14.1
Austria	1999–2001	Mainly Whites	0–14	8	0.25
Hong Kong	1984–1996	Chinese and non-Chinese	0–14	18	0.1
Japan	1976–1980	Japanese	6–12		0.2
Japan	1976–1980	Japanese	13–15		7.3
Japan	1981–1985	Japanese	6–12		1.6
Japan	1981–1985	Japanese	13–15		12.1
Japan	1991–1995	Japanese	6–12		2.0
Japan	1991–1995	Japanese	13–15		13.9
Taiwan	1999	Chinese	6–18	137	6.5
Montana and Wyoming	1997–2001	American Indians	0–19	16	23.3

Data from Refs. [9,13,14,17,22–28].

pared with whites (11.2/100,000). The 1990 to 1994 incidence for African Americans was two- and threefold higher than that reported in 1985 to 1989 and 1980 to 1984, respectively. Such findings may be explained by the potential inclusion of non-T1DM cases in this age group [29,30]. Among black adolescents with DM, 42% had no evidence of autoantibodies compared with only 10% of white adolescents, which further suggests the presence of a non-autoimmune type of diabetes in blacks [31].

In the United States, T2DM seems to account for 8% to 45% of all patients with DM and its prevalence seems to be on the rise. In the Cincinnati, Ohio experience, the annual incidence of T2DM in the 10- to 19-year-old age group jumped from 0.7 per 100,000 in 1982 to 7.2 per 100,000 in 1994. Among 0- to 19-year-old patients, T2DM accounted for 2% to 4% of all new cases of diabetes in the years 1982 to 1992 but accounted for 16% of new cases in 1994 [32]. In Arkansas Children's Hospital, just 1 to 3 patients were diagnosed annually with T2DM between 1988 and 1991, but between 1992 and 1995, the annual figure rose to 6 to 17 [33]. A report from Charleston, South Carolina stated that of 97 African Americans diagnosed with diabetes in 1997, 46% had T2DM [34]. In San Diego, California at two referral hospitals, 8% of all new diabetic cases identified between 1993 and 1994 were T2DM [35]. In Ventura, California, T2DM accounted for 45% of the incidence cases of diabetes between the years 1990 and 1994 [36]. In San Antonio, Texas, 18% of new cases diagnosed between 1990 and 1997 involved T2DM [37]. Another study in Florida school children showed an increase from 8.4% to 23.7% between the years 1994 and 1998 [38].

Outside the United States, clinic-based studies also have evaluated the percentage of diabetes cases labeled as T2DM. In Bangkok, Thailand, newly diagnosed cases of T2DM in children increased from 5% between 1986 and 1995 to 17.9% between 1996 and 1999 [39]. In Europe, however, studies from Austria, Germany, and Sweden have reported that only 0.5% of children with diabetes have been classified as having T2DM [8,10]. In Paris, France, 1% of children aged 1 to 16 years have been diagnosed with T2DM during 1993 to 1998 [6]. In the United Kingdom, the crude minimum prevalence of T2DM under age 16 years was reported as 0.21/100 000 based on a cross-sectional survey of all pediatric diabetes centers [5]. In conclusion, since its initial description approximately 26 years ago, cases of T2DM in childhood and adolescence have been increasing. Further studies are needed, especially population-based, to assess the whole impact of the disease.

Pathophysiology

Insulin resistance and insulin secretion in type 2 diabetes mellitus

Glucose homeostasis is maintained by a delicate balance between insulin secretion from the pancreatic beta cells and insulin sensitivity of the peripheral tissues (eg, muscle, liver, and adipose tissue) [40]. In healthy individuals, the relationship between insulin sensitivity and secretion is nonlinear and best described by a hyperbolic function [40], which indicates that the product of insulin sensitivity and beta-cell function is constant for a given glucose tolerance in any one individual. This hyperbolic relationship implies that a feedback loop governs the interaction between the beta cells and the peripheral tissues. When insulin sensitivity decreases, insulin secretion must increase for glucose tolerance to remain constant (Fig. 1) [41]. An impairment in this compensatory increase in insulin secretion paves the way to glucose intolerance.

Decreased insulin sensitivity and impaired beta-cell function are the two key components in T2DM pathogenesis based on long-term experience in adults [41,42]. The sequence of development of these abnormalities has been debated extensively. The concept of "insulin insensitivity" in DM originally was described by Himsworth in 1936 [43]. Further studies in adults documented that resistance to insulin-stimulated glucose uptake is a characteristic finding in patients who have T2DM and impaired glucose tolerance (IGT) [44]. Several studies in adults proposed that insulin resistance with compensatory hyperinsulinemia is the initial step in T2DM pathogenesis [18,41]. The subsequent step in T2DM pathogenesis is impairment in early insulin secretion, which initially leads to postprandial and later fasting hyperglycemia, at which time clinical DM becomes evident. This sequence also has been documented by

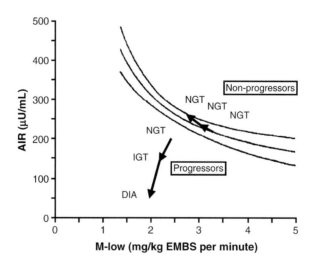

Fig. 1. The hyperbolic relationship between insulin sensitivity and beta cell function. AIR, acute insulin response to glucose; M-low, low insulin concentration; NGT, normal glucose tolerance; IGT, impaired glucose tolerance; DIA, diabetes; EMBS, estimated metabolic body size or fat free mass. (*From* Kahn SE. The importance of β-cell failure in the development and progression of type 2 diabetes. J Clin Endocrinol Metab 2001;86:4051; with permission.)

longitudinal studies in populations at high risk for developing T2DM, such as the Pima Indians of Arizona [45]. In the former study, the progression from normal glucose tolerance (NGT) to IGT was associated with an increase in body weight, worsening in insulin sensitivity, and a decline in the acute insulin secretory response to intravenous glucose. Progression from IGT to diabetes required further increase in body weight, impairment in insulin sensitivity and beta-cell function, and an increase in basal endogenous glucose output [45]. Similar observations were reported in insulin-sensitive and insulin-resistant African-American adults with T2DM who showed a marked decrease in insulin secretion as they progressed from near normoglycemia to frank hyperglycemia [46].

Metabolic studies of T2DM in youth are scarce in the literature. In a study by Umpaichitra and associates [47], 24 patients who had T2DM and 24 control subjects (aged 9–20 years, matched for body mass index [BMI] and pubertal stage) were evaluated for their insulin and glucagon response to a mixed liquid meal tolerance test. In children who had T2DM, relative hypoinsulinemia and hyperglucagonemia represented the pancreatic beta- and alpha-cell dysfunctions, and the severity seemed to depend on duration. Insulin deficiency was not expressed relative to the degree of insulin resistance, however, which was not measured.

A Japanese study evaluated obese adolescents who did not have diabetes, obese adolescents who had T2DM, and nonobese control subjects using the minimal model analysis of insulin-modified, frequently sampled intravenous glucose tolerance test [48]. Obese nondiabetic and obese diabetic groups were significantly and equally insulin resistant compared with the nonobese group. The diabetic group had lower first-phase insulin release compared with the nondiabetic group, however, which resulted in lower glucose disposition index (the product of first-phase insulin secretion and insulin sensitivity). Body composition and body fat topography were not evaluated.

Our group recently demonstrated that insulin sensitivity and insulin secretion are impaired in adolescents with T2DM using the glucose clamp technique, which is considered the gold standard for assessment of in vivo insulin sensitivity and secretion [19]. Adolescents who had T2DM were compared with matched (age, BMI, body composition, and pubertal development) obese controls [19]. Insulin sensitivity was evaluated with a 3-hour hyperinsulinemic euglycemic clamp and first- and second-phase insulin secretion with a 2-hour hyperglycemic clamp. Fasting glucose rate of appearance (hepatic glucose production) was determined with the use of $[6,6-^2H_2]$ glucose. In youth with T2DM compared with obese controls, in vivo insulin sensitivity was approximately 50% lower, first-phase insulin secretion was approximately 74% lower and second-phase insulin secretion was approximately 53% lower, glucose disposition index was approximately 86% lower, and hepatic glucose output was approximately 1.3 times higher [19] (Fig. 2). Our findings were in agreement with the literature in adults with T2DM [41], but we also showed a significant inverse relationship between insulin secretion and HbA1c in T2DM youth (r = −0.61;

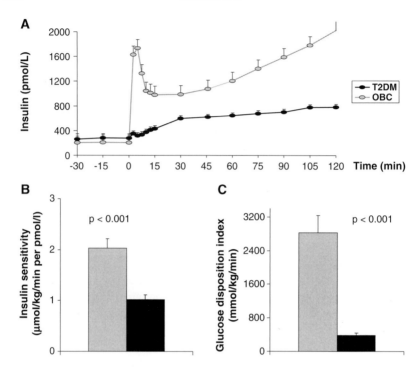

Fig. 2. (*A*) Insulin levels during the hyperglycemic clamp. (*B*) Insulin sensitivity during a 3-hour hyperinsulinemic (80 mu/m²/min)–euglycemic clamp in adolescents with T2DM versus obese controls. (*C*) Glucose disposition index in adolescents who have T2DM and obese controls. (*Adapted from* Gungor N, Bacha F, Saad R, et al. Youth type 2 diabetes: insulin resistance, beta-cell failure, or both? Diabetes Care 2005;28:641–2; with permission.)

$P = 0.025$). This relationship may either reflect the impact of deficient insulin secretion on the outcome of glycemic control or be viewed as a glucotoxic phenomenon of poor glycemic control on insulin secretion. Intensive glycemic control may be important to prevent further deterioration in beta-cell function. These findings of severe impairment in insulin secretion at such an early age could imply the potential need of starting insulin replacement therapy early in youth T2DM to maintain glycemic control and prevent hyperglycemia-driven complications.

Impairments in insulin biosynthetic process have been described in adults with T2DM. Levels of circulating proinsulin and its cleavage intermediate des-31, 32 proinsulin are disproportionately elevated [41]. In our study of youth who have T2DM, fasting proinsulin/insulin ratio was significantly higher compared with controls, similar to findings in adult T2DM [19,49]. This is another metabolic phenotype of impaired beta-cell function in youth who have T2DM.

In summary, when T2DM is clinically present, insulin action and insulin secretion are impaired. The proposed pathophysiology of T2DM in youth is outlined in Fig. 3 [50].

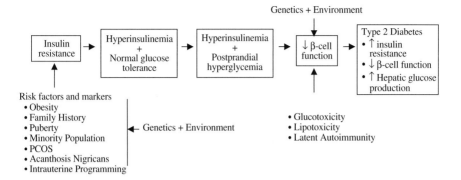

Fig. 3. Proposed pathophysiology of youth-onset T2DM. (*Adapted from* Arslanian SA. Type 2 diabetes mellitus in children: clinical aspects and risk factors. Horm Res 2002;57(Suppl 1):23; with permission.)

Natural history of youth type 2 diabetes mellitus

There are no longitudinal studies in children to follow the evolution of T2DM in high-risk individuals. Studies in adults suggest that the metabolic determinant of the progression from NGT to IGT to T2DM is pancreatic beta-cell function. Observations in insulin-resistant Pima Indian adults demonstrated progressive loss of acute insulin response to intravenous glucose throughout transition from NGT to IGT to T2DM [45]. The Botnia cross-sectional study of T2DM pathogenesis in at-risk European populations depicted a lower insulin sensitivity, using the homeostasis model assessment, when comparing IGT to NGT and T2DM to IGT [51]. This study further demonstrated a markedly impaired insulin secretion in T2DM subjects who no longer could compensate for insulin resistance and elevated glucose levels.

The United Kingdom Prospective Diabetes Study (UKPDS) found that beta-cell function was 50% of normal at the time of clinical diagnosis of T2DM [52]. The UKPDS and the Belfast diet intervention study reaffirmed the progressive nature of adult T2DM as an ongoing decline in beta-cell function without a change in insulin sensitivity [52–54]. In a recent case report of an adolescent with T2DM followed over 6 years, we demonstrated approximately 15% decline in beta-cell function with no substantial changes in insulin sensitivity [55]. This is almost a threefold faster decline in beta-cell function compared with adult UKPDS data. Because this is only a case report, additional studies are needed to explore whether this observation of an accelerated loss of beta-cell function is generalizable to all youth who have T2DM. If the early and severe impairment in insulin secretion in youth with T2DM is followed by an accelerated decline in beta-cell function, insulin therapy early in the course of the disease rather than "insulin as the last resort" should be considered carefully. Further studies are needed to investigate not only the natural history of beta-cell function in youth with T2DM but also strategies to retard or prevent its progressive failure.

Risk factors of youth type 2 diabetes mellitus

The risk factors for youth T2DM are discussed under the following four broad categories: (1) genetics, (2) environment, (3) ethnicity, and (4) insulin resistance phenotype.

Genetics: family history of type 2 diabetes mellitus

The cause of T2DM is heterogeneous, including social, behavioral, and environmental risk factors in addition to a strong hereditary component [42,56]. Although few susceptibility genes have been identified thus far [57], the genetic component of T2DM is evidenced by the strong heritability of the disease [56]. Studies in adult twins demonstrate a 50% to 76% concordance rate of T2DM in monozygotic twins, 37% in dizygotic twins, and a heritability estimate for T2DM of 26% and for abnormal glucose tolerance of 61% [58,59]. A 40% lifetime risk of developing T2DM has been reported in first-degree relatives of persons with T2DM [60].

A strong family history of T2DM is present in most pediatric patients regardless of ethnic background [2,32,33]. Markers of insulin resistance and beta-cell dysfunction are present in adult members of high-risk populations one to two decades before the diagnosis of the disease [56,61,62] and predict the progression to T2DM [63]. In adults, insulin secretion adjusted for the degree of insulin sensitivity is a highly heritable trait, more familial than either insulin sensitivity or insulin secretion alone [64]. Our studies demonstrate that family history of T2DM is associated with approximately 25% lower insulin sensitivity in prepubertal healthy African-American children compared with their peers without a family history of T2DM [65]. Similarly, white children who do not have diabetes but have a positive family history for T2DM have lower insulin sensitivity with an inadequate compensation in insulin secretion, which results in a lower glucose disposition index compared with youth without a family history of diabetes [66]. The superimposition of environmental factors, such as obesity and sedentary lifestyle, on this familial phenotype of an impaired balance between insulin secretion and insulin resistance may lead to T2DM over time.

Environment: behavior and lifestyle translate into a risk for obesity and altered body fat distribution

The increased prevalence of T2DM in childhood has been linked to the epidemic of childhood obesity in the United States and around the world [67,68]. The increasing prevalence of obesity [69] over a relatively short time span has been attributed to environmental factors that promote energy surplus [70,71] and sedentary lifestyle [72,73], rather than a change in the genetic pool

[74,75]. The effects of obesity on glucose metabolism are evident early in childhood. Percent body fat and BMI are proportional directly to fasting insulin levels (as a surrogate marker of insulin resistance) and inversely to glucose disposal in children and adolescents [76–78].

In a recent investigation of youth who do not have diabetes, our group demonstrated that obesity is associated with approximately 50% lower levels of the protective adipocytokine adiponectin in white adolescents [78]. Hypoadipo-nectinemia was a strong and independent correlate of insulin resistance, beta-cell dysfunction, and increased abdominal adiposity [78]. Adiponectin levels were approximately 50% lower in adolescents who had T2DM than obese non-diabetic controls, despite similar body composition and visceral adiposity [19]. Weyer and associates [79] reported lower plasma adiponectin levels in adult Pima Indians with IGT and T2DM than in individuals with NGT.

Independent of total body adiposity and ethnicity, abdominal fat deposition (visceral adiposity) is considered a risk factor for insulin resistance in children [77,80,81] and T2DM in adults [82]. Obese children with IGT were found to have peripheral insulin resistance without compensatory insulin secretion [83] and higher visceral and intramuscular fat [83].

Ethnicity

Most pediatric patients with T2DM in the United States belong to minority ethnic populations, which encompass Native Americans, Pima Indians, Mexican Americans, and African Americans [1,84,85]. Among the Pima Indians, more than 5% of the 15- to 19-year old children are affected [85]; the pathogenesis of T2DM is attributed to a genetic predisposition to insulin resistance modified by lifestyle changes [86]. Epidemiologic and clinical studies indicate that black children are more hyperinsulinemic and insulin resistant than their white peers [87–90]. A study that used genetic admixture analysis suggested a genetic and environmental basis to these differences [91]. We recently showed that despite 30% lower visceral adiposity in black adolescents, insulin sensitivity was not better than that of their white peers [81]. Black obese adolescents with high visceral fat manifested suboptimal compensatory increase in insulin secretion, which resulted in a lower glucose disposition index [81]. The levels of the anti-diabetogenic hormone adiponectin are lower in African-American compared with white healthy children of similar body composition [92]. These findings suggest racial differences in diabetogenic profile, with higher risk of progression to T2DM in blacks. Similarly, insulin sensitivity was found to be significantly lower in Hispanic compared with non-Hispanic white children [93].

Insulin resistance phenotype

Insulin resistance is a major feature of the conditions discussed in association with higher risk for type 2 diabetes.

Puberty

Most youth who have T2DM present at a mean age of 13.5 years, around the time of puberty [56,85]. Puberty is associated with transient insulin resistance that manifests as hyperinsulinemia in response to an oral glucose tolerance test [94] and to intravenous glucose tolerance test [95]. Measurement of in vivo insulin sensitivity using the hyperinsulinemic-euglycemic clamp technique demonstrated that insulin sensitivity is on average 30% lower in adolescents between Tanner stages II and IV of puberty, compared with prepubertal children and young adults [96–98]. In the presence of normally functioning pancreatic beta-cells, puberty-related insulin resistance is compensated by increased insulin secretion [99], which leads to peripheral hyperinsulinemia. The transient increase in growth hormone secretion during normal puberty, but not sex steroids, seems to be the most probable cause of the transient insulin resistance of puberty [89,100].

Polycystic ovary syndrome

Insulin resistance and hyperinsulinemia are major components of polycystic ovary syndrome (PCOS) in obese and lean adult women and in adolescent girls [101,102]. PCOS affects 5% to 10% of women in the reproductive age group and is characterized by hyperandrogenism and amenorrhea or oligomenorrhea secondary to chronic anovulation [102]. Thirty percent to 40% of women with PCOS have IGT, and 7.5% to 10% have T2DM by the fourth decade [103,104]. A recent study of screening PCOS adolescents with oral glucose tolerance test showed IGT in approximately 30% and diabetes in approximately 4% [105]. Our studies revealed that insulin sensitivity is approximately 50% lower in obese adolescents who have PCOS versus matched controls [106]. Adolescents who have PCOS and IGT have 40% lower first-phase insulin secretion and lower glucose disposition index compared with adolescents with NGT [107]. The presence of this metabolic profile in the early course of PCOS significantly increases the risk of progression to T2DM.

Acanthosis nigricans

Acanthosis nigricans is a diffuse hyperplasia of the spinous layer of the skin that manifests as a velvety, hyperkeratotic darkening of the skin. It involves the intertriginous regions, including the base of the neck, the axillae, the antecubital areas, and the beltline. It is associated with obesity, insulin resistance, and hyperinsulinemia. It is present in up to 90% of children and adolescents who have T2DM [1,85]. Its prevalence is 25-fold higher in African Americans compared with other populations [108]. The prevalence of T2DM is six times higher in African-American individuals with acanthosis nigricans [108]. A study in which subjects were preselected for the presence of acanthosis found that the prevalence of IGT was 24% in individuals with acanthosis nigricans [109]. Adiposity, rather than acanthosis nigricans, is a better clinical predictor of insulin resistance in African-American, white, and Hispanic children [110,111]. Obese individuals without acanthosis nigricans should not be presumed to have normal insulin sensitivity.

Exposure to gestational diabetes or intrauterine growth retardation

Both extremes of overnutrition and undernutrition of a fetus during critical time of growth seem to have long-term effects on obesity and glucose tolerance [112,113]. Offspring of mothers with diabetes during pregnancy have a higher frequency of childhood obesity and earlier onset of diabetes [113,114]. A prospective study found that the prevalence of IGT in the offspring of mothers with a diabetic pregnancy increased with time from 1.2% at < 5 years of age to 19.3% at 10.6 years of age [115,116]. Conversely, low birth weight reflective of in utero growth deprivation has been linked to insulin resistance, which leads to adult-onset obesity, T2DM, and cardiovascular disease [112,117]. The intrauterine programming hypothesis has been supported by some clinical studies [118,119]; others have challenged it [120]. Studies in young adults and in the pediatric age group have been few and conflicting, with some studies suggesting decreased insulin resistance in children born small for gestational age [121–123] and others suggesting that the major defect is in insulin secretion [124]. Other studies suggest that obesity is a more powerful determinant of insulin resistance than size at birth [125,126]. In studies of Indian and British children, the highest levels of insulin resistance were in children of low birth weight but high BMI and fat mass in childhood [122,127]. A major deficiency in many of these studies is the absence of body composition and body fat topography evaluation, especially because a recent study showed a negative association between abdominal fat and birth weight [128].

Clinical indicators of insulin resistance include hypertension [129] and dyslipidemia [88,129,130]. Triglyceride levels and triglyceride/high density lipoprotein ratio are simple clinical markers that may help to identify overweight adolescents with insulin resistance. We have found that a triglyceride level ≥ 130 mg/dL and triglyceride/high density lipoprotein > 3 predicts in vivo insulin resistance, as measured by hyperinsulinemic-euglycemic clamp, in white, overweight adolescents [130].

Clinical presentation and diagnosis of youth type 2 diabetes mellitus

Criteria for the diagnosis of diabetes

The criteria for the diagnosis of diabetes, based on standard values of fasting blood glucose, random blood glucose, and the oral glucose tolerance test, are the same for adults and children (Table 2) [131]. Normal fasting plasma glucose is less than 100 mg/dL subsequent to the 2003 revision by the ADA that lowered the threshold separating normal from elevated fasting plasma glucose from 110 mg/dL to 100 mg/dL [132]. Based on revised criteria, patients with fasting

Table 2
Criteria for the diagnosis of impaired glucose tolerance and diabetes

	Normal		Diabetes
Plasma glucose			
Fasting	< 100 mg/dL	100–125 mg/dL (IFG)	≥ 126 mg/dL
OGTT: 2 h PG	< 140 mg/dL	140–199 mg/dL (IGT)	≥ 200 mg/dL
Random			≥ 200 mg/dL + symptoms[a]

Abbreviations: IFG, impaired fasting glucose; IGT, impaired glucose tolerance; OGTT, oral glucose tolerance test; 2 h PG, plasma glucose at 2 hours after ingestion of glucose.

   [a] Polyuria, polydipsia, weight loss.

Data from American Diabetes Association. Report of the expert committee on the diagnosis and classification of diabetes mellitus: follow-up report on the diagnosis of diabetes mellitus. Diabetes Care 2003;26(11):3161.

plasma glucose levels between 100 and 125 mg/dL have impaired fasting glucose. Patients with fasting plasma glucose levels ≥ 126 mg/dL have diabetes. A random or "casual" plasma glucose value ≥ 200 mg/dL indicates diabetes if the patient has additional symptoms, such as polyuria and polydipsia. During an oral glucose tolerance test, a 2-hour plasma glucose value of < 140 mg/dL is considered normal, ≥ 140 and < 200 mg/dL is considered IGT, and ≥ 200 mg/dL indicates diabetes.

Screening of children and adolescents at risk for type 2 diabetes mellitus

T2DM in adults may be asymptomatic for years, yet findings of microangiopathic damage in newly diagnosed patients with T2DM indicate that complications of diabetes often predate the diagnosis of clinical diabetes [133,134]. Aggressive treatment of diabetes has been shown to retard the development of vascular complications [135], thus early identification of children with T2DM may prevent or lessen the severity of comorbidities. Criteria for screening children and adolescents at risk for developing T2DM have been put forth by the ADA (Box 1) [2]. BMI should be plotted by health care providers annually on the Centers for Disease Control and Prevention BMI growth charts, which are specific for age and sex. Screening for diabetes among children with a BMI at or above the eighty-fifth percentile for age and sex with two additional risk factors for T2DM should be part of routine pediatric care.

Screening should commence at 10 years of age or at onset of puberty, if it occurs at a younger age, and should be performed every 2 years. The ADA recommends fasting plasma glucose as a screening tool because of its lower cost and greater convenience [2]. This recommendation is in contrast to the World Health Organization recommendation of an oral glucose tolerance test based on evidence from adult populations that shows that approximately 30% of all persons with undiagnosed diabetes have a nondiabetic fasting glucose [136] but are nevertheless at high cardiovascular risk [137]. A study in obese children with IGT showed that the prevalence of impaired fasting glucose (based on the

---

Box 1. Screening guidelines for type 2 diabetes mellitus in children and adolescents

- BMI > eighty-fifth percentile for age and gender or
- Body weight for height > eighty-fifth percentile or
- Body weight > 120% of ideal for height

Plus any two of the following risk factors:

- Family history of type 2 diabetes in first- or second-degree relatives
- Race/ethnicity (American Indian, African American, Hispanic, Asian/Pacific Islander)
- Signs/symptoms of insulin resistance (acanthosis nigricans, hypertension, dyslipidemia, polycystic ovary syndrome)

When to screen: age 10 or at onset of puberty, if puberty occurs at a younger age
Frequency of screening: every 2 years
Screening test: fasting plasma glucose[a]
Clinical judgment should be used to test for diabetes in high-risk patients who do not meet these criteria. We agree with authorities who recommend a 2-hour postprandial glucose value as a more sensitive index of evolving diabetes mellitus. Fasting hyperglycemia is a late manifestation of failing glucose homeostasis.

[a] Fasting plasma glucose is the test recommended by the American Diabetes Association.
Data from American Diabetes Association. Type 2 diabetes in children and adolescents. Diabetes Care 2000;23:381–9.

---

former threshold of >110 mg/dL) was low (<0.08%) [138]. A report from our institution revealed that the new ADA criteria for impaired fasting glucose (100–125 mg/dL) not only yield a higher number of overweight children at risk for abnormalities of glucose metabolism but also suggest that even at a young age, youth with impaired fasting glucose have worse cardiovascular risk profiles than youth with normal fasting glucose [139]. The prevalence of IGT and T2DM in children varies depending on the population studied. An obesity clinic–based study found 25% IGT in 4- to 10-year-old patients and 21% IGT in 11- to 18-year-old patients and approximately 4% T2DM [138]. Other studies have found much lower rates of IGT that range from 4.1% to 4.5% in children recruited from the community [140,141].

Additional studies are needed to compare diabetes diagnostic categories in pediatric populations according to the ADA versus the World Health Organization diagnostic criteria before arriving at valid conclusions.

Presentation of type 2 diabetes mellitus and ketosis-prone diabetes

T2DM in children and adults may present in various ways that represent a spectrum of severity. On one end of the spectrum is asymptomatic presentation with diagnosis of glucosuria/incidental hyperglycemia on routine screening. In the Japanese experience, from among more than 7 million school children, 188 were detected by routine screening for glucosuria followed by an oral glucose tolerance test [142]. Symptomatic patients may have candidal vulvovaginitis, polyuria, polydipsia, weight loss, headaches, or fatigue. The severe end of the spectrum harbors manifestations of insulin deficiency, however. As is in patients with T1DM, the relative deficiency of insulin in patients with T2DM can lead to diabetic ketosis/ketoacidosis (DKA). In its extreme form, DKA or hyperglycemic hyperosmolar nonketotic state/coma may be the initial presenting picture.

Approximately 5% to 25% of adolescents who are subsequently classified as having T2DM have ketoacidosis at presentation. These patients may have ketoacidosis without any associated stress, other illness, or infection [2]. Pinhas-Hamiel and colleagues [143] reported that 42% of African-American adolescents with T2DM had ketonuria and 25% had DKA. On the contrary, none of the 12 American white adolescents diagnosed with T2DM within the same period had ketonuria. Another study reported that approximately 30% of Hispanic youth with T2DM may present with ketosis [36].

Genetic pancreatic beta-cell defects may predispose to the development of insulinopenia and ketosis, which lead to atypical diabetes in some populations, particularly African Americans [144–146]. Such patients are insulin resistant with acute, severe defects in insulin secretion that are not immune mediated [147,148]. After the institution of therapy, some endogenous insulin secretory capacity may be recovered [149], and normoglycemic remission may occur [150].

Pancreatic autoantibodies in youth type 2 diabetes mellitus

Once the diagnosis of diabetes is established, it is important to distinguish between T1DM and T2DM to optimize therapy. Given the heterogeneity of clinical presentation of T2DM in children, especially when DKA is present, classification into type 1 or type 2 diabetes cannot always be made reliably on the basis of clinical presentation. Additional testing has been proposed by the ADA Consensus Group using the obesity phenotype as the starting point [2]. Clinical signs helpful in distinguishing T2DM from T1DM are obesity, signs of insulin resistance, and elevated C-peptide levels. It should be noted that the prevalence of obesity in children diagnosed with T1DM is increasing [151], which makes it more difficult to distinguish T2DM from T1DM.

Markers of the cellular-mediated immune destruction of the beta-cell, such as islet cell antibodies (ICA), glutamic acid decarboxylase antibodies (GADA), tyrosine phosphatase-like protein autoantibodies, and insulin autoantibodies, are usually identifiable in individuals with or at risk for autoimmune T1DM. One or more of these autoantibodies are present in 85% to 90% of children with T1DM at initial diagnosis, compared with less than 5% of nondiabetic controls [152–154]. T2DM is not considered an autoimmune disease; however, as many as 10% to 15% of adults with apparent T2DM develop a clinical condition characterized by progression into insulin-dependent DM and autoimmune markers, referred to as latent autoimmune diabetes of adulthood [60,155,156]. Data from the UKPDS, which measured ICA and GADA at diagnosis of T2DM in 3672 patients of European background who were between 25 and 65 years of age, revealed that 12% of patients had either ICA or GADA, and 4% had both. At all ages, but more in the younger age group, the presence of these autoantibodies suggested an increased likelihood that insulin therapy would be required [157]. Other studies suggest that the patients with evidence of autoimmunity have a lower BMI and present more commonly symptomatic with polyuria and polydipsia than patients who are antibody negative [158].

Currently, absence of diabetes autoimmune markers is a prerequisite for the diagnosis of T2DM in children and adolescents [2]. Some contradictory data exist in the literature, however. Observations of First Nation youth of Manitoba with T2DM revealed positive ICA titers in 4 of 14 children who have not required insulin during 10 years of follow-up [159]. A study from Loma Linda, California analyzed 48 children and adolescents with T2DM and 39 with T1DM for the presence of ICA, GADA, and insulin antibodies at diagnosis [160]. The group with T2DM had positive ICA in 8.1%, positive GADA in 30.3%, and positive insulin autoantibodies in 34.8%, in comparison to 71.1%, 75.7%, and 76.5%, respectively, in the T1DM group. One additional study from New York also demonstrated that as evidenced by fasting and 90-minute standard liquid meal stimulated serum C-peptide levels of >0.2 and >0.5 nmol/L, respectively, 11 of 37 patients (29.7%) with T2DM tested positive for at least one autoantibody (8.1%, 8.1%, and 27% for GADA, tyrosine phosphatase-like protein autoantibodies, and insulin autoantibodies, respectively). It should be mentioned, however, that nine of ten patients who tested positive for insulin autoantibodies were on insulin treatment at time of testing, which influenced the result. Therefore, 10.8% were considered truly positive (for either GADA or tyrosine phosphatase-like protein autoantibodies or both) [161].

The clinical significance of the presence of autoantibodies in some youth with what seems to be T2DM is uncertain. It is also important to note that currently, pancreatic autoantibody testing methodology is not standardized among commercial and research laboratories. In our research experience we have encountered inconsistencies in pancreatic autoantibodies reported on the same serum sample by various laboratories (S. Arslanian, N. Gungor, unpublished observations) and these issues need clarification. These observations may be interpreted as a reflection of the broad spectrum of T2DM of youth as a nonuniform disease. Longer prospective studies are needed for definitive conclusions.

Comorbidities and complications of youth type 2 diabetes mellitus

The medical literature on complications of childhood-onset T2DM is scanty. Data that pertain to early morbidities indicate that T2DM of youth is not a benign entity, however. In some series, 17% to 34% of the youth who had T2DM had hypertension [32,33], and 4% to 32% had high triglyceride concentrations at diagnosis [32,162]. Pima Indian children who had diabetes were found to have a high prevalence of cardiovascular risk factors, including hypercholesterolemia (7%), hypertension (18%), and microalbuminuria (22%) at diagnosis [162]. Further follow-up of these children between 20 and 29 years of age revealed poor diabetes control (median glycated HbA1c, 12%), with progression of renal impairment, microalbuminuria in 60%, and macroalbuminuria in 17%. In the Northland New Zealand Maori population, microalbuminuria was present at diagnosis in 14% of patients with T2DM diagnosed before the age of 30 years [163]. In Hong Kong Chinese patients with T2DM diagnosed before age 35, hypertension was present in 18% and abnormal albuminuria was present in 27% [164]. Similarly there is a high risk for early nephropathy among Japanese persons who develop T2DM before age 30 [165]. Japanese patients with early-onset T2DM developed severe diabetic vascular complications in their thirties, such as blindness or end-stage renal failure [166]. In Manitoba and Northwestern Ontario, follow-up data in youth diagnosed with T2DM before age 17 revealed alarming observations of high mortality rate (9%), morbidity (eg, dialysis, blindness, amputation), pregnancy loss (38%), and poor glycemic control [167].

Youth with T2DM may present with DKA or hyperglycemic hyperosmolar state (HHS), which are associated with high morbidity and mortality [2]. DKA and HHS may be the presentation of new-onset T2DM or may develop as a complication of inadequate control. Acute decompensation with DKA has been recognized to occur at the time of diagnosis in as many as 25% of children with T2DM [2]. HHS was previously considered a complication in elderly patients with T2DM [168]. Two recent case series, however, brought this condition to attention as an uncommon presentation in T2DM in pediatric patients that can lead to multisystemic organ failure or death [169,170]. The criteria for HHS include plasma glucose concentration >600 mg/dL, serum carbon dioxide concentration >15 μmol/L, small ketonuria, absent to low ketonemia, effective serum osmolality >320 mOsm/kg, and stupor or coma [168]. HHS may not always present with its typical diagnostic criteria, however, and there may be considerable overlap with DKA. Cerebral edema and rhabdomyolysis may accompany HHS or DKA. (See the article by Glaser elsewhere in this issue). The ADA guidelines for fluid rehydration of hyperglycemic crises in patients who have diabetes prescribe a slower fluid resuscitation (48 hours) for patients younger than 20 years with DKA or HHS [168]. Timely diagnosis and prompt and appropriate treatment are the keys for recovery [169,170].

Pediatric patients who have T2DM occasionally may present with the skin manifestation of necrobiosis lipoidica diabeticorum, the incidence of which is 0.3% to 1.2% in patients who have diabetes [171]. Necrobiosis lipoidica diabeticorum lesions start as painless, reddish brown papules that slowly enlarge to waxy yellow plaques with a depressed central area and elevated purple peripheral ring [171]. Necrobiosis lipoidica diabeticorum lesions may predate the diagnosis of diabetes. The pathogenesis is believed to be unrelated to the adequacy of metabolic control. Recurrent necrobiosis lipoidica diabeticorum that required extensive medical and surgical treatment was reported recently in a 16-year-old morbidly obese girl with poorly controlled T2DM [172]. Despite its rare occurrence, clinicians should be aware of this skin condition and its possible association with T2DM of youth.

Atherosclerotic cardiovascular disease is the major cause of mortality and morbidity in adults who have T2DM [173]. The origin of atherosclerosis is early in childhood with progression toward clinically significant lesions in young adulthood [174,175]. Carotid artery intima media thickness and aortic pulse wave velocity, a measure of arterial stiffness, are noninvasive measures of subclinical atherosclerosis that have been used as surrogate measures of cardiovascular events in various adult studies [176–178]. Data regarding intima media thickness and arterial stiffness in children are limited despite the increasing tide of obesity and T2DM. We recently demonstrated significantly higher aortic pulse wave velocity measurements in adolescents with T2DM compared with obese and normal weight controls, with no differences in intima media thickness among the three groups [179].The elevated aortic pulse wave velocity in our T2DM youth, which reflects increased arterial stiffness, was comparable to values reported in 41- to 59-year-old obese adults [180] and in approximately 40-year-old men in the Baltimore Longitudinal Study of Aging [177]. Such an observation would be consistent with the premature aging of the cardiovascular system in youth who have T2DM. These findings may reflect early functional changes in the vasculature in the absence of ultrasonographically detectable structural changes. With increasing age and duration of diabetes, these functional changes may progress to structural changes if left without intervention. This and similar observations would lend further support to the American Heart Association guidelines of primary prevention of atherosclerotic cardiovascular disease beginning in childhood [181].

Management of type 2 diabetes mellitus in children

Team approach and goals of treatment

Ideally, the care of a child with T2DM is shared among a physician, diabetes nurse educator, nutritionist, physical activity leader, and behavioral specialist [135]. Conscientious involvement by family members also is necessary for children to reach therapeutic goals. Components of the comprehensive diabetes evaluation are updated annually by the ADA [182]. The goals of treatment of T2DM are to reverse acute metabolic abnormalities, achieve and maintain near-normoglycemic states (fasting blood glucose < 126 mg/dL, HbA1c 7% or less), eliminate symptoms of hyperglycemia, improve insulin sensitivity and secretion, promote achievement of a healthy body weight, screen for and treat comorbidities, and prevent complications of DM [2,19]. The ultimate goal is to decrease the acute and chronic complications associated with DM. The UKPDS and the Kumamoto Study demonstrated that intensive treatment of adults with T2DM improved metabolic control and decreased the risk of microvascular disease [183,184]. In the UKPDS study, for each 1% reduction in mean HbA1c, a 21% reduction in risk for any end point related to diabetes (ie, 21% for deaths, 14% for myocardial infarction, and 37% for microvascular complications) was seen [185].

Lifestyle modification

Two recent randomized, controlled clinical trials on the prevention of diabetes among adults have demonstrated the benefits of lifestyle intervention on the prevention of progression from IGT to T2DM [186,187]. The impact of such interventions on prevention and treatment of T2DM in children is underway in a national, multicenter, clinical trial. Currently, aggressive lifestyle modification is widely recommended for all children who have risk factors for T2DM, have IGT, or have been diagnosed with T2DM. Lifestyle modification should encompass medical nutrition therapy and increased activity habits.

Pharmacologic therapy

Insulin

Patients who present with severe hyperglycemia (≥ 200 mg/dL), HbA1c more than 8.5%, or severe manifestations of insulin deficiency (eg, ketosis/DKA) should be treated initially with insulin to achieve metabolic control rapidly. Once a child recovers from ketosis after hydration and treatment with insulin, metformin should be started and insulin may be gradually weaned if normoglycemia is maintained. Deterioration in pancreatic beta-cell function occurs with increasing duration in individuals with T2DM, which necessitates the introduction of insulin to achieve metabolic control [19,52,55]. Evidence in adult patients suggests that the early introduction of insulin therapy may reverse some of the damage imparted by hyperglycemia on pancreatic beta-cells and insulin-sensitive tissues and facilitate glucose control in the long-term [188]. Short-term insulin therapy (≤ 4 months) with premixed insulin (70/30) in adolescents who have early T2DM (duration 8.7 ± 4.3 weeks) has been shown to improve glycemic control [189]. It is possible that T2DM is more aggressive in certain populations, including children or persons with islet cell autoantibodies, and serious consideration should be given to starting insulin early [19,55].

New insulin analogs allow for enhanced, more flexible dosing. Ultra–short-acting analogs (eg, insulin lispro, insulin aspart) allow for immediate insulin action and relatively rapid clearance from the blood stream. The ultra–long-acting analog (eg, insulin glargine) is systemically absorbed from the subcutaneous tissues slowly, has a relatively smooth blood concentration profile, and has a prolonged duration of action (approximately 24 hours), which makes it useful as a once-a-day basal insulin [190]. Clinical trials in adults with T2DM have shown insulin glargine to promote optimal glycemic control effectively [191]. Clinical therapeutic studies are needed to examine the optimal combinations of oral agents or insulin preparations for treatment of T2DM in pediatric populations. (See the article by Jacobson-Dickman and Levitsky elsewhere in this issue).

Metformin

Children and adolescents who present with mild hyperglycemia (fasting plasma glucose, 126–199 mg/dL) and HbA1c less than 8.5% can be treated initially with therapeutic lifestyle change in combination with metformin, which has been shown to be safe and effective for use in pediatric patients [192]. Metformin, a biguanide, decreases hepatic glucose production and increases insulin-mediated glucose uptake in peripheral tissues, primarily muscle tissue [67,193], and is the only drug approved by the US Food and Drug Administration for pediatric patients who have T2DM. Metformin is prescribed to non-ketotic patients at a low dose (500 mg twice a day or 850 mg once a day, given with meals) and increased as tolerated (in increments of 500 mg or 850 mg every 2 weeks, up to a total of 2000 mg/d). Side effects associated with metformin include gastrointestinal discomfort and, on rare occasion, lactic acidosis [67,193]. Metformin should not be given to a child who has T2DM and ketosis, renal impairment, abnormal liver enzymes, cardiopulmonary insufficiency, or is undergoing evaluation with radiographic contrast materials, because it may precipitate lactic acidosis. Therapy should be intensified whenever glucose control is not achieved after 3 to 6 months. Fig. 4 provides a working algorithm for the management of youth who have T2DM, based on our current knowledge and approved therapies (Fig. 4) [194].

Other oral agents

Sulfonylureas (eg, glimepiride, glyburide, glipizide) and meglitinides (eg, repaglinide, nateglinide) are insulin secretagogues that exert their effect in the presence of glucose [195]. Unlike metformin, sulfonylureas are associated with hypoglycemia and weight gain [195], which can be particularly troublesome for children and adolescents. Thiazolidinediones (eg, rosiglitazone, pioglitazone) reduce hepatic glucose production, increase glucose uptake by muscle, and inhibit lipolysis in adipose tissue [196]. Edema, weight gain, anemia, and liver damage may occur with thiazolidinediones [197]. Clinical trials are under way with thiazolidinediones and sulfonylureas in pediatric patients who have T2DM. Clinical trials in adult patients who have T2DM demonstrate that all four classes of oral glucose-lowering agents improve HbA1c similarly (reduction of 1%–2%) [198].

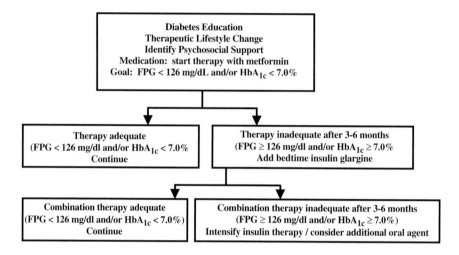

Fig. 4. Proposed algorithm for the management of youth with T2DM. (*Adapted from* Hannon TS, Rao G, Arslanian SA. Childhood obesity and type 2 diabetes mellitus. Pediatrics 2005;116(2):477.)

Approval of these drugs for use in children will greatly expand the armament of treatment options for T2DM in the pediatric population.

Monitoring glycemic control

Children who have T2DM and their families, regardless of whether they are receiving insulin treatment, should receive intensive diabetes education, including education regarding routine self-monitoring of blood glucose. Glucose levels should be monitored frequently, especially when medications are being adjusted, when symptoms of diabetes are present, and during acute illness. As with individuals who have T1DM, patients who have T2DM should check urinary ketones with a dipstick at such times. Routine glucose self-monitoring should include fasting and postprandial measurements. Diabetes therapy should be prescribed and titrated to maintain fasting glucose levels between 70 and 126 mg/dL. We recommend the same follow-up regimen for individuals who have T2DM as for persons with T1DM: clinical follow-up every 3 months with measurement of HbA1c and monitoring of complications as outlined later. The ADA recommends a goal HbA1c of less than 7% [135], whereas the American College of Endocrinology recommends a more stringent goal of $\leq 6.5\%$, based on evidence that shows that there is no minimum level of HbA1c at which complications of diabetes and mortality do not occur [199].

Management of complications

Acute complications

Acute complications of T2DM, including DKA and hyperosmolar coma (ie, hyperglycemia, hyperosmolarity, and an absence of significant ketosis), can be life threatening. The clinical features of DKA and hyperosmolar coma overlap and often are observed simultaneously. Patients who present with either of these complications should be managed in an inpatient setting by a medical team with expertise in the appropriate fluid replacement, insulin therapy, correction and replacement of electrolytes, neurologic/mental status evaluation, and airway management for youth who have DKA [2,169,170].

Hypertension

Blood pressure should be monitored regularly. Height- and age-specific population-based blood pressure percentiles for boys and girls are available [200]. A systolic and diastolic blood pressure less than the ninetieth percentile, adjusted for age, sex, and height, is normal. Prehypertension is defined as either systolic or diastolic blood pressure between the ninetieth and ninety-fifth percentile for age, sex, and height. Stage 1 hypertension is either systolic or diastolic blood pressure more than or equal to the ninety-fifth percentile for age, sex, and height. Stage 2 hypertension is present if either the systolic or diastolic blood pressure is more than the ninety-ninth percentile plus 5 mm Hg.

Lifestyle modifications in the form of weight loss, dietary changes, and increased physical activity form the foundation of initial therapy for children with hypertension. Angiotensin-converting enzyme inhibitors, angiotensin receptor blockers, calcium channel blockers, beta blockers, and diuretics have been used to treat children who have hypertension who do not respond to lifestyle modification. We recommend that all children who have stage 2 hypertension undergo additional renal evaluation, and our preference for medical therapy is initiation of angiotensin-converting enzyme inhibitors.

Dyslipidemia

Fasting lipid profile should be obtained upon diagnosis, after glucose control has been established, and annually thereafter. Target lipid levels and treatment recommendations for youth who have diabetes have been established by the ADA consensus for the treatment of diabetes in youth (Table 3) [201]. Separate and somewhat different target levels for children were recommended recently by the American Heart Association [181]. Recommended lipid levels were as follows: total cholesterol < 170 mg/dL (170–200 mg/dL borderline), low density lipoprotein (LDL) < 130 mg/dL (110–130 mg/dL borderline), triglycerides < 150 mg/dL, and high density lipoprotein > 35 mg/dL [181]. Because diabetes is a major risk factor for cardiovascular disease, the more stringent ADA guidelines seem appropriate for youth who have T2DM.

Therapeutic dietary changes and increased physical activity are the first-line treatment for dyslipidemia in children. Lipid-lowering medications can be considered if lipids remain elevated after 6 months of lifestyle modification [199,201]. HMG-CoA reductase inhibitors (statins) are the most commonly used lipid-lowering agents in pediatric patients. Statins (eg, atorvastatin, lovastatin, pravastatin) are currently indicated for use after an adequate trial of lifestyle

Table 3
Management of dyslipidemia in youth with type 2 diabetes mellitus

Goals		
LDL	< 100 mg/dL	
HDL	> 35 mg/dL	
TG	< 150 mg/dL	
Treatment strategies		
LDL	100–129 mg/dL	Maximize nonpharmacologic therapy
LDL	130–159 mg/dL	Consider pharmacologic therapy based on other risk factors (blood pressure, family history, smoking)[a]
LDL	≥ 160 mg/dL	Start pharmacologic treatment
Pharmacologic therapy		
LDL	≥ 160 mg/dL	Statins ± resins
TG	> 1000 mg/dL	Fibric acid derivatives

Abbreviations: HDL, high density lipoprotein; LDL, low density lipoprotein; TG, triglyceride.

[a] Continue ongoing management of other risk factors, including therapy for hypertension and smoking cessation.

Data from American Diabetes Association. Management of dyslipidemia in children and adolescents with diabetes. Diabetes Care 2003;26(7):2195.

modification with nutritional therapy in boys over the age of 10 and in post-menarchal girls with familial hypercholesterolemia.

Microvascular complications

Primary evaluation and routine follow-up of children who have T2DM should include monitoring for signs of microvascular complications. Urinary micro-albumin excretion and renal function should be checked after the diagnosis is established and annually. A dilated retinal examination to look for retinopathy should be performed annually by a qualified physician. It is not clear how soon this examination should be implemented, however. Currently it is left to the clinician's discretion to decide when to start this screening process. Because T2DM in youth is a relatively new entity, these recommendations are not evidence based but rather stem from our experience with children who have T1DM.

Summary

T2DM has emerged as a serious public health problem in the pediatric population, with its escalating rates paralleling the epidemic of childhood obesity. A high index of suspicion is important to prompt screening in the clinical setting of high-risk youth. Screening helps in the early diagnosis and initiation of therapy in subclinical or silent cases of T2DM in youth. The objective and theory behind early diagnosis are the preservation of pancreatic beta-cell function and the prevention of the relentless decline in insulin secretion. In our efforts to treat hyperglycemia and its associated complications, however, we must remember to treat the patient as a whole, including obesity, insulin resistance, dyslipidemia, hypertension, and psychosocial disorders—all conditions frequently present in youth who have T2DM. Finally, as we gain more experience—both clinical and research—our approaches to some of these problems and recommendations may change over time. In addition to research, public health measures to increase activities of children and youth, along with public education campaigns for healthy eating may have a profound influence in curbing the epidemic of obesity and its related complications.

Acknowledgments

We are indebted to the children and their parents who participated in our research studies that facilitated our understanding of T2DM and related conditions.

References

[1] Fagot-Campagna A, Pettitt D, Engelgau MM, et al. Type 2 diabetes among North American children and adolescents: an epidemiologic review and a public health perspective. J Pediatr 2000;136(5):664–72.

[2] American Diabetes Association. Type 2 diabetes in children and adolescents. Diabetes Care 2000;23(3):381–9.

[3] Ehtisham S, Barrett TG, Shaw NJ. Type 2 diabetes mellitus in UK children: an emerging problem. Diabet Med 2000;17(12):867–71.

[4] Ehtisham S, Kirk J, McEvilly A, et al. Prevalence of type 2 diabetes in children in Birmingham. BMJ 2001;322(7299):1428.

[5] Ehtisham S, Hattersley AT, Dunger DB, et al, British Society for Paediatric Endocrinology and Diabetes Clinical Trials Group. First UK survey of paediatric type 2 diabetes and MODY. Arch Dis Child 2004;89(6):526–9.

[6] Ortega-Rodriguez E, Levy-Marchal C, Tubiana N, et al. Emergence of type 2 diabetes in an hospital based cohort of children with diabetes mellitus. Diabetes Metab 2001;27(1):574–8.

[7] Drake AJ, Smith A, Betts PR, et al. Type 2 diabetes in obese white children. Arch Dis Child 2002;86(3):207–8.

[8] Holl RW, Grabert M, Krause U, et al. Prevalence and clinical characteristics of patients with non-type 1 diabetes in the pediatric age range: analysis of a multicenter database including 20,410 patients from 148 center in Germany and Austria. Diabetologia 2003;46(Suppl 2):A26.

[9] Rami B, Schober E, Nachbauer E, et al, Austrian Diabetes Incidence Study Group. Type 2 diabetes mellitus is rare but not absent in children under 15 years of age in Austria. Eur J Pediatr 2003;162(12):850–2.

[10] Zachrisson I, Tibell C, Bang P, et al. Prevalence of type 2 diabetes among known cases of diabetes aged 0–18 years in Sweden. Diabetologia 2003;46(Suppl 2):A25.

[11] Chan JC, Hawkins BR, Cockram CS. A Chinese family with non-insulin-dependent diabetes of early onset and severe diabetic complications. Diabet Med 1990;7(3):211–4.

[12] Kitagawa T, Owada M, Urakami T, et al. Epidemiology of type 1 (insulin-dependent) and type 2 (non-insulin-dependent) diabetes mellitus in Japanese children. Diabetes Res Clin Pract 1994;24(Suppl 1):S7–13.

[13] Kitagawa T, Owada M, Urakami T, et al. Increased incidence of non-insulin dependent diabetes mellitus among Japanese school children correlates with an increased intake of animal protein and fat. Clin Pediatr 1998;37(2):111–5.

[14] Tajima N. Type 2 diabetes in children and adolescents in Japan. International Diabetes Monitor 2002;14:1–5.

[15] Wei JN, Sung FC, Lin CC, et al. National surveillance for type 2 diabetes mellitus in Taiwanese children. JAMA 2003;290(10):1345–50.

[16] Kadiki O, Reddy M, Marzouk A. Incidence of insulin-dependent diabetes (IDDM) and non insulin-dependent diabetes (NIDDM) (0–34 years at onset) in Benghazi, Libya. Diabetes Res Clin Pract 1996;32(3):165–73.

[17] Braun B, Zimmermann MB, Kretchmer N, et al. Risk factors for diabetes and cardiovascular disease in young Australian aborigines: a 5-year follow-up study. Diabetes Care 1996;19(5):472–9.

[18] Saad MF, Knowler WC, Pettitt DJ, et al. A two-step model for development of non-insulin-dependent diabetes. Am J Med 1991;90(2):229–35.

[19] Gungor N, Bacha F, Saad R, et al. Youth type 2 diabetes: insulin resistance, beta-cell failure, or both? Diabetes Care 2005;28(3):638–44.

[20] Reisman D. Mild diabetes in children. Am J Med Sci 1916;151:40–5.

[21] Savage PJ, Bennett PH, Senter RG, et al. High prevalence of diabetes in young Pima Indians: evidence of phenotypic variation in a genetically isolated population. Diabetes 1979;28(10):937–42.

[22] Freedman D, Serdula M, Percy C, et al. Obesity, levels of lipids and glucose and smoking among Navajo adolescents. J Nutr 1997;127(Suppl 10):2120–7.

[23] Dabelea D, Hanson RL, Bennett PH, et al. Increasing prevalence of type 2 diabetes in American Indian children. Diabetologia 1998;41(8):904–10.

[24] Moore KR, Harwell TS, McDowall JM, et al. Three-year prevalence and incidence of diabetes among American Indian youth in Montana and Wyoming, 1999 to 2001. J Pediatr 2003;143(3):368–71.

[25] Acton KJ, Burrows NR, Moore K, et al. Trends in diabetes prevalence among American Indian and Alaska native children, adolescents, and young adults. Am J Public Health 2002;92(9):1485–90.

[26] Dean HJ, Young TK, Flett B, et al. Screening of non-type 2 diabetes in aboriginal children in northern Canada [letter]. Lancet 1998;352(9139):1523–4.

[27] Huen KF, Low LC, Wong GW, et al. Epidemiology of diabetes mellitus in children in Hong Kong: the Hong Kong childhood diabetes register. J Pediatr Endocrinol Metab 2000;13(3):297–302.

[28] Jung-Nan W, Fung-Chang S, Chau-Ching L, et al. National surveillance for type 2 diabetes mellitus in Taiwanese children. JAMA 2003;290(10):1345–50.

[29] Libman IM, LaPorte RE, Becker D, et al. Was there an epidemic of diabetes in nonwhite adolescents in Allegheny County, Pennsylvania? Diabetes Care 1998;21(8):1278–81.

[30] Libman IM, Pietropaolo M, Trucco M, et al. Islet cell autoimmunity in white and black children and adolescents with IDDM. Diabetes Care 1998;21(11):1824–7.

[31] Libman IM, Pietropaolo M, Arslanian SA, et al. Evidence for heterogeneous pathogenesis of insulin-treated diabetes in black and white children. Diabetes Care 2003;26(10):2876–82.

[32] Pinhas-Hamiel O, Dolan LM, Daniels SR, et al. Increased incidence of non-insulin dependent diabetes mellitus among adolescents. J Pediatr 1996;128(5):608–15.

[33] Scott C, Smith J, Cradock M, et al. Characteristics of youth-onset non-insulin dependent diabetes mellitus and insulin-dependent diabetes mellitus at diagnosis. Pediatrics 1997;100(1):84–91.

[34] Willi SM, Kennedy A, Wojciechowski B, et al. Insulin resistance and defective glucose-insulin coupling in ketosis-prone type 2 diabetes of African-American youth. Diabetes 1998;47(Suppl 1):A306.

[35] Glaser NS, Jones KL. Non-insulin dependent diabetes mellitus in Mexican-American children. West J Med 1998;168(1):11–6.

[36] Neufeld N, Raffel L, Landon C, et al. Early presentation of type 2 diabetes in Mexican-American youth. Diabetes Care 1998;21(1):80–6.

[37] Hale DE, Danney KM. Non-insulin dependent diabetes in Hispanic youth (type 2Y). Diabetes 1998;47(Suppl 1):A82.

[38] Silverstein JH, Rosenbloom AL. Treatment of type 2 diabetes mellitus in children and adolescents. J Pediatr Endocrinol Metab 2000;13(Suppl 6):1403–9.

[39] Likitmaskul S, Kiattisathavee P, Chaichan-Watanakul K, et al. Increasing prevalence of type 2 diabetes mellitus in Thai children and adolescents associated with increasing prevalence of obesity. J Pediatr Endocrinol Metab 2003;16(1):71–7.

[40] Kahn SE. Regulation of β-cell function in vivo: from health to disease. Diabetes Reviews 1996;4:372–89.

[41] Kahn SE. The importance of β-cell failure in the development and progression of type 2 diabetes. J Clin Endocrinol Metab 2001;86(9):4047–58.

[42] Stumvoll M, Goldstein B, van Haeften TW. Type 2 diabetes: principles of pathogenesis and therapy. Lancet 2005;365(9467):1333–46.

[43] Himsworth H. Diabetes mellitus: a differentiation into insulin-sensitive and insulin-insensitive types. Lancet 1936;i:127–30.

[44] Reaven GM. Role of insulin resistance in the pathophysiology of non-insulin dependent diabetes mellitus. Diabetes Metab Rev 1993;9(Suppl 1):5S–12S.

[45] Weyer C, Bogardus C, Mott DM, et al. The natural history of insulin secretory dysfunction and insulin resistance in the pathogenesis of type 2 diabetes mellitus. J Clin Invest 1999;104(6):787–94.

[46] Banerji MA, Lebovitz HE. Insulin action in black Americans with NIDDM. Diabetes Care 1992;15(10):1295–302.

[47] Umpaichitra V, Bastian W, Taha D, et al. C-peptide and glucagon profiles in minority children with type 2 diabetes mellitus. J Clin Endocrinol Metab 2001;86(4):1605–9.

[48] Kobayashi K, Amemiya S, Higashida K, et al. Pathogenic factors of glucose intolerance in obese Japanese adolescents with type 2 diabetes. Metabolism 2000;49(2):186–91.

[49] Roder ME, Dinesen B, Hartling SG, et al. Intact proinsulin and β-cell function in lean and obese subjects with and without type 2 diabetes. Diabetes Care 1999;22(4):609–14.

[50] Arslanian SA. Type 2 diabetes mellitus in children: clinical aspects and risk factors. Horm Res 2002;57(Suppl 1):19–28.

[51] Tripathy D, Carlsson M, Almgren P, et al. Insulin secretion and insulin sensitivity in relation to glucose tolerance: lessons from the Botnia study. Diabetes 2000;49(6):975–80.

[52] Matthews DR, Cull CA, Stratton IM, et al. UKPDS 26: sulfonylurea failure in non-insulin dependent diabetic patients over six years. Diabet Med 1998;15(4):297–303.

[53] Holman RR. Assessing the potential for alpha-glucosidase inhibitors in prediabetic states. Diabetes Res Clin Pract 1998;40(Suppl):S21–5.

[54] Levy J, Atkinson AB, Bell PM, et al. Beta-cell deterioration determines the onset and rate of progression of secondary dietary failure in type 2 diabetes mellitus: the 10-year follow-up of the Belfast Diet Study. Diabet Med 1998;15(4):290–6.

[55] Gungor N, Arslanian S. Progressive beta cell failure in type 2 diabetes mellitus of youth. J Pediatr 2004;144(5):656–9.

[56] Kahn CR. Banting lecture: insulin action, diabetogenes, and the cause of type II diabetes. Diabetes 1994;43(8):1066–84.

[57] Hansen L, Pedersen O. Genetics of type 2 diabetes mellitus: status and perspectives. Diabetes Obes Metab 2005;7(2):122–35.

[58] Poulsen P, Kyvik KO, Vaag A, et al. Heritability of type II (non-insulin-dependent) diabetes mellitus and abnormal glucose tolerance: a population-based twin study. Diabetologia 1999;42(2):139–45.

[59] Medici F, Hawa M, Ianari A, et al. Concordance rate for type II diabetes mellitus in monozygotic twins: actuarial analysis. Diabetologia 1999;42(2):146–50.

[60] Zimmet P, Turner R, McCarty D, et al. Crucial points at diagnosis: type 2 diabetes or slow type 1 diabetes. Diabetes Care 1999;22(Suppl 2):B59–64.

[61] Martin BC, Warram JH, Krolewski AS, et al. Role of glucose and insulin resistance in development of type 2 diabetes mellitus: results of a 25-year follow up study. Lancet 1992;340(8825):925–9.

[62] Goldfine AB, Bouche C, Parker RA, et al. Insulin resistance is a poor predictor of type 2

diabetes in individuals with no family history of disease. Proc Natl Acad Sci U S A 2003; 100(5):2724–9.

[63] Lillioja S, Mott DM, Spraul M, et al. Insulin resistance and insulin secretory dysfunction as precursors of non-insulin-dependent diabetes mellitus: prospective studies of Pima Indians. N Engl J Med 1993;329(27):1988–92.

[64] Elbein SC, Hasstedt SJ, Wegner K, et al. Heritability of pancreatic β-cell function among nondiabetic members of Caucasian familial type 2 diabetic kindreds. J Clin Endocrinol Metab 1999;84(4):1398–403.

[65] Danadian K, Balasekaren G, Lewy V, et al. Insulin sensitivity in African-American children with and without family history of type 2 diabetes. Diabetes Care 1999;22(8):1325–9.

[66] Arslanian SA, Bacha F, Saad R, et al. Family history of type 2 diabetes is associated with decreased insulin sensitivity and an impaired balance between insulin sensitivity and insulin secretion in white youth. Diabetes Care 2005;28(1):115–9.

[67] Rosenbloom AL, Joe JR, Young RS, et al. Emerging epidemic of type 2 diabetes in youth. Diabetes Care 1999;22(2):345–54.

[68] Dietz WD, Robinson TN. Overweight children and adolescents. N Engl J Med 2005;352(20): 2100–9.

[69] Ogden C, Flegal K, Carroll M, et al. Prevalence and trends in overweight among US children and adolescents, 1999–2000. JAMA 2002;288(14):1728–32.

[70] Ludwig DS, Peterson KE, Gortmaker SL. Relation between consumption of sugar-sweetened drinks and childhood obesity: a prospective observational analysis. Lancet 2001;357(9255): 505–8.

[71] Morton JF, Guthrie JF. Changes in children's total fat intakes and their food group sources of fat, 1989–91 versus 1994–95: implications for diet quality. Family Economics and Nutrition Review 1998;11:44–57.

[72] Kimm SY, Glynn NW, Kriska AM, et al. Longitudinal changes in physical activity in a biracial cohort during adolescence. Med Sci Sports Exerc 2000;32(8):1445–54.

[73] Andersen RE, Crespo CJ, Bartlett SJ, et al. Relationship of physical activity and television watching with body weight and level of fatness among children: results from the third National Health and Nutrition Examination Survey. JAMA 1998;279(12):938–42.

[74] Sorensen TIA. The changing lifestyle in the world: body weight and what else? Diabetes Care 2000;23:B1–4.

[75] Hill JO, Peters JC. Environmental contributions to the obesity epidemic. Science 1998; 280(5368):1371–4.

[76] Arslanian S, Danadian K. Insulin secretion, insulin sensitivity and diabetes in black children. Trends Endocrinol Metab 1998;9:194–9.

[77] Caprio S, Tamborlane WV. Metabolic impact of obesity in childhood. Endocrinol Metab Clin North Am 1999;28(4):731–47.

[78] Bacha F, Saad R, Gungor N, et al. Adiponectin in youth: relationship to visceral adiposity, insulin sensitivity, and beta-cell function. Diabetes Care 2004;27(2):547–52.

[79] Weyer C, Funahashi T, Tanaka S, et al. Hypoadiponectinemia in obesity and type 2 diabetes: close association with insulin resistance and hyperinsulinemia. J Clin Endocrinol Metab 2001; 86(5):1930–5.

[80] Gower BA, Nagy TR, Goran MI. Visceral fat, insulin sensitivity and lipids in prepubertal children. Diabetes 1999;48(8):1515–21.

[81] Bacha F, Saad R, Gungor N, et al. Obesity, regional fat distribution and syndrome X in obese black vs white adolescents: race differential in diabetogenic and atherogenic risk factors. J Clin Endocrinol Metab 2003;88(6):2534–40.

[82] Kissebah AH. Central obesity: measurement and metabolic effects. Diabetes Review 1997;5:8–20.

[83] Weiss R, Dufour S, Taksali SE, et al. Prediabetes in obese youth: a syndrome of impaired glucose tolerance, severe insulin resistance, and altered myocellular and abdominal fat partitioning. Lancet 2003;362(9388):951–7.

[84] Dean H. NIDDM-Y in first nation children in Canada. Clin Pediatr 1998;37(2):89–96.

[85] Dabelea D, Pettitt DJ, Jones KL, et al. Type 2 diabetes mellitus in minority children and adolescents: an emerging problem. Endocrinol Metab Clin North Am 1999;28(4):709–29.

[86] Knowler WC, Pettitt DJ, Saad MF. Diabetes mellitus in the Pima Indians: incidence, risk factors and pathogenesis. Diabetes Metab Rev 1990;6(1):1–27.

[87] Svec F, Nastasi K, Hilton C, et al. Black-white contrasts in insulin levels during pubertal development: the Bogalusa Heart Study. Diabetes 1992;41(3):313–7.

[88] Arslanian S, Suprasongsin C. Differences in the in vivo insulin secretion and sensitivity in healthy black vs white adolescents. J Pediatr 1996;129(3):440–4.

[89] Arslanian S, Suprasongsin C. Testosterone treatment in adolescents with delayed puberty: changes in body composition, protein, fat and glucose metabolism. J Clin Endocrinol Metab 1997;82(10):3213–20.

[90] Arslanian SA, Saad R, Lewy V, et al. Hyperinsulinemia in African-American children: decreased insulin clearance and increased insulin secretion and its relationship to insulin sensitivity. Diabetes 2002;51(10):3014–9.

[91] Gower BA, Fernandez JR, Beasley TM, et al. Using genetic admixture to explain racial differences in insulin-related phenotypes. Diabetes 2003;52(4):1047–51.

[92] Bacha F, Saad R, Gungor N, et al. Does adiponectin explain the lower insulin sensitivity and hyperinsulinemia of African-American children? Pediatr Diabetes 2005;6(2):100–2.

[93] Goran MI, Bergman RN, Cruz ML, et al. Insulin resistance and associated compensatory responses in African American and Hispanic children. Diabetes Care 2002;25(12):2184–90.

[94] Lestradet H, Deschamps I, Giron B. Insulin and free fatty acid levels during oral glucose tolerance tests and their relation to age in 70 healthy children. Diabetes 1976;25(6):505–8.

[95] Smith CP, Williams AJ, Thomas JM, et al. The pattern of basal and stimulated insulin responses to intravenous glucose in first degree relatives of type 1 (insulin-dependent) diabetic children and unrelated adults aged 5 to 50 years. Diabetologia 1988;31(7):430–4.

[96] Amiel SA, Caprio S, Sherwin RS, et al. Insulin resistance of puberty: a defect restricted to peripheral glucose metabolism. J Clin Endocrinol Metab 1991;72(2):277–82.

[97] Bloch CA, Clemons P, Sperling MA. Puberty decreases insulin sensitivity. J Pediatr 1987; 110(3):481–7.

[98] Arslanian SA, Kalhan SC. Correlations between fatty acid and glucose metabolism: potential explanation of insulin resistance of puberty. Diabetes 1994;43(7):908–14.

[99] Caprio S, Plewe G, Diamond MP, et al. Increased insulin secretion in puberty: a compensatory response to reductions in insulin sensitivity. J Pediatr 1989;114(6):963–7.

[100] Saad RJ, Keenan BS, Danadian K, et al. Dihydrotestosterone treatment in adolescents with delayed puberty: does it explain insulin resistance of puberty? J Clin Endocrinol Metab 2001; 86(10):4881–6.

[101] Dunaif A. Insulin action in the polycystic ovary syndrome. Endocrinol Metab Clin North Am 1999;28(2):341–59.

[102] Arslanian SA, Witchel SF. Polycystic ovary syndrome in adolescents: is there an epidemic? Current Opinion in Endocrinology and Diabetes 2002;9:32–42.

[103] Legro RS, Kunselman AR, Dodson WC, et al. Prevalence and predictors of risk for type 2 diabetes mellitus and impaired glucose tolerance in polycystic ovary syndrome: a prospective, controlled study in 254 affected women. J Clin Endocrinol Metab 1999;84(1):165–9.

[104] Ehrmann DA. Polycystic ovary syndrome. N Engl J Med 2005;352(12):1223–36.

[105] Palmert MR, Gordon CM, Kartashov AI, et al. Screening for abnormal glucose tolerance in adolescents with polycystic ovary syndrome. J Clin Endocrinol Metab 2002;87(3):1017–23.

[106] Lewy VD, Danadian K, Witchel SF, et al. Early metabolic abnormalities in adolescent girls with polycystic ovarian syndrome. J Pediatr 2001;138(1):38–44.

[107] Arslanian SA, Lewy VD, Danadian K. Glucose intolerance in obese adolescents with polycystic ovary syndrome: roles of insulin resistance and beta-cell dysfunction and risk of cardiovascular disease. J Clin Endocrinol Metab 2001;86(1):66–71.

[108] Stuart CA, Gilkison CR, Smith MM, et al. Acanthosis nigricans as a risk factor for non-insulin dependent diabetes mellitus. Clin Pediatr 1998;37(2):73–9.

[109] Brickman WJ, Howard JC, Metzger BE. Abnormal glucose tolerance in children with acanthosis nigricans: a chart review. Diabetes 2002;51(2):A429.

[110] Nguyen TT, Keil MF, Russell DL, et al. Relation of acanthosis nigricans to hyperinsulinemia and insulin sensitivity in overweight African American and white children. J Pediatr 2001; 138(4):474–80.

[111] Hirschler V, Aranda C, Oneto A, et al. Is acanthosis nigricans a marker of insulin resistance in obese children? Diabetes Care 2002;25(12):2353.

[112] Hales CN, Barker DJ. The thrifty phenotype hypothesis. Br Med Bull 2001;60:5–20.

[113] Pettitt DJ, Baird HR, Aleck KA, et al. Diabetes mellitus in children following maternal diabetes during gestation. Diabetes 1982;31:66A.

[114] Pettitt DJ, Baird HR, Aleck KA, et al. Excessive obesity in offspring of Pima Indian women with diabetes during pregnancy. N Engl J Med 1983;308(5):242–5.

[115] Silverman BL, Metzger BE, Cho NH, et al. Impaired glucose tolerance in adolescent offspring of diabetic mothers: relationship to fetal hyperinsulinism. Diabetes Care 1995;18(5):611–7.

[116] Silverman BL, Rizzo TA, Cho NH, et al. Long-term effects of the intrauterine environment: the Northwestern University Diabetes in Pregnancy Center. Diabetes Care 1998;21(Suppl 2): B142–9.

[117] Barker DJP, Hales CN, Fall CHD, et al. Type 2 (non-insulin-dependent) diabetes mellitus, hypertension and hyperlipidaemia (syndrome X): relation to reduced fetal growth. Diabetologia 1993;36(1):62–7.

[118] Robinson S, Walton RJ, Clark PM, et al. The relation of fetal growth to plasma glucose in young men. Diabetologia 1992;35(5):444–6.

[119] Jaquet D, Gaboriau A, Czernichow P, et al. Insulin resistance early in adulthood in subjects born with intrauterine growth retardation. J Clin Endocrinol Metab 2000;85(4):1401–6.

[120] Hattersley A, Tooke J. The fetal insulin hypothesis: an alternative explanation of the association of low birth weight with diabetes and vascular disease. Lancet 1999;353(9166):1789–92.

[121] Hofman PL, Cutfield WS, Robinson EM, et al. Insulin resistance in short children with intrauterine growth retardation. J Clin Endocrinol Metab 1997;82(2):402–6.

[122] Ong K, Petry C, Emmett P, et al. Insulin sensitivity and secretion in normal children related to size at birth, postnatal growth, and plasma insulin-like growth factor-I levels. Diabetologia 2004;47(6):1064–70.

[123] Veening MA, van Weissenbruch MM, Delemarre-van de Waal HA. Glucose tolerance, insulin sensitivity, and insulin secretion in children born small for gestational age. J Clin Endocrinol Metab 2002;87(10):4657–61.

[124] Jensen CB, Storgaard H, Dela F, et al. Early differential defects of insulin secretion and action in 19-year-old Caucasian men who had low birth weight. Diabetes 2002;51(4):1271–80.

[125] Whincup PH, Cook DG, Adshead F, et al. Childhood size is more strongly related than size at birth to glucose and insulin levels in 10–11 year old children. Diabetologia 1997;40(3):319–26.

[126] Wilkin TJ, Metcalf BS, Murphy MJ, et al. The relative contributions of birth weight, weight change, and current weight to insulin resistance in contemporary 5-year-olds. Diabetes 2002; 51(12):3468–72.

[127] Bavdekar A, Yajnik CS, Fall CHD, et al. Insulin resistance syndrome in 8-year-old Indian children. Diabetes 1999;48(12):2422–9.

[128] Garnett SP, Cowell CT, Baur LA, et al. Abdominal fat and birth size in healthy prepubertal children. Int J Obes 2001;25(11):1667–73.

[129] Weiss R, Dziura J, Burgert TS, et al. Obesity and the metabolic syndrome in children and adolescents. N Engl J Med 2004;350(23):2362–74.

[130] Hannon T, Arslanian S. Can we use simple clinical markers to identify overweight youth with insulin resistance? Diabetes 2005;54(Suppl 1):A52.

[131] American Diabetes Association. Report of the expert committee on the diagnosis and classification of diabetes mellitus. Diabetes Care 2005;28(Suppl 1):S37–42.

[132] American Diabetes Association. Report of the expert committee on the diagnosis and classification of diabetes mellitus: follow-up report on the diagnosis of diabetes mellitus. Diabetes Care 2003;26(11):3160–7.

[133] Hollander P. The case for tight control in diabetes. Postgrad Med 1984;75(4):80–7.
[134] McGill H, McMahan CA. Determinants of atherosclerosis in the young: pathobiological determinants of atherosclerosis in youth (PDAY) research group. Am J Cardiol 1998;82(10B):30T–6T.
[135] The Diabetes Control and Complications Trial Research Group. The effect of intensive treatment of diabetes on the development and progression of long-term complications in insulin-dependent diabetes mellitus. N Engl J Med 1993;329:977–86.
[136] Shaw J, Zimmet P, McCarty D, et al. Type 2 diabetes worldwide according to the new classification and criteria. Diabetes Care 2000;23(Suppl 2):B5–10.
[137] Shaw J, Hodge A, de Courten M, et al. Isolated post-challenge hyperglycaemia confirmed as a risk factor for mortality. Diabetologia 1999;42(9):1050–4.
[138] Sinha R, Fisch G, Teague B, et al. Prevalence of impaired glucose tolerance among children and adolescents with marked obesity. N Engl J Med 2002;346(11):802–10.
[139] Libman I, Marcus M, Kalarchian M, et al. Impaired fasting glucose according to the new ADA criteria: does it identify more youth at risk for cardiovascular disease? Diabetes 2004;53(Suppl 2):294.
[140] Uwaifo GI, Elberg J, Yanovski JA. Impaired glucose tolerance in obese children and adolescents. N Engl J Med 2002;347(4):290–2.
[141] Invitti C, Gilardini L, Viberti G. Impaired glucose tolerance in obese children and adolescents [author's reply]. N Engl J Med 2002;347(4):290–2.
[142] Kitagawa T, Mano T, Fujita H. The epidemiology of childhood diabetes mellitus in Tokyo metropolitan area. Tohoku J Exp Med 1983;141:171–9.
[143] Pinhas-Hamiel O, Dolan LM, Zeitler PS. Diabetic ketoacidosis among obese African-American adolescents with NIDDM. Diabetes Care 1997;20(4):484–6.
[144] Maldonado M, Hampe CS, Gaur LK, et al. Ketosis-prone diabetes: dissection of a heterogeneous syndrome using an immunogenetic and beta-cell functional classification, prospective analysis, and clinical outcomes. J Clin Endocrinol Metab 2003;88(11):5090–8.
[145] Mauvais-Jarvis F, Smith SB, Le May C, et al. PAX4 gene variations predispose to ketosis-prone diabetes. Hum Mol Genet 2004;13(24):3151–9.
[146] Winter WE, Maclaren NK, Riley WJ, et al. Maturity-onset diabetes of youth in black Americans. N Engl J Med 1987;316(6):285–91.
[147] Banerji MA, Chaiken RL, Huey H, et al. GAD antibody negative NIDDM in adult black subjects with diabetic ketoacidosis and increased frequency of human leukocyte antigen DR3 and DR4: flatbush diabetes. Diabetes 1994;43(6):741–5.
[148] Umpierrez GE, Casals MM, Gebhart SP, et al. Diabetic ketoacidosis in obese African-Americans. Diabetes 1995;44(7):790–5.
[149] Rasouli N, Elbein SC. Improved glycemic control in subjects with atypical diabetes results from restored insulin secretion, but not improved insulin sensitivity. J Clin Endocrinol Metab 2004;89(12):6331–5.
[150] McFarlane SI, Chaiken RL, Hirsch S, et al. Near-normoglycaemic remission in African-Americans with type 2 diabetes mellitus is associated with recovery of beta cell function. Diabet Med 2001;18(1):10–6.
[151] Libman IM, Pietropaolo M, Arslanian SA, et al. Changing prevalence of overweight children and adolescents at onset of insulin-treated diabetes. Diabetes Care 2003;26(10):2871–5.
[152] Bingley PJ, Bonifacio E, Shattock M, et al. Can islet cell antibodies predict IDDM in the general population? Diabetes Care 1993;16(1):45–50.
[153] Hagopian WA, Sanjeevi CB, Kockum I, et al. Glutamate decarboxylase-, insulin-and islet cell-antibodies and HLA typing to detect diabetes in a general population-based study of Swedish children. J Clin Invest 1995;95(4):1505–11.
[154] Knip M, Karjalainen J, Akerbloom HK. Islet cell antibodies are less predictive of IDDM among unaffected children in the general population than in sibs of children with diabetes: the Childhood Diabetes in Finland Study Group. Diabetes Care 1998;21(10):1670–3.
[155] Tuomi T, Groop LC, Zimmet PZ, et al. Antibodies to glutamic acid decarboxylase reveal latent autoimmune diabetes mellitus in adults with a non-insulin-dependent onset of disease. Diabetes 1993;42(2):359–62.

[156] Seissler J, de Sonnaville JJ, Morgenthaler NG, et al. Immunological heterogeneity in type I diabetes: presence of distinct autoantibody patterns in patients with acute onset and slowly progressive disease. Diabetologia 1998;41(8):891–7.

[157] Turner R, Stratton I, Horton V, et al. UKPDS 25: autoantibodies to islet-cell cytoplasm and glutamic acid decarboxylase for prediction of insulin requirement in type 2 diabetes. Lancet 1997;350(9087):1288–93.

[158] Juneja R, Hirsch IB, Naik RG, et al. Islet cell antibodies and glutamic acid decarboxylase antibodies, but not the clinical phenotype, help to identify type 1 1/2 diabetes in patients presenting with type 2 diabetes. Metabolism 2001;50(9):1108–13.

[159] Dean HE, Mandy RLL, Miffed M. Non-insulin dependent diabetes mellitus in Indian children in Manitoba. Can Med Assoc J 1992;147(1):52–7.

[160] Hathout EH, Thomas W, El-Shahawy M, et al. Diabetic autoimmune markers in children and adolescents with type 2 diabetes. Pediatrics 2001;107(6):E102.

[161] Umpaichitra V, Banerji MA, Castells S. Autoantibodies in children with type 2 diabetes mellitus. J Pediatr Endocrinol Metab 2002;15(Suppl 1):525–30.

[162] Fagot-Campagna A, Knowler WC, Pettitt DJ. Type 2 diabetes in Pima Indian children: cardiovascular risk factors at diagnosis and 10 years later [abstract]. Diabetes 1998;47(Suppl 1):A155.

[163] McGrath NM, Parker GN, Dawson P. Early presentation of type 2 diabetes mellitus in young New Zealand Maori. Diabetes Res Clin Pract 1999;43(3):205–9.

[164] Chan JC, Cheung CK, Swaminathan R, et al. Obesity, albuminuria and hypertension among Hong Kong Chinese with non-insulin-dependent diabetes mellitus (NIDDM). Postgrad Med 1993;69(809):204–10.

[165] Yokoyama H, Okudaira M, Otani T, et al. High incidence of diabetic nephropathy in early-onset Japanese NIDDM patients: risk analysis. Diabetes Care 1998;21(7):1080–5.

[166] Yokoyama H, Okudaira M, Otani T, et al. Existence of early-onset NIDDM Japanese demonstrating severe diabetic complications. Diabetes Care 1997;20(5):844–7.

[167] Dean H, Flett B. Natural history of type 2 diabetes diagnosed in childhood: long-term follow-up in young adult years. Diabetes 2002;51(S2):A24.

[168] American Diabetes Association. Position statement: hyperglycemic crises in patients with diabetes mellitus. Diabetes Care 2001;24(Suppl):S83–90.

[169] Morales AE, Rosenbloom AL. Death caused by hyperglycemic hyperosmolar state at the onset of type 2 diabetes. J Pediatr 2004;144(2):270–9.

[170] Carchman RM, Dechert-Zeger M, Calikoglu AS, et al. A new challenge in pediatric obesity: pediatric hyperglycemic hyperosmolar syndrome. Pediatr Crit Care Med 2005;6(1):20–4.

[171] Sibbald RG, Landolt S, Toth D. Skin and diabetes. Endocrinol Metab Clin North Am 1996;25(2):463–72.

[172] Yigit S, Estrada E. Recurrent necrobiosis lipoidica diabeticorum associated with venous insufficiency in an adolescent with poorly controlled type 2 diabetes mellitus. J Pediatr 2002;141(2):280–2.

[173] Meigs JB. Epidemiology of cardiovascular complications in type 2 diabetes mellitus. Acta Diabetol 2003;40(Suppl 2):S358–61.

[174] Zieske AW, Malcom GT, Strong JP. Natural history and risk factors of atherosclerosis in children and youth: the PDAY study. Pediatr Pathol Mol Med 2002;21(2):213–37.

[175] Berenson GS. Childhood risk factors predict adult risk associated with subclinical cardiovascular disease: the Bogalusa Heart Study. Am J Cardiol 2002;90(10C):3L–7L.

[176] Salonen R, Salonen JT. Progression of carotid atherosclerosis and its determinants: a population-based ultrasonography study. Atherosclerosis 1990;81(1):33–40.

[177] Vaitkevicius PV, Fleg JL, Engel JH, et al. Effects of age and aerobic capacity on arterial stiffness in healthy adults. Circulation 1993;88(4 Pt 1):1456–62.

[178] Woodman RJ, Watts GF. Measurement and application of arterial stiffness in clinical research focus on new methodologies and diabetes mellitus. Med Sci Monit 2003;9(5):RA81–9.

[179] Gungor N, Thompson T, Sutton-Tyrrell K, et al. Early signs of cardiovascular disease in youth with obesity and type 2 diabetes. Diabetes Care 2005;28(5):1219–21.

[180] Wildman RP, Mackey RH, Bostom A, et al. Measures of obesity are associated with vascular stiffness in young and older adults. Hypertension 2003;42(4):468–73.

[181] Kavey RE, Daniels SR, Lauer RM, et al. American Heart Association guidelines for primary prevention of atherosclerotic cardiovascular disease beginning in childhood. J Pediatr 2003; 142(4):368–72.
[182] American Diabetes Association. Standards of medical care in diabetes. Diabetes Care 2004; 27(Suppl 2):S4–36.
[183] UK Prospective Diabetes Study (UKPDS) Group. Intensive blood glucose control with sulfonylureas or insulin compared with conventional treatment and risk of complications in patients with type 2 diabetes: UKPDS. BMJ 1998;317:703–13.
[184] Ohkubo Y, Kishikawa H, Araki E, et al. Intensive insulin therapy prevents the progression of diabetic microvascular complications in Japanese patients with noninsulin-dependent diabetes mellitus: a randomized prospective 6-year study. Diabetes Res Clin Pract 1995;28(2):103–17.
[185] Stratton IM, Adler AI, Neil HA, et al. Association of glycaemia with macrovascular and microvascular complications of type 2 diabetes (UKPDS 35): prospective observational study. BMJ 2000;321(7258):405–12.
[186] Tuomilehto J, Lindstrom J, Eriksson JG, et al. Prevention of type 2 diabetes mellitus by changes in lifestyle among subjects with impaired glucose tolerance. N Engl J Med 2001; 344(18):1343–50.
[187] Knowler WC, Barrett-Connor E, Fowler SE, et al. Reduction in the incidence of type 2 diabetes with lifestyle intervention or metformin. N Engl J Med 2002;346(6):393–403.
[188] Glaser B, Cerasi E. Early intensive insulin treatment for induction of long-term glycaemic control in type 2 diabetes. Diabetes Obes Metab 1999;1(2):67–74.
[189] Sellers EA, Dean HJ. Short-term insulin therapy in adolescents with type 2 diabetes mellitus. J Pediatr Endocrinol Metab 2004;17(11):1561–4.
[190] Lepore M, Pampanelli S, Fanelli C, et al. Pharmacokinetics and pharmacodynamics of subcutaneous injection of long-acting human insulin analog glargine, NPH insulin, and ultralente human insulin and continuous subcutaneous infusion of insulin lispro. Diabetes 2000;49(12): 2142–8.
[191] Yki-Jarvinen H, Dressler A, Ziemen M. Less nocturnal hypoglycemia and better post-dinner glucose control with bedtime insulin glargine compared with bedtime NPH insulin during insulin combination therapy in type 2 diabetes: HOE 901/3002 Study Group. Diabetes Care 2000;23(8):1130–6.
[192] Jones KL, Arslanian S, Peterokova VA, et al. Effect of metformin in pediatric patients with type 2 diabetes: a randomized controlled trial. Diabetes Care 2002;25(1):89–94.
[193] DeFronzo RA. Pharmacologic therapy for type 2 diabetes mellitus. Ann Intern Med 2000; 133(1):73–4.
[194] Hannon TS, Rao G, Arslanian SA. Childhood obesity and type 2 diabetes mellitus. Pediatrics 2005;116(2):473–80.
[195] Zimmerman BR. Sulfonylureas. Endocrinol Metab Clin North Am 1997;26(3):511–22.
[196] Schwartz S, Raskin P, Fonseca V, et al. Effect of troglitazone in insulin-treated patients with type II diabetes mellitus: Troglitazone and Exogenous Insulin Study Group. N Engl J Med 1998;338(13):861–6.
[197] Schoonjans K, Auwerx J. Thiazolidinediones: an update. Lancet 2000;355(9208):1008–10.
[198] Feinglos MN, Bethel MA. Oral agent therapy in the treatment of type 2 diabetes. Diabetes Care 1999;22(Suppl 3):C61–4.
[199] Khaw KT, Wareham N, Luben R, et al. Glycated haemoglobin, diabetes, and mortality in men in Norfolk cohort of European prospective investigation of cancer and nutrition (EPIC-Norfolk). BMJ 2001;322(7277):15–8.
[200] National High Blood Pressure Education Program Working Group on High Blood Pressure in Children and Adolescents. The fourth report on the diagnosis, evaluation, and treatment of high blood pressure in children and adolescents. Pediatrics 2004;114(2 Suppl):555–76.
[201] American Diabetes Association. Management of dyslipidemia in children and adolescents with diabetes. Diabetes Care 2003;26(7):2194–7.

ELSEVIER
SAUNDERS

Pediatr Clin N Am 52 (2005) 1611–1635

PEDIATRIC CLINICS

OF NORTH AMERICA

Pediatric Diabetic Ketoacidosis and Hyperglycemic Hyperosmolar State

Nicole Glaser, MD

Department of Pediatrics, University of California Davis, School of Medicine,
2516 Stockton Boulevard, Sacramento, CA 95817, USA

Diabetic ketoacidosis (DKA) is an important complication of childhood diabetes mellitus and the most frequent diabetes-related cause of death in children [1,2]. In various population-based studies, reported rates of DKA at presentation of type 1 diabetes have ranged from as low as 15% to as high as 83% [3–7], with most North American and European studies reporting rates of approximately 40%. Although DKA occurs less frequently in children with type 2 diabetes, case series have documented frequencies of DKA at diagnosis of type 2 diabetes in children ranging from 6% to 33% [8–11]. A diagnosis of type 2 diabetes cannot be excluded based on the occurrence of DKA.

Young children with new onset of type 1 diabetes are more likely to present with DKA [4,6,12], as are children who reside in countries with a low overall prevalence of type 1 diabetes [5]. The higher frequency of DKA at presentation in these groups likely reflects the greater difficulty in recognizing symptoms of diabetes in these populations. In a European study, an educational program directed at parents and primary care pediatricians was shown to decrease the frequency of DKA at diagnosis of type 1 diabetes from almost 80% to just 12.5%, which supported the concept that the frequency of DKA at presentation of diabetes is related to recognition of symptoms of diabetes in the population studied [7].

In children who have established diabetes, DKA may occur with episodes of infection or other illnesses or with insulin omission or malfunction of diabetes care equipment, such as insulin pumps. In children who have established diabetes, DKA occurs at a rate of approximately 1% to 8% per year [4,13–15]. DKA in patients who have established diabetes occurs more frequently in persons with

E-mail address: nsglaser@ucdavis.edu

doi:10.1016/j.pcl.2005.09.001   *pediatric.theclinics.com*

lower socioeconomic status, lack of adequate health insurance, higher HbA1c levels, and psychiatric disorders [13]. Insulin omission is the most frequent cause of DKA in children who have known diabetes. One study investigated the frequency of viral and bacterial infections in children who have DKA. Among all children who presented with DKA, bacterial infections were present in only 13% and viral infections in 18% [16]. In the subgroup of children who have known diabetes, bacterial infections were present in 17% and viral infections in 20%. These data contrast with data for adult populations, in which higher frequencies of infection or other illnesses as precipitating factors for DKA have been reported [17,18].

Although the risk of mortality from childhood DKA is less than 0.5%, DKA is still the most frequent diabetes-related cause of death in children [1,2]. Most of these DKA-related deaths are caused by cerebral edema (62%–87%), a complication that is discussed in more detail later.

Pathophysiology of diabetic ketoacidosis

The physiologic abnormalities in patients who have DKA may be viewed as an exaggeration of the normal physiologic mechanisms responsible for maintaining adequate fuel supply to the brain and other tissues during periods of fasting and physiologic stress. The relative concentration of insulin in relation to glucagon and other counterregulatory hormones or stress hormones (eg, epinephrine, norepinephrine, cortisol, and growth hormone) primarily mediates these physiologic abnormalities rather than the absolute concentration of insulin itself [19,20].

Pathophysiologic abnormalities early in the development of diabetic ketoacidosis

In a child who has new onset of type 1 diabetes, declining insulin production lowers the ratio of insulin to glucagon. This decrease in relative insulin concentration leads to excess hepatic glucose production (Fig. 1A). Early in the course of evolving DKA, when levels of epinephrine and other stress hormones are normal or minimally elevated, increased hepatic glucose output is mainly caused by stimulation of glycogenolysis, with a smaller contribution from increased gluconeogenesis [21–23]. Low serum insulin concentrations also contribute to hyperglycemia by decreasing peripheral glucose uptake in muscle and adipose tissue. This effect is mediated by diminished translocation of glucose transporter (GLUT)4 glucose transporters to the cell membrane [24,25]. Increased hepatic glucose output and decreased peripheral glucose use contribute to hyperglycemia [26]. When the serum glucose concentration rises above approximately 180 to 200 mg/dL, which exceeds the renal threshold for glucose reabsorption [27,28], osmotic diuresis results, with an increase in urine output. Fluid losses then stimulate compensatory oral intake of fluids, which leads to polydipsia.

Low insulin concentrations also stimulate the release of free fatty acids (FFA) from adipose tissue by allowing activation of hormone-sensitive lipase (Fig. 2). This increase in FFA delivery to the liver is necessary but not sufficient for the stimulation of ketone body formation [29]. For ketogenesis to occur, activation of the hepatic β-oxidative enzyme sequence is also necessary [20,30,31]. It is mainly a further decline in insulin concentration relative to glucagon that allows this activation to occur. A larger decline in insulin concentration relative to counter-regulatory hormones is necessary to promote lipolysis and ketogenesis, compared with that required to cause hyperglycemia [32]. These findings in part explain the lesser tendency toward the development of DKA in patients who have type 2 diabetes, despite the occurrence of substantial hyperglycemia.

Under fasting conditions in a normal individual, modest ketosis occurs, but marked ketoacidosis is prevented by direct ketone-induced stimulation of insulin, which limits further release of FFAs from adipose tissue [33]. In children who have type 1 diabetes, however, this "hormonal brake" is lacking and ketone production proceeds unchecked, eventually resulting in acidosis with an elevated anion gap.

Pathophysiologic abnormalities later in the development of diabetic ketoacidosis

Physiologic stress caused by acidosis and progressive dehydration eventually stimulates release of the counterregulatory hormones, cortisol, catecholamines, and growth hormone (see Fig. 1B) [26,34,35] Coexisting infection or other illness or injury likewise can accelerate the development of ketosis via further elevations in counterregulatory hormone concentrations. Elevated cortisol concentrations augment FFA release from adipose tissue to fuel ketogenesis and decrease peripheral glucose uptake via effects on insulin-dependent mechanisms of glucose uptake and insulin-independent mechanisms (Fig. 2) [36–38]. Increased epinephrine concentrations directly increase glycogenolysis and stimulate release of gluconeogenic precursors from muscle, which allows gluconeogensis to make a more substantial contribution to hyperglycemia [22,23,39]. Epinephrine and norepinephrine also stimulate lipolysis and β-oxidation of FFAs to form ketone bodies [40,41]. Catecholamines also may inhibit insulin secretion directly via stimulation of α-adrenergic receptors and cause a further decline in serum insulin concentrations [42,43]. Although this effect is inconsequential in children who have longstanding type 1 diabetes (and absent or minimal endogenous insulin production), it may accelerate the development of DKA in patients with a new diagnosis of type 1 diabetes in whom some insulin-producing capacity remains, and it likely contributes more substantially to the development of DKA in children who have type 2 diabetes. Elevated growth hormone concentrations likewise contribute to worsening hyperglycemia, mainly via further decreasing peripheral glucose uptake, and enhance ketone production by increasing FFA release [23,44]. Growth hormone effects occur over a longer time course than those of other counterregulatory hormones that lead to more acute elevations in glucose and FFAs.

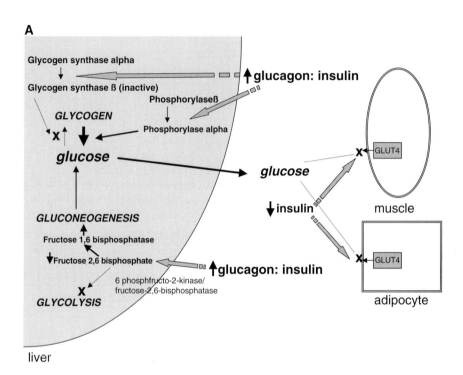

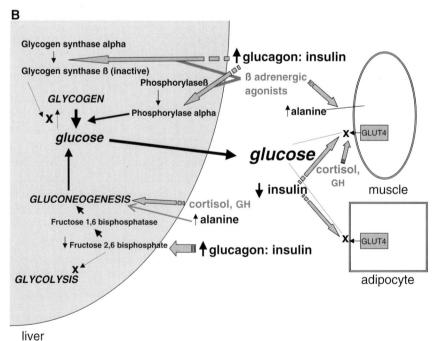

With the increase in hepatic glucose production, ketogenesis, and peripheral insulin resistance stimulated by elevations in counterregulatory hormone concentrations, acidosis and dehydration worsen. These changes then accelerate the development of DKA by stimulating further increases in the concentrations of counterregulatory hormones. A vicious cycle is created and is responsible for the eventual development of severe ketoacidosis.

Other physiologic processes also contribute to worsening acidosis and dehydration (Fig. 3). Intestinal ileus occurs as a consequence of acidosis, potassium depletion, and diminished splanchnic perfusion caused by dehydration. Intestinal ileus causes abdominal pain and vomiting, which impairs a patient's ability to compensate for osmotic diuresis by increased intake of fluids. More substantial dehydration eventually leads to diminished tissue perfusion, which enhances acidosis via accumulation of lactic acid [45,46]. Severe dehydration eventually compromises renal function and diminishes the capacity for clearance of glucose and ketones, which causes concentrations of both to rise further. Ongoing osmotic diuresis and ketonuria in the setting of acidosis also result in urinary losses of electrolytes, particularly potassium, sodium, chloride, calcium, phosphate, and magnesium. Urinary losses of sodium and potassium as ketone salts may result in excess chloride retention, such that hyperchloremic acidosis is superimposed on the increased anion gap acidosis [47]. Elevated aldosterone concentrations that result from dehydration also serve to further enhance potassium loss [46]. Typical electrolyte deficits in patients who have DKA include approximately 5 to 13 mmol/kg of sodium, 3 to 5 mmol/kg of potassium, and 0.5 to 1.5 mmol/kg of phosphate [48,49].

Clinical manifestations of diabetic ketoacidosis

Classic symptoms of DKA include polyuria, polydipsia, weight loss, abdominal pain, nausea, and vomiting. Abdominal tenderness, absence of bowel sounds, and guarding may be present and may mimic the acute abdomen [50].

Fig. 1. (*A*) Early in the development of DKA, a decrease in the concentration of insulin relative to glucagon results in stimulation of glycogenolysis by promoting conversion of glycogen synthase α to inactive glycogen synthase β and conversion of phosphorylase β to active phosphorylase α. Gluconeogenesis is also stimulated but plays a lesser role in the increase in hepatic glucose output at this stage than does glycogenolysis. An increase in the ratio of glucagon to insulin stimulates a decrease in fructose 2,6 bisphosphate concentrations mediated by phosphorylation of 6-phosphofructo-2-kinase/ fructose-2,6-bisphosphatase. The decreased concentration of fructose 2,6 bisphosphate inactivates the rate-limiting enzyme for glycolysis (6-phosphofructo-1-kinase) and stimulates gluconeogenesis via activation of fructose-2,6-bisphosphatase. Decreased insulin concentrations also result in a lower peripheral glucose uptake by muscle and adipose tissue with diminished transport of GLUT4 to the cell membrane. (*B*) Later in the development of DKA, elevated concentrations of other counterregulatory hormones (eg, cortisol, noripinephrine, epinephrine, growth hormone) further increase hepatic glucose output and decrease peripheral glucose uptake. β-Adrenergic agonists enhance glycogenolysis and promote release of gluconeogenic substrate from muscle. Elevated cortisol and growth hormone concentrations cause further declines in peripheral glucose uptake and augment gluconeogenesis.

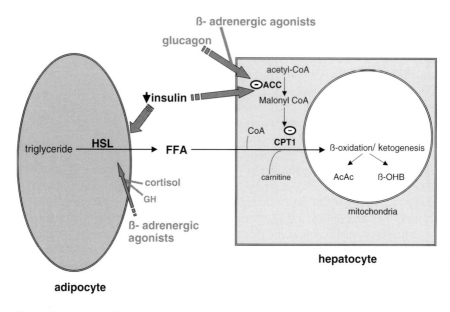

Fig. 2. Decreased insulin concentrations result in increased activity of hormone-sensitive lipase in adipose tissue with release of FFA. As concentrations of stress hormones (eg, cortisol, growth hormone (GH), catecholamines) increase later in the course of DKA, hormone-sensitive lipase activity is further stimulated. FFAs are taken up by the liver, where they are esterified to fatty acyl-CoA. Transport of the CoA ester across the mitochondrial membrane for β-oxidation requires transesterification with carnitine, which is accomplished by carnitine palmityl transferase 1 (CPT-1). Once inside the mitochondria, esterification to carnitine is reversed, and fatty acyl-CoA undergoes β-oxidation to form ketones (AcAc) and (β-OHB). CPT-1 is regulated by the concentration of malonyl CoA, which inhibits CPT-1 activity. Malonyl CoA is produced from acetyl-CoA by acetyl-CoA carboxylase (ACC), whose activity is increased by insulin and decreased by glucagon and β-adrenergic agents. Glucagon also decreases the concentration of malonyl CoA by diminishing the rate of glycolysis and the rate of production of citrate, the substrate for malonyl CoA production.

Tachycardia is frequent, and signs of hypoperfusion, such as delayed capillary refill time and cool extremities, are also common. Other signs of dehydration also may be present, including dry mucous membranes, absence of tears, and poor skin turgor. Hypothermia also has been described [51]. Although profound acidosis may depress myocardial contractility and vascular smooth muscle tone, the occurrence of these effects to a clinically relevant degree has not been demonstrated in DKA [52], and hypotension in children who have DKA is rare. Tachypnea occurs in response to metabolic acidosis as a result of stimulation of chemoreceptors in the central nervous system (CNS). Tachypnea may be extreme and may cause DKA to be initially misdiagnosed as respiratory illness. Acetone (produced from nonenzymatic decarboxylation of acetoacetate [AcAc]) typically causes a fruity breath odor, which may be a helpful initial clue to the diagnosis of DKA. Despite profound systemic acidosis, most children who have DKA present with normal mentation or only minimal depression of mental status. The lack of substantial neurologic depression reflects the fact that brain pH in patients who

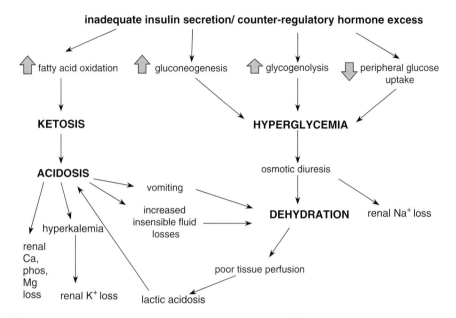

Fig. 3. Pathophysiology of diabetic ketoacidosis. (*From* Glaser NS, Styne DM. Endocrine disorders. In: Behrman R, Kliegman R, editors. Nelson essentials of pediatrics. 3rd edition. Philadelphia: WB Saunders; 1997; with permission.)

present with DKA is generally preserved within the normal range because of the impermeability of the blood-brain barrier to hydrogen ions [53,54].

Laboratory abnormalities in diabetic ketoacidosis

Hyperglycemia

A diagnosis of DKA can be made when the serum glucose concentration is more than 200 mg/dL and venous pH is less than 7.30 (or the serum bicarbonate concentration is less than 15 mmol/L) in the presence of elevated urine or serum ketone concentrations. DKA with near-normal glucose concentrations also has been described but occurs infrequently [55–57]. This euglycemic DKA may occur in pregnancy and in patients who have known diabetes who have administered insulin before coming to the emergency department. Children who have DKA who have prolonged vomiting and minimal oral intake before presentation also may present with lower initial glucose concentrations. Much of the variability in serum glucose concentrations at presentation may be explained by differences in hydration and nutritional status [35]. Prolonged fasting or poor nutrient intake before the development of DKA decreases substrate availability and results in lower serum glucose concentrations at presentation, whereas more severe dehydration favors higher glucose concentrations. In the absence of pre-existing renal disease or unusually high carbohydrate intake, blood glucose concentrations of 500 to 600 mg/dL imply that dehydration is of sufficient severity to diminish the glomerular filtration rate by approximately 30% to 40%. Blood glucose concentrations more than 800 mg/dL suggest that the glomerular filtration rate is decreased by 50% or more [58].

Acidosis

Concentrations of ketone bodies (beta-hydroxybutyrate [βOHB] and AcAc) are elevated in DKA. The serum bicarbonate concentration is low because bicarbonate is used as a buffer against metabolic acidosis, which results in increased anion gap acidosis. Some degree of hyperchloremic acidosis frequently coexists with increased anion gap acidosis in DKA [47], and the anion gap reflects the combination of these processes. Although concentrations of βOHB and AcAc are elevated in patients who have DKA, the ratio of βOHB:AcAc is increased during DKA as a result of changes in the redox potential (NADH/NAD$^+$ ratio) in hepatic mitochondria [59]. Although the ratio of βOHB:AcAc is typically 1:1 in a normal individual, this ratio rises to as high as 10:1 in persons who have DKA. These changes are important mainly because the nitroprusside reaction used to test urine ketone concentrations detects only AcAc and not βOHB. Although urine testing can be relied on to help diagnose DKA, the urine ketone concentration should not be relied on as an indication of DKA severity or treatment response, particularly because the ratio of βOHB:AcAc decreases during DKA treatment. Bedside blood ketone meters recently were developed and provide a rapid means for accurately measuring βOHB rather than AcAc in children who have DKA [60]. How these measurements might best be used to enhance diagnosis and treatment of DKA, however, remains to be determined.

Metabolic acidosis stimulates chemoreceptors in the CNS, which results in partial correction of the metabolic acidosis via hyperventilation and a decrease in the partial pressure of CO_2. There is a linear relationship between serum bicarbonate concentration and pCO_2, and this relationship suggests that end-tidal CO_2 measurements may be used as a rapid screen for acidosis in children who have suspected DKA or to follow the course of acidosis in children who have DKA (Fig. 4) [61].

Electrolyte abnormalities

Hyperglycemia results in fluid movement from the extravascular to the intravascular space and a decrease in the serum sodium concentration. This decrease can be calculated as a 1.6 mEq/L decrease in sodium concentration for every 100 mg/dL increase in serum glucose more than 100 mg/dL [62]. Hyperlipidemia caused by lipolysis also may affect serum sodium measurements and result in a decrease in measured serum sodium concentrations [63].

Typically, serum potassium concentrations at presentation are in the high-normal range or even above the normal range. Redistribution of potassium ions

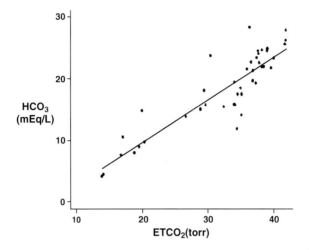

Fig. 4. End-tidal CO_2 levels versus serum bicarbonate concentrations in children with diabetic ketoacidosis. (*From* Fearon DM, Steele DW. End-tidal carbon dioxide predicts the presence and severity of acidosis in children with diabetes. Acad Emerg Med 2002;9:1373–8; with permission.)

from the intracellular to the extracellular space in DKA results from a combination of factors, including direct effects of low insulin concentrations, intracellular protein and phosphate depletion, and buffering of hydrogen ions in the intracellular fluid compartment [64]. Despite normal or elevated initial potassium concentrations, total body potassium concentrations are depleted, often profoundly, and serum potassium concentrations usually drop rapidly with insulin treatment. The initial serum potassium concentration should not be taken as an indication of total body potassium stores. Serum phosphate concentrations are similarly elevated or normal at presentation but tend to decrease during treatment.

Other biochemical abnormalities

White blood cell counts are frequently elevated in children who have DKA, and the differential may be left shifted. The precise mechanism responsible for leukocytosis in DKA is not fully understood, but elevated catecholamine concentrations may play a role [65,66]. Another contributing factor may be an elevation in proinflammatory cytokines (eg, tumor necrosis factor-α, interleukin-6, interleukin-8, interleukin-1β) and C-reactive protein caused by DKA. [67–69] Cytokine concentrations are substantially increased during DKA and decrease promptly with the initiation of insulin therapy. C-reactive protein concentrations, although also frequently elevated in patients who have DKA, show a less consistent decrease with treatment [68]. Infection is infrequently the cause of DKA in children [16], and an elevated or left-shifted white blood cell count need not prompt a search for an infectious process unless fever or other symptoms or signs of infection are present.

Serum amylase or lipase concentrations are elevated in 40% of children who have DKA and in 40% to 80% of adults who have DKA [70–72]. The cause and significance of these elevations, however, are not known. Clinical pancreatitis in children who have DKA is rare, and elevated amylase or lipase concentrations need not prompt further investigation for pancreatitis unless abdominal pain persists after resolution of ketosis.

Treatment of diabetic ketoacidosis

Fluids

Intravenous fluids (0.9% saline or other isotonic fluids) should be administered as soon as possible to restore adequate perfusion and hemodynamic stability. An intravenous fluid bolus of 10 to 20 mL/kg is often required. In patients who are well perfused and hemodynamically stable, an initial fluid bolus may not be necessary. A recent study indicated that physicians' clinical assessments of the degree of dehydration in children who have DKA correlate poorly with the actual percentage dehydration and often underestimate dehydration severity [73]. Difficulties in clinical estimation of dehydration may result in part from osmotically mediated water movement from the tissues to the intravascular space. This fluid movement results in preservation of intravascular volume and may obscure some of the clinical signs of dehydration. Because severity of dehydration is difficult to estimate clinically, it may be most appropriate to assume an average degree of dehydration for most patients (approximately 7%–9% of body weight [73,74]). This estimated fluid deficit, along with maintenance fluid requirements, should be replaced evenly over a 36- to 48-hour period using 0.45% to 0.9% saline. Because the serum glucose concentration typically decreases to levels near the renal threshold for glucose reabsorption within a few hours of initiating treatment, replacement of ongoing fluid losses from osmotic diuresis is usually unnecessary. Ongoing fluid losses caused by profuse vomiting or diarrhea may need to be replaced on rare occasion.

The serum glucose concentration often decreases substantially with rehydration alone as a result of improvements in the glomerular filtration rate and decreased concentrations of counterregulatory hormones [46,75]. This decline in glucose concentration early in treatment should not be interpreted as an indication of excessive insulin administration.

Insulin and dextrose

Insulin is required to resolve acidosis and hyperglycemia via suppression of ketogenesis, gluconeogenesis, and glycogenolysis and promotion of peripheral glucose uptake and metabolism. Insulin should be administered intravenously at a rate of 0.1 U/kg/h [75]. An initial bolus or loading dose of insulin is unnecessary because maximal reductions in ketogenesis and lipolysis are achieved rapidly with the insulin infusion rate specified previously [26,32]. More rapid declines in serum glucose concentration may be achieved with insulin administered at rates in excess of 0.1 U/kg/h, but these higher insulin dosages may increase the frequency of hypoglycemia during therapy [32,75]. The risk of hypokalemia also is greater at higher insulin infusion rates [32,75]. Thus, there seems to be no benefit to higher insulin dosages, and the potential for adverse effects may increase. The use of insulin dosages less than 0.1 U/kg/h have not been studied extensively, but available data suggest that these lower dosages may not suppress ketogenesis adequately [76].

With insulin treatment, serum glucose concentrations often normalize before ketosis and acidosis have resolved. When the serum glucose concentration declines to approximately 250 to 300 mg/dL, dextrose should be added to the intravenous fluids to avoid hypoglycemia as the insulin infusion is continued to promote resolution of ketosis and acidosis. The two-bag system is an effective and efficient method for administering dextrose in children who have DKA. This system allows a more rapid response to changes in serum glucose concentration and is more cost effective than single-bag methods [77]. Two bags of intravenous fluids with identical electrolyte content but varying dextrose concentrations (usually 0% and 10%) are administered simultaneously. The relative rates of administration of the two fluids can be adjusted to vary the dextrose concentration while maintaining a constant overall rate of administration of fluid and other electrolytes (Fig. 5). Once this system is established, the blood glucose concentration should be maintained between 150 and 250 mg/dL to strike a balance between avoidance of hypoglycemia during treatment and prevention of ongoing fluid losses from osmotic diuresis.

Electrolytes

With insulin treatment and resolution of acidosis, there is substantial movement of potassium from the extracellular space to the intracellular space, and serum potassium concentrations may decrease precipitously. Intravenous administration of potassium is essential, and concentrations of 30 to 40 mEq/L intravenous fluids are usually required. Adequate renal function should be ensured before administration of potassium. Potassium chloride may be used alone or in combination with potassium phosphate or potassium acetate. Use of combinations of potassium salts may help to diminish the risk of development of hyperchloremic acidosis by decreasing the chloride load.

Studies have demonstrated that some degree of hyperchloremic acidosis develops during treatment of DKA in most patients, and the severity of hyperchloremic acidosis correlates with serum urea nitrogen concentrations [47]. Patients who are less dehydrated and have better preservation of renal function have a greater tendency to develop hyperchloremic acidosis during treatment. This tendency is likely caused by the increased urinary loss of bicarbonate precursors (ketoacid and lactic acid anions) and diminished conversion of these precursors to bicarbonate with insulin administration [47,78].

Whether phosphate replacement should be given routinely in children who
have DKA is controversial. It is known that 2,3-diphosphoglycerate levels in red
blood cells are decreased in patients who have DKA, and hypophosphatemia may
result in persistence of low 2,3-diphosphoglycerate levels. This situation theoretically may lead to reduced tissue oxygen delivery, particularly during therapy
when correction of acidosis increases the affinity of hemoglobin for oxygen,

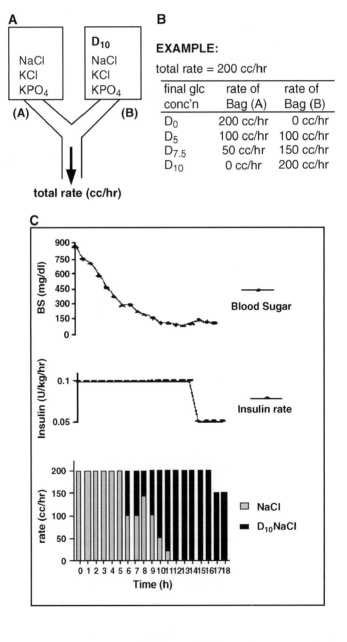

reversing the Bohr effect [79,80]. Occurrence of this effect to a degree that would be clinically relevant, however, has been difficult to demonstrate [80,81]. Conversely, although hypocalcemia can result from phosphate replacement, symptomatic hypocalcemia has been documented mainly with aggressive or rapid phosphate replacement and is uncommon when phosphate is administered slowly in more modest concentrations [81,82]. It is difficult to make a strong case either in favor of or against phosphate replacement. Case reports, however, have documented rhabdomyolysis and hemolytic anemia as results of severe hypophosphatemia during DKA [83,84]. Therefore, regardless of whether phosphate replacement is given routinely, it is necessary to monitor serum phosphate concentrations during treatment and administer phosphate replacement if severe hypophosphatemia develops.

Hypomagnesemia is common during DKA treatment and may contribute to hypocalcemia by inhibition of parathyroid hormone secretion [85,86]. Although monitoring of serum calcium and magnesium concentrations is recommended to detect rare cases of severe hypomagnesemia or hypocalcemia, decreases in the concentrations of these electrolytes are usually mild and asymptomatic and rarely require treatment.

Bicarbonate

Bicarbonate should not be administered routinely in children who have DKA because acidosis usually can be corrected with insulin and fluids alone, and hemodynamic instability that results from acidosis is rare [52]. Most studies have found minimal or no differences in the rapidity of correction of acidosis in patients who have DKA treated with or without bicarbonate [87–89]. One reason for the apparent lack of effect of bicarbonate on rapidity of resolution of acidosis is that bicarbonate administration may cause an increase in hepatic ketone production [90]. It is believed that this increase results from pH-dependent stimulation of ketogenesis via increased mitochondrial uptake of fatty acyl-CoA.

Bicarbonate administration also increases the likelihood of hypokalemia during DKA treatment [91] and theoretically may increase tissue hypoxia as a result of leftward shifts in the hemoglobin-oxygen dissociation curve [79]. Bicarbonate

Fig. 5. Two-bag system and illustrative typical course. (*A*) Two-bag system allows independent manipulation of glucose and total fluid volume, because electrolyte content of two bags is identical except for dextrose. (*B*) Differential rates of two bags modulate glucose delivery, which can be any concentration ranging from 0% to 10%. Total fluid volume is based on a patient's degree of dehydration and ongoing fluid requirement. (*C*) In this typical course, insulin therapy is instituted as continuous infusion of 0.1 U/kg/h, and total fluid rate is set at 200 mL/h. Because patient is markedly hyperglycemic, no dextrose is given initially. As insulin action lowers patient's glucose level, dextrose is titrated into intravenous fluid without changing administered fluid volume. Glucose titration aims to control rate of blood glucose decline (possible risk factor for cerebral edema) and prevent hypoglycemia in the face of continued insulin requirement. Later, when a patient's dehydration and ketosis become partially corrected, insulin and total fluid can be independently adjusted. (*From* Grimberg A, Cerri RW, Satin-Smith M, et al. The "two bag system" for variable intravenous dextrose and fluid administration: benefits in diabetic ketoacidosis management. J Pediatr 1999;134:377; with permission.)

treatment also may lead to paradoxic acidosis of the cerebrospinal fluid [53,92]. This phenomenon likely occurs because administration of bicarbonate results in diminished respiratory drive and a rise in the partial pressure of CO_2. Although the blood-brain barrier is impermeable to bicarbonate, CO_2 crosses the blood-brain barrier readily and generates carbonic acid and cerebrospinal fluid acidosis. Bicarbonate administration also has been associated with an increased risk of cerebral edema in childhood DKA [93]. Routine administration of bicarbonate is not recommended. In rare cases in which hemodynamic instability is believed to be caused by severe acidosis and does not respond to standard measures or in rare cases of symptomatic hyperkalemia, however, bicarbonate administration should be considered.

Monitoring

Specific recommendations for monitoring of children who have DKA are outlined in the report of the European Society for Pediatric Endocrinology/Lawson Wilkins Pediatric Endocrine Society international DKA consensus conference [94,95]. Most patients who have DKA should be treated in a pediatric intensive care unit or other unit with similar capacities for managing children who have DKA. Blood glucose concentrations should be measured hourly and electrolyte concentrations should be monitored every 2 to 4 hours. Venous pH measurements are helpful because serum bicarbonate concentrations may not increase over the first several hours despite improvements in acidosis. Arterial blood gas measurements, however, are generally unnecessary. Lack of appropriate improvement in acidosis with treatment suggests inadequate insulin infusion, inadequate rehydration, renal failure, sepsis, or other intercurrent condition.

Vital signs and mental status should be monitored hourly, and fluid intake and output should be recorded accurately. Cardiac monitoring is recommended because cardiac arrhythmias may occur during treatment, albeit infrequently. Recent data demonstrated a high frequency of prolonged QT interval corrected for heart rate (QTc) in children who have DKA (N. Kuppermann, MD, personal communication, 2005).

Complications

The most frequent complications of DKA treatment are hypoglycemia and hypokalemia. With adequate monitoring of serum glucose and potassium concentrations, however, these complications are usually detected at an early stage, are easily treated, and rarely result in permanent morbidity or mortality. More serious complications of DKA are rare but may be life threatening, including cerebral edema [93,96], pulmonary edema [97–99], CNS hemorrhage or thrombosis [100], other large vessel thromboses [101], cardiac arrhythmias caused by electrolyte disturbances [93,102,103], pancreatitis [104], renal failure [105], and intestinal necrosis [106–108]. Patients who have DKA are also uniquely susceptible to rhinocerebral and pulmonary mucormycosis, a rare fungal infection [109]. Acidosis interferes with an important host defense mechanism against this fungus by disrupting the capacity of transferrin to bind iron. Mucormycosis occurs most frequently in children with longstanding poor blood glucose control. This infection carries a poor prognosis with high mortality rates. Aggressive treatment with antifungal agents and early resection of involved tissue is recommended [110].

Although severe dehydration and electrolyte depletion likely cause some of the complications of DKA, the mechanisms responsible for several others are not well understood. Recent studies have suggested that β-OHB may cause pulmonary vascular endothelial dysfunction and that perfusion of rabbit lungs with either β-OHB or AcAc results in edema and hemorrhage [111]. DKA also may cause a prothrombotic state, which may predispose children to CNS and other thromboses [101,112]. Studies have reported increased levels of von Willibrand factor and decreased free protein S and protein C activity in DKA and enhanced platelet aggregation associated with hyperglycemia [112–114]. Case series have suggested that deep venous thromboses may develop in as many as 50% of children with femoral central venous catheters [101,115]. Central venous catheters, particularly femoral venous catheters, should therefore be used with caution in children who have DKA.

Cardiac arrhythmias occur infrequently during DKA treatment and generally have been attributed to electrolyte disturbances. Recent data, however, documented a consistent increase in the QT interval corrected for heart rate (QTc) in children during acute DKA, with 47% of children having a QTc above 450 msec, the threshold generally considered to indicate prolongation of QTc [96]. In the recent study, the increase in QTc did not correlate with electrolyte concentrations, and the frequency of abnormal electrolyte concentrations in the study group was low, which raised the possibility that ketosis per se might have an effect on the myocardium. QTc intervals normalized after treatment of DKA.

The most frequent serious complication of DKA is cerebral edema, which occurs in 0.3% to 1% of pediatric DKA episodes [93,96,116,117]. Symptoms and signs of cerebral edema include headache, altered mental status, recurrence of vomiting, hypertension, inappropriate slowing of the heart rate, and other signs of increased intracranial pressure. Recent studies have documented a 21% to 24% mortality rate for DKA-related cerebral edema and a 21% to 26% rate of permanent neurologic morbidity [93,96].

Although less than 1% of children who have DKA develop symptomatic cerebral edema, studies that used sequential CT scans or other imaging technologies in children who have DKA showed that mild, asymptomatic cerebral edema is likely present in most children who have DKA (Fig. 6) [118–120]. The pathophysiologic mechanisms that cause cerebral edema during DKA remain unclear and have been the source of much controversy. Many investigators have attributed cerebral edema to rapid changes in serum osmolality or overly vigorous fluid resuscitation during DKA treatment. This hypothesis, however, has not been supported by data from clinical studies. In studies that used appropriate multi-

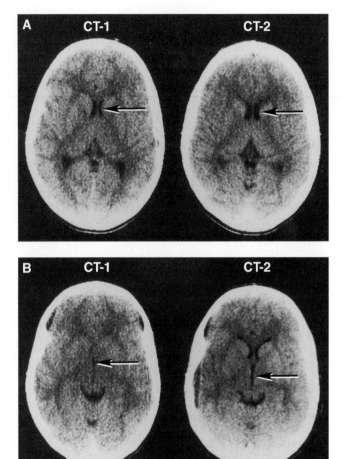

Fig. 6. CT scans of the same patient during DKA treatment (*A*) and after recovery from DKA (*B*). Narrowing of the ventricles during DKA indicates cerebral edema, although the patient was asymptomatic. (*From* Krane EJ, Rockoff MA, Wallman JK, et al. Subclinical brain swelling in children during treatment of diabetic ketoacidosis. N Engl J Med 1985;312:1147–51; with permission.)

variate statistical techniques to adjust for DKA severity, an association between the rate of change in serum glucose concentration or the volume or sodium content of fluid infusions and risk for cerebral edema was not demonstrated [93,121,122]. Several case reports also described symptomatic and even fatal cerebral edema that occurred before hospital treatment for DKA [1,123,124]. This information suggests that DKA-related cerebral edema likely cannot be explained simply by osmotically mediated fluid shifts. More recent data suggested that cerebral edema during DKA may be predominantly vasogenic and may result from activation of ion transporters in the blood-brain barrier [118,125]. Cerebral hypoperfusion during DKA or direct effects of ketosis or inflammatory cytokines on blood-brain barrier endothelial cell function might play a role in stimulating this process [69,118,126].

Epidemiologic studies have shown that children at greatest risk for symptomatic cerebral edema are children with high blood urea nitrogen concentrations [93] at presentation and children who present with more profound hypocapnia [93,122]. A lesser rise in the measured serum sodium concentration during treatment (as the serum glucose concentration falls) also indicates increased risk for cerebral edema [93,127]. More intensive monitoring of neurologic state and vital signs for children who present with these risk factors is recommended.

Clinical studies have not demonstrated a clear beneficial effect of any pharmacologic agent in treating DKA-related cerebral edema. Case reports, however, suggest that prompt administration of mannitol (0.25–1 g/kg) may be beneficial [128,129]. Intubation with associated hyperventilation has been correlated with poorer outcomes of DKA-related cerebral edema [130]. Therapeutic hyperventilation that attempts to decrease pCO_2 below a patient's own compensation for metabolic acidosis likely should be avoided in intubated children who have DKA except when absolutely necessary to treat clinically overt elevated intracranial pressure. CNS imaging in patients with suspected cerebral edema is recommended to rule out other causes of altered mental status, such as CNS thromboses; however, treatment for suspected cerebral edema should not be delayed while awaiting imaging studies.

Differential diagnosis

In children, findings of hyperglycemia, increased anion gap acidosis, and ketonuria or ketonemia generally indicate a diagnosis of DKA, and other disorders that result in this constellation of biochemical abnormalities are rare. Occasionally, however, other disorders may have a similar presentation. Rare metabolic defects may cause ketoacidosis, including succinyl-CoA: 3-ketoacid coenzyme A transferase deficiency, a defect in ketolysis, and beta-ketothiolase deficiency, a defect in L-isoleucine catabolism. These conditions, however, are most frequently associated with hypoglycemia or normoglycemia rather than hyperglycemia [30,131–133].

In the setting of gastroenteritis, hyperglycemia may occur when stress hormone concentrations are markedly elevated in response to dehydration. Lactic acidosis results from dehydration, and the combination of hyperglycemia with acidosis initially may suggest a diagnosis of DKA. FFA concentrations also may be elevated, and modest ketonemia occasionally occurs [134–138]. These findings have been documented most frequently in infants and toddlers. In rare cases, extreme elevations in serum glucose concentration (> 800–1000 mg/dL) have been reported in infants with gastroenteritis without diabetes mellitus [139]. Rapid resolution of hyperglycemia with hydration alone can be helpful in differentiating this situation from DKA [134].

Hyperglycemic hyperosmolar state without ketosis

Extreme hyperglycemia and hyperosmolality can occur without ketosis in patients who have diabetes (hyperglycemic hyperosmolar state [HHS]). This condition occurs much more frequently in adults than in children and more frequently in patients who have type 2 diabetes than in persons who have type 1 diabetes. Among pediatric patients, case series have suggested that obese African-American children who have type 2 diabetes may be at greatest risk for HHS [140,141]. HHS also has been documented to occur with increased frequency in patients who are predisposed to dehydration because of limited access to fluids, including infants and children with cognitive deficits [139, 142]. Although HHS has been viewed as a condition separate from DKA, it may be more appropriate to view HHS as one extreme in the various presentations of altered glucose and fat metabolism in patients who have diabetes. DKA with near-normal glucose concentrations (euglycemic DKA) may be viewed as the opposite extreme on this continuum. Where a particular patient falls in this spectrum is determined by the relative concentrations of insulin and counterregulatory hormones and by the states of hydration and nutrition of the patient. The clinical picture in many patients may have elements of DKA and HHS [143].

The pathogenesis of HHS is similar to that of DKA; however, some important differences should be noted. Hyperglycemia without ketosis generally occurs in patients who retain some ability to produce insulin, most commonly persons who have type 2 diabetes. Ketogenesis and lipolysis are suppressed at lower serum insulin concentrations than the levels required to suppress hepatic glucose production, and patients develop hyperglycemia without ketosis [32,144]. In patients who do not develop ketoacidosis, osmotic diuresis with electrolyte and water loss may persist for prolonged periods and result in profound dehydration. Without ketosis, urinary cation excretion is not necessary to balance ketoanion excretion, and less electrolyte loss relative to free water loss occurs in HHS than in DKA, which contributes to the hyperosmolar state. Nonetheless, because the duration of osmotic diuresis in HHS may be lengthy, patients who have HHS may have greater electrolyte deficits than patients who have DKA [145]. Diminished renal function that results from severe dehydration is particularly important in the pathogenesis of HHS because diminished capacity for glucose excretion is necessary for the development of marked hyperglycemia.

The criteria for diagnosis of HHS include blood glucose concentration more than 600 mg/dL, serum osmolality more than 330 mOsm/kg, and lack of significant ketosis [146]. The serum sodium concentration, when corrected for the blood glucose concentration, is generally above the normal range [146,147]. The clinical presentation of HHS is otherwise similar to that of DKA, with some exceptions. Children who have HHS often have a more prolonged history of polyuria and polydipsia than children who have DKA [140,142]. Because of the absence of ketosis, fruity breath odor is not present, and tachypnea is not a prominent feature, except in patients in whom substantial lactic acidosis occurs.

In adults, approximately 10% to 20% of patients who have HHS present in coma, and other mental status abnormalities at presentation are more frequent than in DKA. Seizures may occur, and focal neurologic deficits (eg, hemiparesis, hemianopsia, chorea-ballismus) also have been described with HHS [139,142, 146,148].

Because HHS occurs infrequently in children, data regarding the optimal approach to treatment are lacking. Some authors have suggested that it may be preferable to delay insulin therapy in patients who have HHS because the serum glucose concentration decreases considerably with rehydration alone [142]. Patients who have HHS are not ketotic, and insulin is not needed for resolution of acidosis [142]. Delaying insulin treatment in these patients may result in more gradual declines in serum glucose concentration and serum osmolality. Use of 0.9% saline for intravenous fluid replacement rather than hypotonic saline also has been recommended to promote a more gradual decline in serum sodium concentration. Because patients with HHS may have had ongoing osmotic diuresis for prolonged periods before presentation, electrolyte deficits may be particularly pronounced. Close monitoring of serum electrolyte concentrations (particularly potassium and phosphate) is recommended [146]. Hypernatremia frequently develops during therapy as the serum glucose concentration declines and water returns to the extravascular tissues. Hypernatremia occasionally may be difficult to treat in patients who have HHS, in part because of ongoing free water losses caused by osmotic diuresis and persistent stimulation of sodium retention by aldosterone [149].

In contrast to DKA, in which complications occur infrequently and the mortality rate is less than 1%, HHS is associated with more frequent complications and a high mortality rate. Although limited epidemiologic data are available on HHS in children, one report documented a mortality rate of 14% [150], similar to the approximately 15% to 20% mortality rate of HHS in adults [143]. Thromboembolic complications, including pulmonary emboli and deep venous thromboses, occur frequently in patients who have HHS as a result of severe dehydration and increased blood viscosity [151]. Routine use of anticoagulant therapy, however, is controversial. A malignant hyperthermia-like syndrome with hyperpyrexia and rhabdomyolysis also was described in several children who had HHS [141]. The cause of this syndrome is unclear. Cardiac arrhythmias caused by severe electrolyte disturbances, cerebral edema, and pulmonary edema also may occur [140,141].

Summary

DKA occurs frequently in children who have diabetes, particularly at the time of diagnosis. Greater efforts are necessary to promote earlier recognition of new onset of diabetes so that DKA can be prevented and to avoid subsequent occurrences of DKA in children who have established diabetes. Further research is also necessary to understand and prevent cerebral edema, the most serious complication of DKA. International recommendations for DKA treatment in children recently were published and will be helpful in standardizing the treatment of this condition [94,95].

References

[1] Edge J, Ford-Adams M, Dunger D. Causes of death in children with insulin-dependent diabetes 1990–96. Arch Dis Child 1999;81:318–23.

[2] Scibilia J, Finegold D, Dorman J, et al. Why do children with diabetes die? Acta Endocrinol Suppl (Copenh) 1986;279:326–33.

[3] Faich G, Fishbein H, Ellis E. The epidemiology of diabetic acidosis: a population-based study. Am J Epidemiol 1983;117:551–8.

[4] Pinkney J, Bingley P, Sawtell P. Presentation and progress of childhood diabetes mellitus: a prospective population-based study. Diabetologia 1994;37:70–4.

[5] Levy-Marchal C, Patterson C, Green A. Geographical variation of presentation at diagnosis of type 1 diabetes in children: the EURODIAB study. Diabetologia 2001;44(Suppl 3):B75–80.

[6] Mallare J, Cordice C, Ryan B, et al. Identifying risk factors for the development of diabetic ketoacidosis in new onset type 1 diabetes mellitus. Clin Pediatr 2003;42:591–7.

[7] Vanelli M, Chiari G, Ghizzoni L, et al. Effectiveness of a prevention program for diabetic ketoacidosis in children. Diabetes Care 1999;22:7–9.

[8] Hathout E, Thomas W, El-Shahawy M, et al. Diabetic autoimmune markers in children and adolescents with type 2 diabetes. Pediatrics 2001;107:e102.

[9] Glaser N, Jones K. Non-insulin dependent diabetes mellitus in Mexican-American children and adolescents. West J Med 1998;168:11–6.

[10] Grinstein G, Muzumdar R, Aponte L, et al. Presentation and 5-year follow-up of type 2 diabetes mellitus in African-American and Caribbean-Hispanic adolescents. Horm Res 2003;60:121–6.

[11] Zdravkovic V, Daneman D, Hamilton J. Presentation and course of type 2 diabetes in youth in a large multi-ethnic city. Diabet Med 2004;21:1144–8.

[12] Blanc N, Lucidarme N, Tubiana-Rufi N. Factors associated with childhood diabetes manifesting as ketoacidosis and its severity. Arch Pediatr 2003;10:320–5.

[13] Rewers A, Chase H, Mackenzie T, et al. Predictors of acute complications in children with type 1 diabetes. JAMA 2002;287:2511–8.

[14] Rosilio M, Cotton J, Wieliczko M, et al. Factors associated with glycemic control: a cross-sectional nationwide study in 2,579 French children with type 1 diabetes. The French Pediatric Diabetes Group. Diabetes Care 1998;21:1146–53.

[15] Norfeldt S, Ludvigsson J. Adverse events in intensively treated children and adolescents with type 1 diabetes. Acta Paediatr 1999;88:1184–93.

[16] Flood R, Chiang V. Rate and prediction of infection in children with diabetic ketoacidosis. Am J Emerg Med 2001;19:270–3.

[17] Umpierrez G, Murphy M, Kitabchi A. Diabetic ketoacidosis and hyperglycemic hyperosmolar syndrome. Diabetes Spectrum 2002;15:28–36.

[18] Azoulay E, Chevret S, Didier J, et al. Infection as a trigger of diabetic ketoacidosis in intensive care-unit patients. Clin Infect Dis 2001;32:30–5.

[19] Gerich J, Lorenzi M, Bier D, et al. Prevention of human diabetic ketoacidosis by somatostatin: evidence for an essential role of glucagon. N Engl J Med 1975;292:985–9.

[20] Schade D, Eaton R. Glucagon regulation of plasma ketone body concentration in human diabetes. J Clin Invest 1975;56:1340–4.

[21] Boden G, Cheung P, Homko C. Effects of acute insulin excess and deficiency on gluconeogenesis and glycogenolysis in type 1 diabetes. Diabetes 2003;52:133–7.

[22] Gustavson S, Chu C, Nishizawa M, et al. Interaction of glucagon and epinephrine in the control

of hepatic glucose production in the conscious dog. Am J Physiol Endocrinol Metab 2002; 284:E695–707.

[23] Gustavson S, Chu C, Nishizawa M, et al. Glucagon's actions are modified by the combination of epinephrine and gluconeogenic precursor infusion. Am J Physiol Endocrinol Metab 2003; 285:E534–44.

[24] Cheatham B, Volchuk A, Kahn R, et al. Insulin-stimulated translocation of GLUT4 glucose transporters requires SNARE-complex proteins. Proc Natl Acad Sci U S A 1996;93:15169–73.

[25] Minokoshi Y, Kahn R, Kahn B. Tissue-specific ablation of the GLUT4 glucose transporter or the insulin receptor challenges assumptions about insulin action and glucose homeostasis. J Biol Chem 2004;278:33609–12.

[26] Luzi L, Barrett E, Groop L, et al. Metabolic effects of low-dose insulin therapy on glucose metabolism in diabetic ketoacidosis. Diabetes 1988;37:1470–7.

[27] Menzel R, Kaisaki P, Rjasanowski I, et al. A low renal threshold for glucose in diabetic patients with a mutation in the hepatocyte nuclear factor-1alpha (HNF-1alpha) gene. Diabet Med 1998;15:816–20.

[28] Ruhnau G, Faber O, Borch-Johnsen K, et al. Renal threshold for glucose in non-insulin-dependent diabetic patients. Diabetes Res Clin Pract 1997;36:27–33.

[29] McGarry J, Foster D. Regulation of ketogenesis and clinical aspects of the ketotic state. Metabolism 1972;21:471–89.

[30] Fukao T, Lopaschuk G, Mitchell G. Pathways and control of ketone body metabolism: on the fringe of lipid biochemistry. Prostaglandins Leukot Essent Fatty Acids 2004;70:243–51.

[31] McGarry J, Wright P, Foster D. Rapid activation of hepatic ketogenic capacity in fed rats by anti-insulin serum and glucagon. J Clin Invest 1975;55:1202–9.

[32] Schade D, Eaton R. Dose response to insulin in man: differential effects on glycose and ketone body regulation. J Clin Endocrinol Metab 1977;44:1038–53.

[33] Madison L, Mebane D, Unger R, et al. The hypoglycemic action of ketones. II. Evidence for a stimulatory feedback of ketones on the pancreatic beta cells. J Clin Invest 1964;43: 408–15.

[34] Umpierrez G, DiGirolamo M, Tuvlin J, et al. Differences in metabolic and hormonal milieu in diabetic and alcohol-induced ketoacidosis. J Crit Care 2000;15:52–9.

[35] Burge M, Garcia N, Qualls CS. Differential effects of fasting and dehydration in the pathogenesis of diabetic ketoacidosis. Metabolism 2001;50:171–7.

[36] Djurhuus C, Gravholt C, Nielsen S, et al. Additive effects of cortisol and growth hormone on regional and systemic lipolysis in humans. Am J Physiol Endocrinol Metab 2003;286: E488–94.

[37] Nolte L, Rincon J, Wahlstrom E, et al. Hyperglycemia activates glucose transport in rat skeletal muscle via a $Ca(2+)$- dependent mechanism. Diabetes 1995;44:1345–8.

[38] Jonhston D, Gill A, Orskov H, et al. Metabolic effects of cortisol in man: studies with somatostatin. Metabolism 1982;31:312–7.

[39] Sacca L, Vigorito C, Cicala M, et al. Role of glyconeogenesis in epinephrine-stimulated hepatic glucose production in humans. Am J Physiol 1983;245:E294–302.

[40] Krentz A, Freedman D, Greene R, et al. Differential effects of physiological versus pathophysiological plasma concentrations of epinephrine and norepinephrine on ketone body metabolism and hepatic portal blood flow in man. Metabolism 1996;45:1214–20.

[41] Avogaro A, Valerio A, Gnudi L, et al. The effects of different plasma insulin concentrations on lipolytic and ketogenic responses to epinephrine in normal and type 1 (insulin-dependent) diabetic humans. Diabetologia 1992;35:129–38.

[42] Porte D. Sympathetic regulation of insulin secretion. Arch Intern Med 1969;123:252–60.

[43] Nonogaki K. New insights into sympathetic regulation of glucose and fat metabolism. Diabetologia 2000;43:533–49.

[44] Butler P, Kryshak E, Rizza R. Mechanism of growth hormone-induced postprandial carbohydrate intolerance in humans. Am J Physiol 1991;260:E513–20.

[45] Zimmet P, Taft P, Ennis G, et al. Acid production in diabetic acidosis: a more rational approach to alkali replacement. BMJ 1970;3:610–2.

[46] Waldhausl W, Kleinberger G, Korn A, et al. Severe hyperglycemia: effects of rehydration on endocrine derangements and blood glucose concentration. Diabetes 1979;28:577–84.

[47] Adrogue H, Wilson H, Boyd A, et al. Plasma acid-base patterns in diabetic ketoacidosis. N Engl J Med 1982;307:1603–10.

[48] Foster D, McGarry J. The metabolic derangements and treatment of diabetic ketoacidosis. N Engl J Med 1983;309:159–69.

[49] Kreisberg R. Diabetic ketoacidosis: new concepts and trends in pathogenesis and treatment. Ann Intern Med 1978;88:681–95.

[50] Valerio D. Acute diabetic abdomen in children. Lancet 1976;1(7950):66–8.

[51] Matz R. Hypothermia in diabetic acidosis. Hormones 1972;3:36–41.

[52] Maury E, Vassal T, Offenstadt G. Cardiac contractility during severe ketoacidosis. N Engl J Med 1999;341:1938.

[53] Assal J, Aoki T, Manzano F, et al. Metabolic effects of sodium bicarbonate in management of diabetic ketoacidosis. Diabetes 1973;23:405–11.

[54] Ohman J, Marliss E, Aoki T, et al. The cerebrospinal fluid in diabetic ketoacidosis. N Engl J Med 1971;284:283–90.

[55] Cullen M, Reece E, Homko C, et al. The changing presentations of diabetic ketoacidosis during pregnancy. Am J Perinatol 1996;13:449–51.

[56] Jenkins D, Close C, Krentz A, et al. Euglycemic diabetic ketoacidosis: does it exist? Acta Diabetol 1993;30:251–3.

[57] Burge M, Hardy K, Schade D. Short term fasting is a mechanism for the development of euglycemic ketoacidosis during periods of insulin deficiency. J Clin Endocrinol Metab 1993;76:1192–8.

[58] Halperin M, Goldstein M, Richardson R, et al. Quantitative aspects of hyperglycemia in the diabetic: a theoretical approach. Clin Invest Med 1980;2(4):127–30.

[59] Laffel L. Ketone bodies: a review of physiology, pathophysiology and application of monitoring to diabetes. Diabetes Metab Res Rev 1999;15:412–26.

[60] Ham M, Okada P, White P. Bedside ketone determination in diabetic children with hyperglycemia and ketosis in the acute care setting. Pediatr Diabetes 2004;5:39–43.

[61] Fearon D, Steele D. End-tidal carbons dioxide predicts the presence and severity of acidosis in children with diabetes. Acad Emerg Med 2002;9:1373–8.

[62] Katz M. Hyperglycemia-induced hyponatremia: calculation of expected serum sodium depression. N Engl J Med 1973;289:843–4.

[63] Kaminska E, Pourmotabbed G. Spurious laboratory values in diabetic ketoacidosis and hyperlipidemia. Am J Emerg Med 1993;11:77–80.

[64] Halperin M, Bear R, Goldstein M, et al. Interpretation of the serum potassium concentration in metabolic acidosis. Clin Invest Med 1979;2(1):55–7.

[65] Yu D, Clements P. Human lymphocyte subpopulations effect of epinephrine. Clin Exp Immunol 1976;25:472–9.

[66] Bessey P, Watters J, Aoki T, et al. Combined hormonal infusion simulates the metabolic response to injury. Ann Surg 1984;200:264–81.

[67] Stentz F, Umpierrez G, Cuervo R, et al. Proinflammatory cytokines, markers of cardiovascular risk, oxidative stress, and lipid peroxidation in patients with hyperglycemic crises. Diabetes 2004;53:2079–86.

[68] Dalton R, Hoffman W, Passmore G, et al. Plasma C-reactive protein levels in severe diabetic ketoacidosis. Ann Clin Lab Sci 2003;33:435–42.

[69] Hoffman W, Burek C, Waller J, et al. Cytokine response to diabetic ketoacidosis and its treatment. Clin Immunol 2003;108:175–81.

[70] Kaergaard J, Salling N, Magid E, et al. Serum amylase during recovery from diabetic ketoacidosis. Diabetes Metab 1984;10:25–30.

[71] Moller-Petersen J, Andersen P, Hjorne N, et al. Hyperamylasemia, specific pancreatic enzymes and hypoxanthine during recovery from diabetic ketoacidosis. Clin Chem 1985;31:2001–4.

[72] Haddad N, Croffie J, Eugster E. Pancreatic enzyme elevations in children with diabetic ketoacidosis. J Pediatr 2004;145:122–4.

[73] Koves I, Neutze J, Donath S, et al. The accuracy of clinical assessment of dehydration during diabetic ketoacidosis in childhood. Diabetes Care 2004;27:2485–7.

[74] Smith L, Rotta A. Accuracy of clinical estimates of dehydration in pediatric patients with diabetic ketoacidosis. Pediatr Emerg Care 2002;18:395–6.

[75] Burghen G, Etteldorf J, Fisher J, et al. Comparison of high-dose and low-dose insulin by continuous intravenous infusion in the treatment of diabetic ketoacidosis in children. Diabetes Care 1980;3:15–20.

[76] Miles J, Gerich J. Glucose and ketone body kinetics in diabetic ketoacidosis. Clin Endocrinol Metab 1983;12:303–19.

[77] Grimberg A, Cerri R, Satin-Smith M, et al. The "two bag system" for variable intravenous dextrose and fluid administration: benefits in diabetic ketoacidosis management. J Pediatr 1999;134:376–8.

[78] Oh M, Banerji M, Carroll H. The mechanism of hypercholoremic acidosis during the recovery phase of diabetic ketoacidosis. Diabetes 1981;30:310–3.

[79] Alberti G, Darley J, Emerson P, et al. 2,3-Diphosphoglycerate and tissue oxygenation in uncontrolled diabetes mellitus. Lancet 1972;2(7774):391–5.

[80] Fisher J, Kitabchi A. A randomized study of phosphate therapy in the treatment of diabetic ketoacidosis. J Clin Endocrinol Metab 1983;57:177–80.

[81] Gibby O, Veale K, Hayes T, et al. Oxygen availability from the blood and the effect of phosphate replacement on erythrocyte 2,3-diposphoglycerate and haemoglobin-oxygen affinity in diabetic ketoacidosis. Diabetologia 1978;15:381–5.

[82] Becker D, Brown D, Steranka B, et al. Phosphate replacement during treatment of diabetic ketoacidosis. Am J Dis Child 1983;137:241–6.

[83] Lord G, Scott J, Pusey C, et al. Diabetes and rhabdomyolysis: a rare complication of a common disease. BMJ 1993;307:1126–8.

[84] Shilo S, Werner D, Hershko C. Acute hemolytic anemia caused by severe hypophosphatemia in diabetic ketoacidosis. Acta Haematol 1985;73:55–7.

[85] Zipf W, Bacon G, Spencer M, et al. Hypocalcemia, hypomagnesemia, and transient hypo-parathyroidism during therapy with potassium phosphate in diabetic ketoacidosis. Diabetes Care 1979;2:265–8.

[86] Ionescu-Tirgoviste C, Bruckner I, Mihalache N, et al. Plasma phosphorus and magnesium values during treatment of severe diabetic ketoacidosis. Med Intern 1981;19:63–8.

[87] Green S, Rothrock S, Ho J, et al. Failure of adjunctive bicarbonate to improve outcome in severe pediatric diabetic ketoacidosis. Ann Emerg Med 1998;31:41–8.

[88] Lever E, Jaspan J. Sodium bicarbonate therapy in severe diabetic ketoacidosis. Am J Med 1983;75:263–8.

[89] Morris L, Murphy M, Kitabchi A. Bicarbonate therapy in severe diabetic ketoacidosis. Ann Intern Med 1986;105:836–40.

[90] Okuda Y, Adrogue H, Field J, et al. Counterproductive effects of sodium bicarbonate in diabetic ketoacidosis. J Clin Endocrinol Metab 1996;81:314–20.

[91] Soler N, Bennet M, Dixon K, et al. Potassium balance during treatment of diabetic ketoacidosis with special reference to the use of bicarbonate. Lancet 1972;30:665–7.

[92] Bureau M, Begin R, Berthiaume Y, et al. Cerebral hypoxia from bicarbonate infusion in diabetic acidosis. J Pediatr 1980;96:968–73.

[93] Glaser N, Barnett P, McCaslin I, et al. Risk factors for cerebral edema in children with diabetic ketoacidosis. N Engl J Med 2001;344:264–9.

[94] Sperling M, Dunger D, Acerini C, et al. ESPE / LWPES consensus statement on diabetic ketoacidosis in children and adolescents. Pediatrics 2003;113:e133–40.

[95] Dunger D, Sperling M, Acerini C, et al. ESPE / LWPES consensus statement on diabetic ketoacidosis in children and adolescents. Arch Dis Child 2003;89:188–94.

[96] Edge J, Hawkins M, Winter D, et al. The risk and outcome of cerebral oedema developing during diabetic ketoacidosis. Arch Dis Child 2001;85:16–22.

[97] Young M. Simultaneous acute cerebral and pulmonary edema complicating diabetic keto-acidosis. Diabetes Care 1995;18:1288–90.

[98] Hoffman W, Locksmith J, Burton E, et al. Interstitial pulmonary edema in children and adolescents with diabetic ketoacidosis. J Diabetes Complications 1998;12:314–20.

[99] Breidbart S, Singer L, St. Louis Y, et al. Adult respiratory distress syndrome in an adolescent with diabetic ketoacidosis. J Pediatr 1987;111:736–7.

[100] Rosenbloom A. Intracerebral crises during treatment of diabetic ketoacidosis. Diabetes Care 1990;13:22–33.

[101] Gutierrez J, Bagatell R, Sampson M, et al. Femoral central venous catheter-associated deep venous thrombosis in children with diabetic ketoacidosis. Crit Care Med 2003;31:80–3.

[102] Malone J, Brodsky S. The value of electrocardiogram monitoring in diabetic ketoacidosis. Diabetes Care 1980;3:543–7.

[103] Tanel R. ECGs in the ED. Pediatr Emerg Care 2004;20:849–51.

[104] Slyper A, Wyatt D, Brown C. Clinical and/or biochemical pancreatitis in diabetic ketoacidosis. J Pediatr Endocrinol 1994;7:261–4.

[105] Murdoch I, Pryor D, Haycock G, et al. Acute renal failure complicating diabetic ketoacidosis. Acta Paediatr 1993;82:498–500.

[106] Todani T, Sato Y, Watanabe Y, et al. Ischemic jejunal stricture developing after diabetic coma in a girl: a case report. Eur J Pediatr Surg 1993;3(2):115–7.

[107] Chan-Cua S, Jones K, Lynch F, et al. Necrosis of the ileum in a diabetic adolescent. J Pediatr Surg 1992;27:1236–8.

[108] Dimeglio L, Chaet M, Quigley C, et al. Massive ischemic intestinal necrosis at the onset of diabetes mellitus with ketoacidosis in a three-year old girl. J Pediatr Surg 2003;38:1537–9.

[109] Khanna S, Soumekh B, Bradley J, et al. A case of fatal rhinocerebral mucormycosis with new onset diabetic ketoacidosis. J Diabetes Complications 1998;12:224–7.

[110] Dokmetas H, Canbay E, Yilmaz S, et al. Diabetic ketoacidosis and rhino-orbital mucormycosis. Diabetes Res Clin Pract 2002;57:139–42.

[111] McCloud L, Parkerson J, Freant L, et al. Beta-hydroxybutyrate induces pulmonary endothelial dysfunction in rabbits. Exp Lung Res 2004;30:193–206.

[112] Carl G, Hoffman W, Passmore G, et al. Diabetic ketoacidosis promotes a prothrombotic state. Endocr Res 2003;29:73–82.

[113] Mustard J, Packham M. Platelets and diabetes mellitus. N Engl J Med 1984;311:665–7.

[114] Timperley W, Preston F, Ward J. Cerebral intravascular coagulation in diabetic ketoacidosis. Lancet 1974;18:952–6.

[115] Worly J, Fortenberry J, Hansen I, et al. Deep venous thrombosis in children with diabetic ketoacidosis and femoral central venous catheters. Pediatrics 2004;113:e57–60.

[116] Bello F, Sotos J. Cerebral oedema in diabetic ketoacidosis in children. Lancet 1990; 336(8706):64.

[117] Cummings E, Lawrence S, Daneman D. Cerebral edema (CE) in pediatric diabetic ketoacidosis (DKA) in Canada. Diabetes 2003;52:A400.

[118] Glaser N, Gorges S, Marcin J, et al. Mechanism of cerebral edema in children with diabetic ketoacidosis. J Pediatr 2004;145:164–71.

[119] Hoffman W, Steinhart C, El Gammal T, et al. Cranial CT in children and adolescents with diabetic ketoacidosis. AJNR Am J Neuroradiol 1988;9:733–9.

[120] Krane E, Rockoff M, Wallman J, et al. Subclinical brain swelling in children during treatment of diabetic ketoacidosis. N Engl J Med 1985;312:1147–51.

[121] Hale P, Rezvani I, Braunstein A, et al. Factors predicting cerebral edema in young children with diabetic ketoacidosis and new onset type I diabetes. Acta Paediatr 1997;86:626–31.

[122] Mahoney C, Vlcek B, Del Aguila M. Risk factors for developing brain herniation during diabetic ketoacidosis. Pediatr Neurol 1999;21:721–7.

[123] Glasgow A. Devastating cerebral edema in diabetic ketoacidosis before therapy. Diabetes Care 1991;14(1):77–8.

[124] Couch R, Acott P, Wong G. Early onset of fatal cerebral edema in diabetic ketoacidosis. Diabetes Care 1991;14:78–9.

[125] Lam T, Anderson S, Glaser N, et al. Bumetanide reduces cerebral edema formation in rats with diabetic ketoacidosis. Diabetes 2005;54:510–6.

[126] Isales C, Min L, Hoffman W. Acetoacetate and B-hydroxybutyrate differentially regulate endothelin-1 and vascular endothelial growth factor in mouse brain microvascular endothelial cells. J Diabetes Complications 1999;13(2):91–7.

[127] Harris G, Fiordalisi I, Harris W, et al. Minimizing the risk of brain herniation during treatment of diabetic ketoacidemia: a retrospective and prospective study. J Pediatr 1990;117:22–31.

[128] Roberts M, Slover R, Chase H. Diabetic ketoacidosis with intracerebral complications. Pediatr Diabetes 2001;2:103–14.

[129] Franklin B, Liu J, Ginsberg-Fellner F. Cerebral edema and ophthalmoplegia reversed by mannitol in a new case of insulin-dependent diabetes mellitus. Pediatrics 1982;69:87–90.

[130] Marcin J, Glaser N, Barnett P, et al. Clinical and therapeutic factors associated with adverse outcomes in children with DKA-related cerebral edema. J Pediatr 2003;141:793–7.

[131] Gibson K, Feigenbaum A. Phenotypically mild presentation in a patient with 2-methylacetoacetyl-coenzyme A (beta-keto) thiolase deficiency. J Inherit Metab Dis 1997;20:712–3.

[132] Longo N, Fukao T, Singh R, et al. Succinyl-CoA:3-ketoacid transferase (SCOT) deficiency in a new patient homozygous for an R217X mutation. J Inherit Metab Dis 2004;27:691–2.

[133] Fukao T, Scriver C, Kondo N. The clinical phenotype and outcome of mitochondrial acetoacetyl-CoA thiolase deficiency (beta-ketothiolase or T2 deficiency) in 26 enzymatically proved and mutation-defined patients. Mol Genet Metab 2001;72:109–14.

[134] Boulware S, Tamborlane W. Not all severe hyperglycemia is diabetes. Pediatrics 1992;89:330–2.

[135] Stevenson R, Bowyer F. Hyperglycemia with hyperosmolal dehydration in nondiabetic infants. J Pediatr 1970;77:818–23.

[136] Mandell F, Fellers F. Hyperglycemia in hypernatremic dehydration. Clin Pediatr 1974;13:367–9.

[137] Perkins K. Hyperglycemia without ketosis or hypernatremia. Am J Dis Child 1974;128:885.

[138] Rabinowitz L, Joffe B, Abkiewicz C, et al. Hyperglycemia in infantile gastroenteritis. Arch Dis Child 1984;59:771–5.

[139] Rother K, Schwenk W. An unusual case of the nonketotic hyperglycemic syndrome during childhood. Mayo Clin Proc 1995;70:62–5.

[140] Morales A, Rosenbloom A. Death caused by hyperglycemic hyperosmolar state at the onset of type 2 diabetes. J Pediatr 2004;144:270–3.

[141] Hollander A, Olney R, Blackett P, et al. Fatal malignant hyperthermia-like syndrome with rhabdomyolysis complicating the presentation of diabetes mellitus in adolescent males. Pediatrics 2003;111:1447–52.

[142] Gottschalk M, Ros S, Zeller W. The emergency management of hyperglycemic-hyperosmolar nonketotic coma in the pediatric patient. Pediatr Emerg Care 1996;12:48–51.

[143] MacIsaac R, Lee L, McNeil K, et al. Influence of age on the presentation and outcome of acidotic and hyperosmolar diabetic emergencies. Int Med J 2002;32:379–85.

[144] Chupin M, Charbonnel B, Chupin F. C-peptide levels in keto-acidosis and in hyperosmolar non-ketotic diabetic coma. Acta Diabetol 1981;18:123–8.

[145] Wachtel T, Silliman R, Lamberton P. Predisposing factors of the diabetic hyperosmolar state. Arch Intern Med 1987;147:499–501.

[146] Kitabchi A, Umpierrez G, Murphy M, et al. Management of hyperglycemic crises in patients with diabetes. Diabetes Care 2001;24:131–53.

[147] Gerich J, Martin M, Recant L. Clinical and metabolic characteristics of hyperosmolar non-ketotic coma. Diabetes 1971;20:228–38.

[148] Lai P, Tien R, Chang M, et al. Chorea-ballismus with nonketotic hyperglycemia in primary diabetes mellitus. AJNR Am J Neuroradiol 1996;17:1957–64.

[149] Tanaka S, Kobayashi T, Kawanami D, et al. Paradoxical glucose infusion for hypernatremia in diabetic hyperglycaemic hyperosmolar syndrome. J Int Med 2000;248:166–7.

[150] Fourtner SH, Weinzimer SA, Levitt-Katz LE. Hyperglycemic hyperosmolar nonketotic syndrome in children with type 2 diabetes. Pediatr Diabetes 2005;6:129–35.

[151] Kian K, Eiger G. Anticoagulant therapy in hyperosmolar non-ketotic diabetic coma. Diabetes Med 2003;20:603.

ELSEVIER
SAUNDERS

PEDIATRIC CLINICS
OF NORTH AMERICA

Pediatr Clin N Am 52 (2005) 1637–1650

Monogenic and Other Unusual Causes of Diabetes Mellitus

Meranda Nakhla, MD, Constantin Polychronakos, MD*

Department of Pediatrics, Division of Pediatric Endocrinology, McGill University Health Center, Montreal Children's Hospital, 2300 Tupper, Suite C-244, Montréal, Québec H3H 1P3, Canada

The latest version of the American Diabetes Association practice guidelines [1] distinguishes no fewer than 59 causes of diabetes mellitus. This array of etiologies can be dazzling even to the specialist but can be made manageable by putting it in statistical perspective and reducing it to the two basic physiologic disruptions responsible for hyperglycemia: insulin deficiency and insulin resistance. First, it is important to know that most (more than 95%) patients can be classified into either type 1 or type 2 diabetes. Second, the clinical management of the rare patient with unusual forms of diabetes does not require a profound understanding of the underlying disorder, just the ability to estimate the relative contributions of insulin resistance versus deficiency. A specific diagnosis is helpful in this regard. This is facilitated by the fact that many of these rare etiologies of diabetes are associated with specific (and often pre-existing) clinical syndromes or characteristic age of onset (ie, neonatal diabetes). In addition, molecular diagnosis is becoming available for an increasing number of these disorders. This article aims to help the practicing pediatrician make such a specific diagnosis and understand its implication in clinical case management.

Maturity-onset diabetes of the young

Maturity-onset diabetes of the young (MODY) is a clinically and genetically heterogeneous group of disorders with autosomal-dominant inheritance [2]. It

---

Dr. Nakhla is the recipient of an Eli Lilly pediatric endocrine fellowship. Dr. Polychronakos' research is supported by the Juvenile Diabetes Foundation, Genome Canada, and Genome Québec.

* Corresponding author.

E-mail address: constantin.polychronakos@mcgill.ca (C. Polychronakos).

pediatric.theclinics.com

accounts for 1% to 5% of all cases of diabetes in the United States and other industrialized countries [3]. MODY is characterized by a nonketotic hyperglycemia, pancreatic β-cell dysfunction, and onset of disease before the age of 25 years [3]. Patients with MODY are similar to patients with type 2 diabetes mellitus in that they have a relatively mild hyperglycemia and usually do not require insulin treatment. In contrast to patients with type 2 diabetes mellitus, however, MODY patients are not obese or insulin resistant, because the primary defect in MODY is that of β-cell dysfunction. When they do require insulin, patients need very small doses (approximately 0.5 U/kg/d) to achieve good glycemic control, indicating incomplete insulin deficiency. MODY should be considered in patients who are not obese and with a two- to three-generation family history of diabetes. MODY can result from mutations in any one of six different genes including the gene encoding the glycolytic enzyme glucokinase (MODY2) and five other genes encoding transcription factors important in β-cell development or function (Table 1).

Physiology of the β-cell and the role of maturity-onset diabetes of the young genes

The dominant inheritance of the loss-of-function mutations that cause MODY suggests that the disease is caused by haploinsufficiency (phenotype resulting from half the normal dose) of the gene involved. This may be any of a number of genes that regulate β-cell development, function, or both.

Table 1
Summary of MODY types and special clinical characteristics

	Gene mutated	Function	Special features	Reference
MODY1	HNF4α	Transcription factor	Decreased levels of triglycerides, apolipoproteins apoAII and apoCIII	[3]
MODY2	Glucokinase (GCK)	Enzyme, glucose sensor	Hyperglycemia early onset but mild and nonprogressive	[4,5]
MODY3	HNF-1α	Transcription factor	Decreased renal absorption of glucose and consequent glycosuria	[3,6,7]
MODY4	IPF-1	Necessary for pancreatic development		[8]
MODY5	HNF-1β	Transcription factor	Nonhyperglycemic renal disease; associated with uterine abnormalities, hypospadias, joint laxity, and learning difficulties	[9–11]
MODY6	NEUROD1	Differentiation factor in the development of pancreatic islets		[12–14]

Abbreviation: MODY, maturity-onset diabetes of the young.

Glucose is transported into the β-cell by a glucose-transporter protein, GLUT-2, which is present in excess and is not a limiting factor (Fig. 1). Once in the cell, glucose is phosphorylated to glucose-6-phosphate, a step catalyzed by gluco-kinase, the gene mutated in MODY2. This step is considered the rate-limiting step in glucose metabolism [2] and results in an increase in the ATP/ADP ratio that closes K^+ channels, resulting in insulin release. A decrease of glucokinase activity to half normal means that a higher glucose level is required to cause these changes, hence the reduced sensitivity of the β-cells to glucose [4]. Furthermore, because glucokinase is also responsible for glucose phosphorylation in hepa-tocytes, its mutation results in a defect in postprandial glycogen synthesis in the liver [5].

The pathophysiology of other forms of MODY is less well understood at the molecular level. Hepatocyte nuclear factors (three of which are MODY genes [see [Table 1]) play a role in the development of the β-cell, regulating both proliferation and metabolism [2]. Insulin promoter factor-1, the gene mutated in MODY4, is a pancreatic transcription factor that regulates early development of both endocrine and exocrine pancreas but persists in the mature β-cell, where it is necessary for the transcription of insulin [6]. Homozygosity for insulin promoter factor-1 mutation in an offspring of consanguineous heterozygous par-ents with MODY4 resulted in pancreatic agenesis that required pancreatic enzyme replacement in addition to insulin [7]. Finally *NEUROD1*, the gene mutated in MODY6, encodes a transcription factor that, in addition to playing a role in neuron development, also regulates insulin gene expression by binding to a critical E-box motif on the insulin promoter [8].

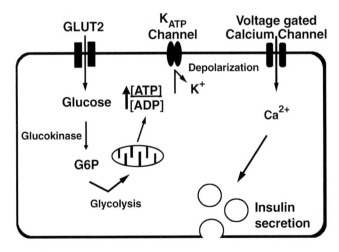

Fig. 1. Glucose enters the β-cell by the glucose transporter protein, Glut-2. Once within the cell, glucose is phosphorylated to glucose-6-phosphate, a rate-limiting step that is catalyzed by the enzyme glucokinase. This results in an increase in the ATP/ADP ratio with resultant closure of the ATP-dependent potassium channel and depolarization of the β-cell. Depolarization results in opening of the voltage-dependent calcium channel and influx of calcium leading to fusion of insulin-secretory granules with the cell membrane and release of insulin. (Courtesy of Z. Punthakee, Montréal, Québec.)

Clinical manifestations and diagnosis

The basic pathophysiology in all forms of MODY is mild, partial, but in most cases progressive, β-cell failure in the face of normal insulin sensitivity. Patients can be mildly hyperglycemic for many years before diagnosis. Although the age of onset and rate of progression can vary among the different types of MODY, the clinical management of the hyperglycemia depends on the metabolic status of the patient, not on the specific molecular diagnosis. Specific diagnosis is helpful in anticipating nonmetabolic features of the particular syndrome, most notably progressive renal disease in MODY5 patients, unrelated to diabetic nephropathy. It consists of renal cysts, oligomeganephronia, and hypoplastic glomerulocystic kidneys that cause renal impairment and end-stage renal failure in 50% of cases by age 45 [9–11].

Specific diagnosis is also helpful in distinguishing between MODY and type 2 or, less commonly but even more significantly, type 1 diabetes. It is neither necessary nor logistically feasible to screen all patients with diabetes for all MODY genes. Common sense dictates, however, to test genetically any nonobese individual with impaired carbohydrate tolerance or overt diabetes, regardless of age of diagnosis, who has either a close relative known to have MODY of any type or who has a parent or offspring with diabetes. To this one should, perhaps, add testing for MODY5 in the presence of dominant coinheritance of diabetes with nondiabetic renal disease. The presence of obesity or insulin resistance, both common phenotypes, does not protect against MODY, so in the presence of a family history strongly suggesting dominant inheritance, insulin-resistant individuals also should be tested.

Molecular diagnosis

Molecular diagnosis based on DNA obtained from a few milliliters of blood is offered by many laboratories, but logistical and financial considerations must be kept in mind. Unless the mutation is already known from the study of an affected family member, an exhaustive search for mutations in six different genes is a time-consuming and expensive proposition, difficult to apply to all patients who meet the criteria. Prior probability may be used to rationalize the use of resources, keeping in mind that some of these forms of MODY are extremely rare. MODY4, for example, has been described in a single family [7]. For diabetes diagnosed in the pediatric age group, most cases are diagnosed with a mutation search in glucokinase and HNF1-α (MODY2 and MODY3, respectively).

Treatment

Treatment should be guided by the patient's metabolic status, not the specific molecular diagnosis. It is helpful, nevertheless, to distinguish between MODY and type 2 diabetes, because insulin sensitizers are of no use in MODY and sulfonylureas should be the first line of treatment. The increased sensitivity of MODY3 patients to sulfonylureas, with consequent need for low doses, should be kept in mind [12]. Some patients go on to need insulin. Even in those patients, significant residual endogenous insulin persists, which makes excellent glycemic control possible in compliant patients, with doses lower than those used in type 1 diabetes [12]. The physician should be aware, however, of the risk that the mild nature of the symptomatology might not motivate compliance. Diabetic complications can certainly be seen in MODY [13–15].

Neonatal diabetes

Both permanent and transient neonatal diabetes are extremely rare entities with an estimated incidence of 1 per 500,000 births [16]. Between 50% and 60% of cases of neonatal diabetes are transient [16].

Transient neonatal diabetes

Transient neonatal diabetes is defined as diabetes beginning in the first 6 weeks of life in term infants with recovery by 18 months of age. Clinically, patients have intrauterine growth retardation, low birth weight, and decreased adipose tissue. Macroglossia is sometimes seen. Patients may present with dehydration, failure to thrive, hyperglycemia, and mild ketosis [17]. Most patients present with diabetes within the first week of life and insulin-dependence disappears by 3 months of age [18]. Endogenous insulin production is low during this time period with the requirements for exogenous insulin. Approximately 40% of patients go on to develop recurrence of diabetes, most commonly during adolescence [18]. It is usually mild and does not require insulin.

In most cases, transient neonatal diabetes seems to be caused by a double dose of a gene on chromosome 6q24 that is normally expressed only from the paternal copy [17,18]. Any one of three distinct molecular pathologies may be responsible for this overexpression. Most sporadic cases are caused by paternal uniparental disomy of chromosome 6 (UPD $_{pat}$ 6), in which both copies of chromosome 6 are inherited from the father, with no contribution from the mother. Familial cases have a paternal duplication of 6q24 [18]. This duplication results in transient neonatal diabetes only when paternally inherited. Rarely, transient neonatal diabetes can be caused by absent or defective methylation of the maternal copy of chromosome 6q24 [19], methylation being the molecular mechanism for silencing the maternal copy of the gene. The maternal copy behaves as if paternal. Two paternally expressed imprinted genes are located in the critical interval: ZAC, encoding a zinc-finger transcription factor that inhibits proliferation and promotes apoptosis; and HYMAI, encoding an untranslated RNA of unknown function (if any). It is widely believed, but not proved, that ZAC is the gene involved.

Permanent neonatal diabetes

In contrast to transient neonatal diabetes, the etiology of permanent neonatal diabetes (PND) is more heterogeneous. PND may be caused by mutations in genes encoding the transcription factors insulin-promoter factor-1, eukaryotic translation initiation factor-2α kinase 3 (EIF2AK3), and forkhead box-P3. In addition, homozygous inactivating mutations in the genes encoding the glucose-sensing enzyme of the β-cell, glucokinase, and activating mutations of the Kir 6.2 subunit of the ATP-sensitive K$^+$ channel of the β-cell, which prevents its closure and hence insulin secretion, may also cause PND.

The most common cause of PND is a heterozygous activating mutation in the gene, KCNJ11, encoding the Kir 6.2 subunit of the ATP-sensitive K$^+$ channel of the β-cell [20]. It has been described to cause both familial and sporadic (usually because of new mutations) PND [21]. The ATP-sensitive K$^+$ channel regulates the release of insulin from the pancreatic β-cell. Activating mutations in the Kir 6.2 subunit increase the number of open channels on the cell membrane, resulting in hyperpolarization of the β-cell and subsequent prevention of insulin release. Most cases reported resulted from sporadic mutations. In addition to diabetes, some patients with mutations in *KCNJ11*, the gene encoding the Kir 6.2 subunit, have been reported to have global developmental delay, muscle weakness, epilepsy, and dysmorphic features [21]. These features include a prominent metopic suture, bilateral ptosis, downturned mouth, and limb contractures [21]. Conversely, homozygous inactivating mutations in the gene KCNJ11 encoding the subunit Kir6.2 cause familial persistent hyperinsulinemic hypoglycemia of infancy [22]. Generally, treatment for PND has been insulin therapy. Recently, however, it has been shown that some patients with PND caused by mutations in Kir 6.2 respond to high-dose oral sulfonylureas [20]. Sulfonylureas stimulate insulin secretion by binding to the sulfonylurea receptor on the β-cell and closing the ATP-sensitive K$^+$ channel, stimulating insulin release. In one study, patients with PND caused by activating mutation of the Kir 6.2 subunit were progressively weaned off of insulin while increasing doses of glibenclamide were instituted [20]. The glibenclamide was initiated at a dose of 0.1 mg/kg/d and increased to 0.4 mg/kg/d after 4 to 6 months of initiation of treatment, at which point insulin was discontinued [20]. Patients studied had either stable or improved A1c on glibenclamide as compared with insulin therapy [20]. Although these findings are still preliminary and long-term follow-up studies are needed, PND caused by *KCNJ11* mutations is an excellent example of molecular diagnosis making a dramatic difference in treatment options.

Cases of PND have also been found to be caused by homozygosity to the MODY genes glucokinase and insulin promoter factor-1 [7,23], the latter associated with pancreatic agenesis [7]. Both are rare causes of PND.

Other associations with PND include a rare autosomal-recessive syndrome known as Wolcott-Rallison syndrome (OMIM # 22698). The syndrome results from mutations in the gene encoding the eukaryotic translation initiation factor-2α kinase 3 (EIF2AK3) [24]. It is characterized by PND and spondyloepiphyseal dysplasia [24]. Another association with PND is the immunodysregulation, polyendocrinopathy, enteropathy, and X-linked disorder (OMIM #304790). This is a rare, x-linked recessive disease caused by mutations in the gene Forkhead Box P3 (FOXP3) [25], a gene essential for the development of regulatory T-cells that prevent autoimmune reaction. In addition to the diabetes, autoimmune manifestations of this syndrome include intractable diarrhea, hemolytic anemia, autoimmune hypothyroidism, eczema, and variable immunodeficiency [25,26]. The onset of diabetes is generally soon after birth [27]. The prognosis is poor and most of the cases reported have been lethal [28].

Wolfram syndrome

Wolfram syndrome is an autosomal-recessive, progressive, neurodegenerative disease. Also referred to as the acronym DIDMOAD, it is characterized by diabetes insipidus, diabetes mellitus, optic atrophy, and deafness. The insulin-dependent diabetes mellitus is a nonautoimmune process. In a United Kingdom nationwide series of 45 patients with Wolfram syndrome, diabetes mellitus presented at a mean age of 6 years with optic atrophy following at 11 years [29]. The optic atrophy is progressive with eventual blindness. Central diabetes insipidus occurred in 73% of patients in the second decade of life and sensorineural deafness in 28% [29]. Genitourinary abnormalities, including incontinence and neuropathic bladder, presented in the third decade of life [29]. The neurologic manifestations are diverse including cerebellar ataxia, peripheral neuropathies, horizontal nystagmus, mental retardation, and a variety of psychiatric illnesses (Box 1) [29,30]. Abnormalities of brain MRI have been reported in patients [29]. Typical abnormalities include generalized cerebral atrophy, absence of posterior pituitary signal, and reduced signal from the optic nerves [29]. The psychiatric illnesses reported in patients with Wolfram syndrome include depression, suicide, and psychosis with a prevalence of approximately 25% in patients [30]. There also has been a reported increased risk of psychiatric illnesses, hear-

---

Box 1. Neurologic manifestations of Wolfram syndrome

Truncal ataxia
Startle myoclonus
Areflexia of lower limbs
Horizontal nystagmus
Loss of taste and smell
Hemiparesis
Cerebellar dysarthria
Central apnea
Autonomic neuropathy

ing loss, and diabetes mellitus in first-degree relatives of patients with Wolfram syndrome [31,32]. Primary gonadal atrophy is common in males and females may have menstrual irregularity [29]. The median age of death is 30 years, often caused by respiratory failure from brainstem atrophy [33]. Wolfram syndrome is caused by a loss-of-function mutation of the gene (*WFS1*) encoding the protein wolframin on chromosome 4p [34]. The human *WFS1* gene is expressed at high levels in the heart, pancreas, placenta, brain, and lung [35] and encodes a transmembrane protein that primarily localizes in the endoplasmic reticulum for which its function has still not been elucidated. A second locus, *WFS2*, mapped to chromosome 4q, was discovered after linkage analysis of four families with Wolfram syndrome [36]. These patients did not have evidence of diabetes insipidus, however, but did have upper gastrointestinal bleeding and ulcerations.

For diagnosis of Wolfram syndrome at a minimum patients must have insulin-dependent diabetes mellitus and progressive, bilateral optic atrophy occurring before 15 years of age [29]. Using these criteria, screening for WFS1 mutations identifies a mutation in 90% and compound heterozygosity for at least two mutations in 78% of patients [37]. The diagnosis of Wolfram syndrome is mainly clinical with genetic analysis used to confirm the diagnosis.

Mitochondrial diabetes

Mitochondria are intracellular organelles that are responsible for generating energy through the process of oxidative phosphorylation. These are the only intracellular organelles apart from the nucleus that has its own DNA. The DNA is exclusively maternally inherited, double-stranded, and encodes proteins involved in the oxidative phosphorylation process. Mutations in mitochondrial DNA have characteristically been associated with neurologic disease, but diabetes can also be a feature. The most common clinical presentation is the syndrome of maternally inherited diabetes and deafness, caused by a point mutation in the A3243G nucleotide pair of mitochondrial DNA [38], encoding the Leucine tRNA. The age of diagnosis of diabetes varies widely, generally occurring in the fourth decade of life, although the onset may be as early as adolescence [39]. At onset, hyperglycemia is usually mild but many patients go on to require insulin treatment because the insulin deficiency is progressive [39]. Carriers of the A3243G mutation characteristically have sensorineural hearing impairment, the onset of which typically precedes the onset of diabetes by several years. Patients also develop pigmentary retinal dystrophy. Some patients may develop neuro-muscular disorder characterized by a cardiomyopathy or muscular weakness [39]. The mutation seems to impair glucose-induced insulin secretion by the pancreas. Patients are treated with insulin, diet, or sulfonylureas. Metformin seems to be contraindicated because of its risk of inducing lactic acidosis and the vulnerability of these patients of developing it. The same mutation may result in the less common disease of mitochondrial encephalopathy with lactic acidosis and stroke-like episodes, which is also associated with diabetes [40]. Drastically different phenotypes on the basis of the same mutation are mainly determined by the degree of heteroplasmy in the mitochondrial DNA. Unlike nuclear DNA, which is restricted to only two copies, mtDNA exists in several hundred copies per cell, any proportion of which can have the mutation while the rest of the copies can be normal; this is referred to as "heteroplasmy."

Two other syndromes, caused by deletions in mitochondrial DNA, tend to be severe and associated with diabetes. One of these, the Kearns-Sayre syndrome, is characterized by cardiomyopathy, pigmentary degeneration of the retina, chronic progressive external ophthalmoplegia, ataxia, and sensorineural hearing loss. In Pearson's syndrome, patients present with exocrine pancreatic dysfunction, sideroblastic anemia, and lactic acidosis [41]. The onset of diabetes is usually in early infancy and requires treatment with insulin. Patients generally do not survive beyond the first decade of life.

Cystic fibrosis–related diabetes

Cystic fibrosis is a multisystem disorder caused by deficiency of the CFTR chloride channel with resultant inspissated secretions of the lungs, pancreas, intestine, and male reproductive tract. Because cystic fibrosis patients are living longer, such complications as glucose intolerance and cystic fibrosis–related diabetes (CFRD) are becoming common. Cystic fibrosis initially affects the exocrine pancreatic function but the pancreatic islet cells are also affected in many patients, with decreasing insulin secretion.

Up to 50% of cystic fibrosis patients develop CFRD [42]. The median age of onset is 20 years. Risk factors for the development of diabetes include pancreatic insufficiency, recurrent pulmonary infections, corticosteroid treatment, and supplemental feeding [43]. Patients with CFRD present with polyuria and polydipsia usually associated with poor growth velocity, failure to gain or maintain weight despite nutritional intervention, unexplained decline in pulmonary function, and failure of pubertal progression [42]. CFRD patients tend to have increased weight loss, more of a decline in lung function, and increased mortality compared with cystic fibrosis patients without diabetes [42]. Retrospective studies have shown that the increase in weight loss and decline in lung function may occur a few years before the onset of CFRD [42]. Because insulin deficiency is usually incomplete, diabetic ketoacidosis is much less common and slower to develop compared with type 1 diabetes. Patients with CFRD develop diabetic microvascular complications with a reported prevalence of 5% to 21% [42].

According to the North American 1998 cystic fibrosis consensus conference report there are four glucose tolerance categories in cystic fibrosis: (1) normal glucose tolerance, (2) impaired glucose tolerance, (3) CFRD without fasting hyperglycemia, and (4) CFRD with fasting hyperglycemia [42]. CFRD may be chronic or intermittent, with or without fasting hyperglycemia [42]. Patients with intermittent CFRD may require insulin therapy at times of stress, with corticosteroid therapy for lung disease or with high-calorie nutritional intervention [42]. Between periods of stress the blood glucose is normal. The consensus report recommends the following criteria for diagnosis of CFRD [42] (1 mmol/L = 18 mg/dL):

- On two or more occasions a fasting plasma glucose ≥ 7 mmol/L
- One fasting plasma glucose ≥ 7 mmol/L and a random plasma glucose ≥ 11.1 mmol/L
- On two or more occasions a random plasma glucose ≥ 11.1 mmol/L with symptoms
- 2-hour plasma glucose ≥ 11 on a 75-g oral glucose tolerance test

For screening, cystic fibrosis patients should have random plasma glucose done annually. Fasting plasma glucose should be done in all patients with a random glucose greater than 7 mmol/L [42]. An oral glucose tolerance test is recommended if cystic fibrosis patients present with symptoms of CFRD.

Insulin therapy is the standard treatment for CFRD. Patients generally require multiple daily injections of short-acting insulin before each meal, with dosage dependent on insulin-to-carbohydrate ratios for the meal. Patients should monitor their blood glucose at least three to four times per day, with occasional 2-hour postprandial tests to assess the mealtime insulin adequately. Screening for diabetic complications should begin at the diagnosis of CFRD, because the diabetes may have been unrecognized for years [42]. These include regular measurement of blood pressure, foot examination, annual ophthalmologic examination, and urinary albumin measurements [42].

Insulin receptor defects

Mutations in the insulin receptor gene result in three syndromes that are characterized by insulin resistance. These include type A severe insulin resistance, Rabson-Mendenhall syndrome, and leprechaunism. The various mutations affect the function of the insulin receptor in a number of ways including (1) interfering with insulin receptor synthesis, (2) impairment of posttranslational processing and intracellular-transport of the receptor to the cell membrane, (3) defective insulin binding to the insulin receptor, (4) decreasing the insulin receptor activation, and (5) increasing degradation of the insulin receptor [44]. Patients with Rabson-Mendenhall syndrome and leprechaunism are homozygous or compound heterozygotes for insulin receptor mutations [45,46]. In both Rabson-Mendenhall syndrome and leprechaunism patients have abnormal glucose homeostasis with problems initially with fasting hypoglycemia, elevated postprandial hyperglycemia, and extremely elevated insulin levels [46].

Leprechaunism (OMIM # 246200) is the most extreme form of insulin resistance, typically characterized by near complete absence of functional insulin receptors [45]. During infancy patients present with intrauterine and postnatal growth retardation, acanthosis nigricans, characteristic facial facies, abdominal distention, bilateral cystic ovaries, and lipoatrophy [46]. Characteristically they have elfin facies, upturned nose, prominent eyes, low-set ears, micrognathia, and hirsutism [46]. Male infants have penile enlargement and female infants have clitoromegaly. Most patients do not survive beyond infancy.

Rabson-Mendenhall syndrome (OMIM#262190) is also caused by severe insulin resistance, although less complete than in leprechaunism. Unlike patients with leprechaunism, patients with Rabson-Mendenhall syndrome over time develop persistent hyperglycemia and severe diabetic ketoacidosis that is refractory to insulin therapy [47]. Classically, patients have coarse facial features, pineal gland hyperplasia, acanthosis nigricans, hirsutism, severe growth retardation, and abnormal early dentition. Patients survive longer than those with leprechaunism to an approximate age of 9 years [46].

Type A insulin resistance is the least severe form of insulin resistance. Age of onset is generally in the adolescent period [48]. Patients typically have acanthosis nigricans and hyperandrogenism in female patients [48]. The hyperandrogenism manifests as hirsutism, polycystic ovaries, virilization, and increased serum testosterone [48]. In some cases removal of the enlarged ovaries has been done to control the hyperandrogenism [48]. In general, patients are not obese. Patients require enormous amounts of exogenous insulin to improve the hyperglycemia, despite which they still have poor glycemic control, with a very high morbidity and mortality [48].

Congenital lipoatrophic diabetes

Lipoatrophic diabetes is a heterogeneous group of disorders characterized by complete or partial absence of adipose tissue associated with diabetes mellitus. This adipose insufficiency results in consequent insulin resistance, diabetes mellitus, and hypertriglyceridemia. The term "lipoatrophy" refers to the characteristic loss of fat, whereas "lipodystrophy" is a generalized term and refers to the abnormal distribution of fat. Two inherited forms exist: congenital generalized lipoatrophy and familial partial lipodystrophy. Congenital generalized lipoatrophy has an autosomal-recessive inheritance, characterized by generalized absence of subcutaneous adipose tissue within the first year of life [49]. Before adolescence patients typically have evidence of acanthosis nigricans, insulin resistance, and diabetes mellitus [49]. Patients also develop severe hypertriglyceridemia resulting in frequent episodes of pancreatitis. Leptin levels are low [50].

Familial partial lipodystrophy, also known as Dunnigan syndrome, is inherited in an autosomal-dominant fashion. It is caused by mutations in the lamin A/C gene located at 1q21-23 [51,52]. How lamin A/C mutations cause lipoatrophy is unclear. Typically, patients are born with normal fat distribution but begin to lose subcutaneous adipose tissue in the extremities and trunk in early puberty [53]. As puberty is completed there is an increase in subcutaneous fat in the face and neck [53]. Patients may develop acanthosis nigricans, hirsutism, and polycystic ovary syndrome. Patients develop diabetes mellitus and hypertriglycer-idemia. In female patients, however, the onset tends to be earlier and more severe as compared with males [49,54].

Summary

This article covers some unusual or rare causes of diabetes mellitus chosen not necessarily on the basis of frequency or rarity, but rather on the basis of how well the disease and its implications in diabetes management is understood. A specific diagnosis is of help in these rare syndromes but not absolutely necessary for optimal management. The basic principles of diabetes management are well-defined, regardless of etiology. What is important in each case is to understand the relative contribution of insulin resistance versus insulin deficiency, regardless of etiology, as the most important guide to management.

References

[1] American Diabetes Association. Diagnosis and classification of diabetes mellitus. Diabetes Care 2005;28(Suppl 1):S37–42.
[2] Fajans SS, Bell GI, Polonsky KS. Molecular mechanisms and clinical pathophysiology of maturity-onset diabetes of the young. N Engl J Med 2001;345:971–80.
[3] Froguel P, Vaxillaire M, Sun F, et al. Close linkage of glucokinase locus on chromosome 7p to early-onset non-insulin-dependent diabetes mellitus. Nature 1992;356:162–4.
[4] Matschinsky FM, Glaser B, Magnuson MA. Pancreatic beta-cell glucokinase: closing the gap between theoretical concepts and experimental realities. Diabetes 1998;47:307–15.
[5] Velho G, Petersen KF, Perseghin G, et al. Impaired hepatic glycogen synthesis in glucokinase-deficient (MODY-2) subjects. J Clin Invest 1996;98:1755–61.
[6] Jonsson J, Carlsson L, Edlund T, et al. Insulin-promoter-factor 1 is required for pancreas development in mice. Nature 1994;371:606–9.
[7] Stoffers DA, Zinkin NT, Stanojevic V, et al. Pancreatic agenesis attributable to a single nucleotide deletion in the human IPF1 gene coding sequence. Nat Genet 1997;15:106–10.
[8] Naya FJ, Stellrecht CM, Tsai MJ. Tissue-specific regulation of the insulin gene by a novel basic helix-loop-helix transcription factor. Genes Dev 1995;9:1009–19.
[9] Lindner TH, Njolstad PR, Horikawa Y, et al. A novel syndrome of diabetes mellitus, renal dysfunction and genital malformation associated with a partial deletion of the pseudo-POU domain of hepatocyte nuclear factor-1beta. Hum Mol Genet 1999;8:2001–8.
[10] Bingham C, Bulman MP, Ellard S, et al. Mutations in the hepatocyte nuclear factor-1beta gene are associated with familial hypoplastic glomerulocystic kidney disease. Am J Hum Genet 2001;68:219–24.
[11] Carbone I, Cotellessa M, Barella C, et al. A novel hepatocyte nuclear factor-1beta (MODY-5) gene mutation in an Italian family with renal dysfunctions and early-onset diabetes. Diabetologia 2002;45:153–4.
[12] Pearson ER, Liddell WG, Shepherd M, et al. Sensitivity to sulphonylureas in patients with hepatocyte nuclear factor-1alpha gene mutations: evidence for pharmacogenetics in diabetes. Diabet Med 2000;17:543–5.
[13] Owen K, Hattersley AT. Maturity-onset diabetes of the young: from clinical description to molecular genetic characterization. Best Pract Res Clin Endocrinol Metab 2001;15:309–23.

[14] Pearson ER, Velho G, Clark P, et al. Beta-cell genes and diabetes: quantitative and qualitative differences in the pathophysiology of hepatic nuclear factor-1alpha and glucokinase mutations. Diabetes 2001;50(Suppl 1):S101–7.

[15] Lehto M, Tuomi T, Mahtani MM, et al. Characterization of the MODY3 phenotype: early-onset diabetes caused by an insulin secretion defect. J Clin Invest 1997;99:582–91.

[16] von Muhlendahl KE, Herkenhoff H. Long-term course of neonatal diabetes. N Engl J Med 1995;333:704–8.

[17] Temple IK, Gardner RJ, Mackay DJ, et al. Transient neonatal diabetes: widening the understanding of the etiopathogenesis of diabetes. Diabetes 2000;49:1359–66.

[18] Temple IK, Shield JP. Transient neonatal diabetes, a disorder of imprinting. J Med Genet 2002;39:872–5.

[19] Gardner RJ, Mackay DJ, Mungall AJ, et al. An imprinted locus associated with transient neonatal diabetes mellitus. Hum Mol Genet 2000;9:589–96.

[20] Sagen JV, Raeder H, Hathout E, et al. Permanent neonatal diabetes due to mutations in KCNJ11 encoding Kir6.2: patient characteristics and initial response to sulfonylurea therapy. Diabetes 2004;53:2713–8.

[21] Gloyn AL, Pearson ER, Antcliff JF, et al. Activating mutations in the gene encoding the ATP-sensitive potassium-channel subunit Kir6.2 and permanent neonatal diabetes. N Engl J Med 2004;350:1838–49.

[22] Thomas P, Ye Y, Lightner E. Mutation of the pancreatic islet inward rectifier Kir6.2 also leads to familial persistent hyperinsulinemic hypoglycemia of infancy. Hum Mol Genet 1996;5:1809–12.

[23] Njolstad PR, Sovik O, Cuesta-Munoz A, et al. Neonatal diabetes mellitus due to complete glucokinase deficiency. N Engl J Med 2001;344:1588–92.

[24] Brickwood S, Bonthron DT, Al-Gazali LI, et al. Wolcott-Rallison syndrome: pathogenic insights into neonatal diabetes from new mutation and expression studies of EIF2AK3. J Med Genet 2003;40:685–9.

[25] Chatila TA, Blaeser F, Ho N, et al. JM2, encoding a fork head-related protein, is mutated in X-linked autoimmunity-allergic disregulation syndrome. J Clin Invest 2000;106:R75–81.

[26] Levy-Lahad E, Wildin RS. Neonatal diabetes mellitus, enteropathy, thrombocytopenia, and endocrinopathy: further evidence for an X-linked lethal syndrome. J Pediatr 2001;138:577–80.

[27] Peake JE, McCrossin RB, Byrne G, et al. X-linked immune dysregulation, neonatal insulin dependent diabetes, and intractable diarrhoea. Arch Dis Child Fetal Neonatal Ed 1996;74:F195–9.

[28] Baud O, Goulet O, Canioni D, et al. Treatment of the immune dysregulation, polyendocrinopathy, enteropathy, X-linked syndrome (IPEX) by allogeneic bone marrow transplantation. N Engl J Med 2001;344:1758–62.

[29] Barrett TG, Bundey SE, Macleod AF. Neurodegeneration and diabetes: UK nationwide study of Wolfram (DIDMOAD) syndrome. Lancet 1995;346:1458–63.

[30] Swift RG, Sadler DB, Swift M. Psychiatric findings in Wolfram syndrome homozygotes. Lancet 1990;336:667–9.

[31] Swift RG, Polymeropoulos MH, Torres R, et al. Predisposition of Wolfram syndrome heterozygotes to psychiatric illness. Mol Psychiatry 1998;3:86–91.

[32] Ohata T, Koizumi A, Kayo T, et al. Evidence of an increased risk of hearing loss in heterozygous carriers in a Wolfram syndrome family. Hum Genet 1998;103:470–4.

[33] Kinsley BT, Swift M, Dumont RH, et al. Morbidity and mortality in the Wolfram syndrome. Diabetes Care 1995;18:1566–70.

[34] Inoue H, Tanizawa Y, Wasson J, et al. A gene encoding a transmembrane protein is mutated in patients with diabetes mellitus and optic atrophy (Wolfram syndrome). Nat Genet 1998;20:143–8.

[35] Strom TM, Hortnagel K, Hofmann S, et al. Diabetes insipidus, diabetes mellitus, optic atrophy and deafness (DIDMOAD) caused by mutations in a novel gene (wolframin) coding for a predicted transmembrane protein. Hum Mol Genet 1998;7:2021–8.

[36] El-Shanti H, Lidral AC, Jarrah N, et al. Homozygosity mapping identifies an additional locus for Wolfram syndrome on chromosome 4q. Am J Hum Genet 2000;66:1229–36.

[37] Khanim F, Kirk J, Latif F, et al. WFS1/wolframin mutations, Wolfram syndrome, and associated diseases. Hum Mutat 2001;17:357–67.

[38] van den Ouweland JM, Lemkes HH, Ruitenbeek W, et al. Mutation in mitochondrial tRNA(Leu)(UUR) gene in a large pedigree with maternally transmitted type II diabetes mellitus and deafness. Nat Genet 1992;1:368–71.

[39] Guillausseau PJ, Massin P, Dubois-LaForgue D, et al. Maternally inherited diabetes and deafness: a multicenter study. Ann Intern Med 2001;134(9 Pt 1):721–8.

[40] Hirano M, Ricci E, Koenigsberger MR, et al. Melas: an original case and clinical criteria for diagnosis. Neuromuscul Disord 1992;2:125–35.

[41] Rotig A, Colonna M, Bonnefont JP, et al. Mitochondrial DNA deletion in Pearson's marrow/pancreas syndrome. Lancet 1989;1:902–3.

[42] Moran A, Hardin D, Rodman D, et al. Diagnosis, screening and management of cystic fibrosis related diabetes mellitus: a consensus conference report. Diabetes Res Clin Pract 1999;45:61–73.

[43] Mackie AD, Thornton SJ, Edenborough FP. Cystic fibrosis-related diabetes. Diabet Med 2003;20:425–36.

[44] Hunter SJ, Garvey WT. Insulin action and insulin resistance: diseases involving defects in insulin receptors, signal transduction, and the glucose transport effector system. Am J Med 1998;105:331–45.

[45] Krook A, Brueton L, O'Rahilly S. Homozygous nonsense mutation in the insulin receptor gene in infant with leprechaunism. Lancet 1993;342:277–8.

[46] Longo N, Wang Y, Smith SA, et al. Genotype-phenotype correlation in inherited severe insulin resistance. Hum Mol Genet 2002;11:1465–75.

[47] Longo N, Wang Y, Pasquali M. Progressive decline in insulin levels in Rabson-Mendenhall syndrome. J Clin Endocrinol Metab 1999;84:2623–9.

[48] Musso C, Cochran E, Moran SA, et al. Clinical course of genetic diseases of the insulin receptor (type A and Rabson-Mendenhall syndromes): a 30-year prospective. Medicine (Baltimore) 2004;83:209–22.

[49] Oral EA. Lipoatrophic diabetes and other related syndromes. Rev Endocr Metab Disord 2003;4:61–77.

[50] Jaquet D, Khallouf E, Levy-Marchal C, et al. Extremely low values of serum leptin in children with congenital generalized lipoatrophy. Eur J Endocrinol 1999;140:107–9.

[51] Peters JM, Barnes R, Bennett L, et al. Localization of the gene for familial partial lipodystrophy (Dunnigan variety) to chromosome 1q21–22. Nat Genet 1998;18:292–5.

[52] Cao H, Hegele RA. Nuclear lamin A/C R482Q mutation in Canadian kindreds with Dunnigan-type familial partial lipodystrophy. Hum Mol Genet 2000;9:109–12.

[53] Garg A, Peshock RM, Fleckenstein JL. Adipose tissue distribution pattern in patients with familial partial lipodystrophy (Dunnigan variety). J Clin Endocrinol Metab 1999;84:170–4.

[54] Garg A. Gender differences in the prevalence of metabolic complications in familial partial lipodystrophy (Dunnigan variety). J Clin Endocrinol Metab 2000;85:1776–82.

ELSEVIER
SAUNDERS

PEDIATRIC CLINICS
OF NORTH AMERICA

Pediatr Clin N Am 52 (2005) 1651–1675

Insulin Analogues in Children and Teens with Type 1 Diabetes: Advantages and Caveats

Marianna Rachmiel, MD, Kusiel Perlman, MD, FRCPC, Denis Daneman, MB, BCh, FRCPC*

Division of Endocrinology, Department of Pediatrics, The Hospital for Sick Children and University of Toronto, 555 University Avenue, Toronto, Ontario, Canada M5G 1X8

Type 1 diabetes mellitus (T1D) is a chronic, metabolic disorder that most commonly presents during childhood and is characterized by absolute insulin deficiency. T1D is caused by selective immune-mediated autoreactive T-cell destruction of beta cells in the pancreatic islets of Langerhans [1]. Insulin deficiency leads to chronic hyperglycemia and other disturbances of intermediary metabolism. As a result, individuals who have diabetes are at risk of developing progressive long-term microvascular (eg, retinopathy, nephropathy, and neuropathy) and macrovascular (eg, cerebral, coronary, and peripheral vascular disease) complications [2]. The seminal trial in T1D, the Diabetes Control and Complications Trial, proved in adults and adolescents that the onset and progression of the microvascular complications can be prevented or delayed by tight control of blood glucose levels [2–4].

Although advanced complications are rare in youth, the demonstration of glycemic memory in follow-up studies of the Diabetes Control and Complications Trial cohort mandates the implementation of meticulous glycemic control in all individuals who have T1D as early as possible in the course of the disease [4]. This goal is particularly difficult to achieve in the pediatric population because of the increased risk for hazardous hypoglycemia [5–9], fluctuating insulin requirements caused by exercise, illness, and variable carbohydrate intake, and psychosocial and physiologic issues related to age, puberty, and weight gain [10,11]. Adolescents who have T1D have higher average HbA1c levels compared with adults [8,11,12], which is probably the result of a combination of biologic

* Corresponding author.
E-mail address: denis.daneman@sickkids.ca (D. Daneman).

0031-3955/05/$ – see front matter © 2005 Elsevier Inc. All rights reserved.
doi:10.1016/j.pcl.2005.07.010
pediatric.theclinics.com

(eg, insulin resistance of puberty) and psychosocial (eg, adolescent noncompliance, eating disorders) factors [10,13,14]. Although potential novel therapies for T1D are being developed (eg, islet transplantation, artificial endocrine pancreas), insulin replacement by injection remains the cornerstone of treatment [15]. For the moment, better outcomes for children and teens who have T1D depend in large part on the ability to more appropriately tailor the insulin regimen for each individual. This article reviews the advantages to and caveats of the use of newer insulin formulations (insulin analogues) and regimens in children and teens who have T1D, their affect on glycemic control, frequency of hypoglycemic events, daily insulin requirements, and adverse affects such as excessive weight gain, which provides a further major challenge in adolescents. We also address briefly the use of adjunctive agents in the treatment of T1D in children and teens.

Development of insulin formulations

Since the discovery of insulin by Banting and Best at the University of Toronto in 1921, there have been important advances in insulin therapy. The first commercial preparations isolated and purified insulin from porcine and bovine pancreata. They were relatively cheap and readily available in many parts of the world. Although not necessarily inferior in clinical efficacy, these preparations had greater immunogenicity, which was believed to alter their pharmacodynamics by the presence of high titer anti-insulin antibodies acting as insulin-binding proteins [16].

In the early 1980s, first purified pork insulin and soon thereafter insulin produced by recombinant DNA technology became available, which dramatically reduced the immune effects (eg, antibody production, insulin allergy, and lipoatrophy) of the porcine and beef products. The production of biosynthetic human insulin largely eliminated the need for animal pancreata in the production process. The pharmacokinetic and pharmacodynamic properties of biosynthetic human insulins were not sufficiently different from those of animal-derived insulins to allow major improvements in the ability to achieve and maintain glycemic control in individuals who have T1D [17]. Over the past 10 years or so, recombinant DNA technology has been used to produce modified human insulins, which are insulin analogues with—at least theoretically—improved pharmacokinetic features. These insulins include rapid-acting and very long-acting analogues.

The ultimate goal of exogenous insulin therapy is to mimic endogenous insulin secretion, which is characterized by continuous basal and meal-related acute increases in insulin secretion [18,19]. Bolus insulins aim to match the meal-related or prandial increases in blood glucose and include short-acting insulins and rapid-acting insulin analogues, both of which have a relatively fast onset and short duration of action. The basal insulins are the intermediate-acting, long-acting insulins and the very long-acting analogues, which have a slower onset and a longer duration of action and are used to suppress lipolysis and hepatic glucose

Table 1
Pharmcodynamics of subcutaneous injections of insulin types*

Insulin type	Appearance	Action characteristics (h)		
		Onset	Peak	Duration
Rapid-acting analogues insulin lispro insulin aspart	Clear	5–10 min	0.5–2	3–4
Fast-acting insulins humulin regular soluble insulin	Clear	0.5–1	2–5	6–8
Intermediate-acting insulins isophane or NPH lente	Cloudy	1–3	5–8	12–18
Long-acting insulin ultralente	Cloudy	3–4	8–15	22–26
Very long-acting analogues detemir glargine	Clear	1.5–4	None	20–24

* The action characteristics provided in this table are averages but can vary greatly from one individual to another and from one day to another in any one individual. Insulin analogues have, on average, shown less inter- and intra-individual variation than either animal source or biosynthetic human insulin preparations. Insulin absorption is also affected by several other factors, including site and depth of injection, exercise of the limb into which the insulin has been injected, and ambient temperature.

production (Table 1). Even the most sophisticated regimens for subcutaneous insulin delivery cannot reproduce physiologic insulin secretion perfectly for two reasons. First, in individuals who do not have diabetes, insulin is delivered into the portal system rather than into the peripheral circulation. Second, meal-related insulin secretion occurs in two distinct phases (first- and second-phase insulin secretion).

The most common insulin regimens used today in children and teens who have T1D include split-mix regimens with two to three injections of rapid- and intermediate-acting insulin, basal-bolus regimens, which consist of multiple (usually four or more) subcutaneous injections per day comprising pre-meal boluses, with one or two injections of basal insulin (also known as multiple daily injections) and continuous subcutaneous insulin infusion (CSII) via a pump, using only rapid-acting insulin at a basal rate with boluses at times of food ingestion [16,20,21].

Pharmacokinetic and pharmacodynamic profile of insulin analogues

Rapid-acting analogues: meal-related (bolus) insulin

Regular (also called soluble) insulin was used as the only meal-related component of most insulin treatment regimens until the emergence of the rapid-acting insulin analogues. It was used either in combination with intermediate-acting insulin in twice- or three-times-daily regimens or as pre-meal bolus injections in the basal-bolus regimens (multiple daily injections), given approximately 30 minutes [15–45] before each meal [16]. Its injection resulted in a plasma insulin profile that was different from the normal prandial insulin response seen in individuals who did not have diabetes. The physiologic prandial response is intraportal, biphasic, and rapid, whereas after the subcutaneous injection of regular insulin there is an initial lag phase followed by an increase in plasma insulin concentrations that peak after 1 to 2 hours and return to basal concentrations only after approximately 6 to 8 hours. Several factors contribute to the differences from the normal physiologic response; primary among these factors are the self-association of the insulin molecules into dimers and hexamers, which impede their absorption, and their subcutaneous rather than intraportal route of delivery. Other factors that contribute to the variability in absorption and serum insulin concentrations are the site and depth of the injection, the concentration of the injected insulin, and variations in degradation and insulin clearance within and between individuals [10,19].

Compared to regular human insulin, the new rapid-acting insulin analogues more closely resemble endogenous insulin secretion by their faster onset and shorter duration of action, which is attributed to their monomeric structure with reduced self-association to form hexamers and the rapid dissociation of the monomers as soon as they are injected subcutaneously [22–24]. This ability has been achieved either by an interchange of a lysine at position 28 and proline at position 29 of the B-chain to decrease nonpolar contacts and B sheet interactions (or by replacing proline with aspartic acid at position 29 of the B-chain thereby introducing charge repulsion (Fig. 1A). Insulin lispro and aspart essentially have identical effects on glucose and fat metabolism, which makes them completely interchangeable [22,25]. Both are more rapidly absorbed from the subcutaneous tissue, show less variability in absorption at the injection site, and possibly have less variation within and between individuals compared to regular human insulin preparations [19,22,26]. Their action starts within 5 to 10 minutes, peaks after 1.5 to 2 hours, and disappears within 4 to 6 hours, as reported in adult and pediatric populations [24,27,28]. The peak insulin action occurs approximately twice as fast with these rapid-acting analogues compared to regular human insulin (Fig. 2A) [26,29]. DeVries and colleagues [30] did report a slightly shorter duration of action of insulin aspart in children and adolescents than in adults, possibly because of a faster turnaround of the circulation in youth [30]. Unlike regular insulin, in which the length of time to peak activity increases with increasing doses, with the rapid-acting insulin analogues the time to peak action is independent of the dose. There is also no alteration to their pharmacokinetics with impaired hepatic or renal function [22,25].

In children, adolescents, and adults, measurement of plasma insulin levels after administration of insulin aspart showed a significantly higher insulin concentration, which appeared and disappeared earlier compared to regular in-

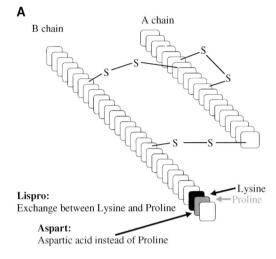

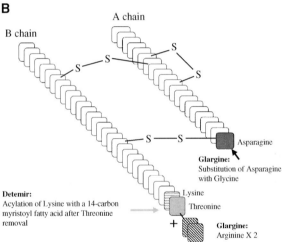

Fig. 1. Amino acid changes from the human insulin to produce insulin analogues. (*A*) Rapid-acting analogues: insulin lispro and insulin aspart. (*B*) Very long-acting analogues: insulin glargine and insulin detemir.

sulin. This was accompanied by a smaller increase in plasma glucose levels [28,31]. Overnight metabolic profiles performed in adults and adolescents demonstrated lower insulin concentrations in the early part of the night with insulin aspart and insulin lispro compared to regular insulin, with an earlier, higher, and briefer increase of insulin after the evening meal [31,32]. This finding suggested that the administration of regular insulin with the evening meal contributes, at least in part, to the over-insulinization of the early part of the night. Similar results have been found in prepubertal children whose blood glucose

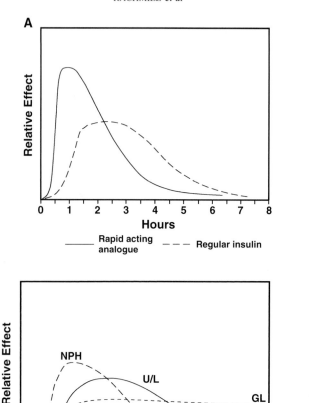

Fig. 2. Approximate pharmacokinetic characteristics of the various insulins. (*A*) Schematic representation of the time course of action of the bolus insulins (regular insulin and rapid-acting insulin
analogues). (*Modified from* Pampanelli S, Torlone E, Lalli C, et al. Improved postprandial metabolic
control after subcutaneous injection of a short-acting insulin analogue in IDDM of short duration
with residual pancreatic β-cell function. Diabetes Care 1995;18(11):1452–9; with permission of the
American Diabetes Association.) (*B*) Schematic representation of the time course of action of the basal
insulins (intermediate-acting, long-acting, and very long-acting insulin). The duration varies within
and between individuals. (*Modified from* Lepore M, Pampanelli S, Fanelli C, et al. Pharmacokinetics
and pharmacodynamics of subcutaneous injection of long acting human insulin analog glargine, NPH
insulin, and Ultralente human insulin and continuous subcutaneous infusion of insulin lispro. Diabetes
2000;49(12):2142–8; with permission of the American Diabetes Association.)

levels tended to be higher in the late night to early morning hours (10:00PM–04:00AM) [33]. Rapid-acting insulin leads to less overlap with the peak action of nighttime intermediate-acting insulin and a smoother glucose profile overnight with less risk of nocturnal hypoglycemia.

Because the rapid-acting analogues were designed to be injected immediately before meals, they are much more acceptable to children who often have difficulty giving their injection 30 minutes before a meal, as required with regular insulin. In some children, the analogues may be injected 15 minutes after the start of a meal without significantly compromising glycemic control. Studies in children and teens who have T1D have failed to show significant difference in the frequency of hypoglycemic episodes, HbA1c, and fructoseamine levels when lispro and aspart were given before or after a meal [27,34–36]. Postprandial injection allows care providers to adjust the insulin dose to the amount eaten, which limits the risk of hypoglycemic episodes. This is of particular importance among infants and preschool-aged children, whose food intake may be inconsistent. The tendency to higher blood glucose levels 30, 60, and sometimes 120 minutes after a meal with postprandial injection indicates that preprandial administration is still preferable when the size of the meal can be predicted accurately [27,34,35].

Basal insulins: (very) long-acting insulin analogues

Until recently, the insulin preparations available that aimed at maintaining constant basal insulin levels during the interprandial and nocturnal periods consisted of the intermediate-acting noncovalent complex of insulin with protamine (neutral protamine Hagedorn [NPH]) and the zinc-containing preparations. These insulins all have reduced solubility at physiologic pH that results in slower absorption from the subcutaneous tissue [19]. Although they remain an essential component of the twice- or three-times-daily regimens and of the pre-bed dosage in basal bolus regimens [16,21], the intermediate-acting insulins have three major disadvantages. First, there is considerable dose-to-dose variation in the amount of insulin absorbed [19]. Second, there is an attenuation of their peak and duration of action with increasing dose administered. Third, they are certainly not peakless. The major part of the variation is attributed to their pharmacokinetic properties and the inaccurate and highly user-dependent variability in their efforts to homogeneously mix the crystal suspension [20,37]. The peak insulin levels contribute substantially to the high frequency of nocturnal hypoglycemia, and the variability in action contributes to the unsatisfactory control of fasting blood glucose concentrations [38].

In response to the shortcomings of intermediate-acting insulin preparations, the very long-acting human insulin analogues, glargine and detemir, have been developed with the aim of providing a constant, flat, and reproducible supply of basal insulin, which better mimics the slow, continuous basal release of pancreatic insulin (Fig. 2B) [18,24,38]. Both preparations are solutions, not suspensions, that should reduce inter- and intra-user variability because they do not require resuspension before administration, Unfortunately, the manufacturers recommend that these long-acting analogues not be mixed with any of the short-acting insulin preparations [18,38–40].

Insulin glargine is synthesized by recombinant DNA technology using *Escherichia coli* plasmid DNA. It results from two modifications of human insulin: (1) the addition of two positive charges (two arginine molecules) to the C terminus of the B chain and (2) the replacement of an asparagine residue at position 21 in the A chain (see Fig. 1B). These modifications shift the isoelectric point to a pH of 5.4 from 6.7, which results in normal solubility in slightly acidic pH but reduced solubility at the neutral subcutaneous pH. Insulin glargine remains stable in the formulated acidic solution. These changes allow more prolonged absorption from the subcutaneous tissue, where it forms a microprecipitate. There is a more consistent diurnal release of insulin into the circulation, with no pronounced peaks over 24 hours. Insulin glargine exhibits an action profile that is flatter and longer and has less nocturnal variability than that of NPH and Ultralente [18,24,38,41–43].

Overnight metabolic profiles of insulin glargine injected at bedtime compared to NPH at bedtime have demonstrated that insulin levels were lower between 1:00 and 2:00AM and higher between 4:00 and 7:30AM among adults treated with insulin glargine, whereas blood glucose levels were higher at 3:00AM and lower before breakfast [43]. Similar results were reported in eight children, who were a small cohort of a larger randomized study of two groups that received either NPH or insulin glargine at bedtime. In the insulin glargine group, insulin levels declined slowly during the night with a peakless pattern, which confirmed a slow rate of absorption, in keeping with the stable blood glucose levels. In the NPH group, insulin levels continued to rise and did not decline until 4:00AM, which caused relative nocturnal hyperinsulinemia, which reflected in the blood glucose levels that dropped during the night to their nadir at 4:00AM [44]. Studies suggest that insulin glargine may be administered before breakfast, at dinner, or at bedtime without a deterioration in blood glucose control [43,45–47].

Insulin detemir is synthesized by removal of the amino acid Threonine[B30] from human insulin (see Fig. 1B), enabling the epsilon amino group of Lys[B29] to be acylated with a 14-carbon myristoyl fatty acid. This allows reversible binding to the fatty acid binding sites of albumin; 98% to 99% of insulin detemir is reversibly bound to albumin in plasma. Its self-association to hexamers and solubility at neutral pH enables insulin detemir to exist as a liquid after subcutaneous injection, when it forms a depot with larger surface area and results in a more stable absorption pattern [40]. In children, adolescents, and adults, insulin detemir provides a consistent, predictable, and protracted pharmacokinetic and pharmacodynamic effect on blood glucose with a lower degree of inter- and intraindividual variability compared with either NPH insulin or insulin glargine [48–51].

Non–diabetes-related side effects

There have been reports of pain at injection sites with the insulins glargine and detemir and local lipodystrophy [41,52–54]. The overall tolerability of insulin glargine, detemir, and NPH are comparable [41,52,53,55]. In all age groups, the quality of life seemed to improve with the new analogues compared to Ultralente or NPH, which was attributed to less fear of hypoglycemia and more flexibility in lifestyle and food intake [39,42].

As a consequence of using *E coli* plasmid DNA in preparation of insulin glargine, there were more individuals in the glargine group with *E coli* antibodies, without known clinical significance [56]. Although insulin detemir is bound to albumin, it has not demonstrated any significant interactions with other albumin-bound medications [40].

Safety of insulin analogues

Molecular modifications may carry the risk of receptor overstimulation and mitogenic potency as reported for a previously studied rapid-acting insulin analogue, (Asp)B10. This analogue was reported to cause mammary, ovarian, and bone tumors in animals. Administration of this analogue also was accompanied by the development and progression of retinopathy and diabetic nephropathy, which was attributed to an increase in its insulin growth factor (IGF)-I receptor affinity. In general, the analogues' metabolic potencies correlate well with insulin receptor affinities, and their mitogenic potencies correlate better with IGF-I receptor affinities. It is difficult to assess to what extent an IGF-I receptor–mediated effect of insulin can add to the biologic response of endogenous IGF-I [57,58]. Insulins aspart, lispro and glargine are equally potent to human insulin in binding to the insulin receptor, whereas insulin detemir has a lower affinity [24,58]. Different results have been reported with respect to IGF-1 receptor affinity compared to human insulin: insulin aspart shows similar affinity, insulin detemir is fivefold less potent, insulin lispro is 1.5-fold more potent and insulin glargine is 6.5-fold more potent. The mitogenic potential of the insulin analogues has been evaluated using different human cells. When osteosarcoma cells were used, insulins aspart, lispro, and detemir were less potent than human insulin in stimulating cell growth, whereas insulin glargine was eightfold more potent [59]. When human cell lines and muscle cells were used, insulin glargine demonstrated similar growth promoting activity as human insulin [59,60]. In summary, modifications in the rapid-acting insulin analogues lispro and aspart and the long-acting analogue insulin detemir had no significant influence on metabolic or mitogenic potency. The clinical safety implications of insulin glargine are not clear, however [58]. One of the major current issues concerning the recombinant DNA–modified products is their long-term safety, because patients with clinically relevant microvascular complications largely have been excluded from most studies [61].

Clinical efficacy of insulin analogues in type 1 diabetes

Rapid-acting insulin analogues

Early evidence suggested that the rapid-acting insulins reduced postprandial hyperglycemia, preprandial hypoglycemia, and nocturnal hypoglycemia [16]. A meta-analytic study and the Cochrane Metabolic and Endocrine Disorders Group recently reviewed 42 randomized controlled trials (RCTs) that compared the effect of intensified therapy regimens with rapid-acting insulins to regular insulin. The analyses demonstrated a small (overall -0.1 to -0.15%) but statistically significant decrease in HbA1c using rapid-acting insulin analogues, with comparable results between these analogues and regular insulin in terms of overall hypoglycemia [61,62]. Although rapid-acting analogues did not achieve marked reductions in HbA1c levels, they may decrease the risk of long-term complications by their impact in reducing postprandial glycemia. The assessment of quality of life (evaluated by the diabetes treatment satisfaction questionnaire) showed significant improvements for analogues compared to regular insulin, which were attributed largely to the difference in the time interval between injection and eating. This was the greatest identified benefit of the rapid-acting analogues despite their questionable objective benefits [27,30,33,63–66].

Insulin lispro in adults who have type 1 diabetes

Multicenter RCTs in adult patients who have T1D using insulin lispro injected at meal time reported lower postprandial blood glucose increases and less frequent hypoglycemia. The effect on metabolic control measured by HbA1c levels in these early studies was not significant, however [63,67,68]. A meta-analysis performed to compare the frequency of severe hypoglycemic events (which required third party intervention, glucagon, or intravenous glucose) during insulin lispro and regular insulin treatment regimens showed a significantly reduced frequency with insulin lispro. There was a 25% reduction in severe hypoglycemia in more than 1400 patient-years studied. This reduction did not result from better glycemic control, however, because there was no difference in HbA1c levels. All studies reviewed in the meta-analysis excluded subjects with a history of recurrent severe hypoglycemia [69].

A prospective audit performed by Lunt and colleagues [64] failed to show an improvement in HbA1c levels 1 year after conversion from regular to preprandial insulin lispro among 190 patients who received routine clinical care. Patients who used insulin lispro reported a decreased frequency of hypoglycemia and improved convenience of use with no change in body mass index, however [64,65].

Insulin aspart in adults who have type 1 diabetes

The efficacy of insulin aspart compared to regular insulin in adults who have T1D has been assessed in several multicenter RCTs [30,31,66,70,71], which compared daily insulin aspart and regular insulin used in a basal bolus regimen together with once or twice daily NPH or Ultralente insulin. In one of the studies, 45 of 187 patients who received aspart and 2 of 181 patients who received regular insulin also received three to four injections per day of NPH, which showed no additional benefit on HbA1c levels or glucose control [30]. The total study periods ranged between 12 and 64 weeks with 362 to 1070 participants in each study. Most studies reported a minor but statistically significant difference in HbA1c of 0.12% to 0.15% between the groups receiving insulin aspart and regular insulin [66,70,71]. A nonsignificant difference of 0.14% was observed in the longest study (64 weeks) [30].

Insulin aspart was more effective than regular insulin at providing 24-hour glycemic control as assessed by blood glucose excursions outside of the normal range. There was an improvement in postprandial glucose concentrations without deterioration of preprandial control [30,31]. Frequency of hypoglycemia differed among these studies. Some studies failed to show any difference between patients treated with insulin aspart and patients treated with regular insulin [25,30,31]. Others researchers, such as Home and colleagues [66], showed a trend for reduced frequency of hypoglycemic events. The relative risk of experiencing a major hypoglycemic episode with insulin aspart compared to human insulin was 0.83 (95% CI 0.59–1.18, NS).

Rapid-acting analogues in children and adolescents who have type 1 diabetes

There are limited data of the use of rapid-acting analogues in children and teens compared to adults who have T1D (Table 2). These studies have been open labeled with smaller groups of participants and short periods of follow-up of 3 to 4 months. All but one of them used insulin lispro [33,35,65,72–74]. Fortunately, most of these studies used a randomized cross-over design that used the same basal insulin, NPH, in all subjects [35,65,72–74]. None showed a significant decrease in HbA1c levels, and only one demonstrated lower rates of hypoglycemic episodes with insulin lispro in total and less nocturnal hypoglycemia [73]. This study also demonstrated significantly higher glucose levels at 3:00AM with insulin lispro compared to regular insulin. Two other studies showed a lower prevalence of low blood sugar during the night (one at 03:00AM, the other between 10:00PM and 4:00AM), although with no difference in frequency of symptomatic hypoglycemic episodes [33,74]. As in adults, three of the studies [33,35,73] showed a significant decrease of postprandial glucose concentrations without deterioration of preprandial control. We found only one report in children that compared treatment with insulin aspart to regular insulin in parallel groups. It reported a total of 123 children aged 7 to 17 years and showed no difference in HbA1c levels or in the frequency of hypoglycemic episodes [72].

Chase and colleagues [12] performed a retrospective analysis of the impact of the introduction of insulin lispro on HbA1c concentrations and the frequency

Table 2
Summary of randomized controlled trials of clinical effectiveness of insulin lispro and insulin aspart in children and adolescents with type 1 diabetes

Study (ref.)	Study design (treatment duration, n, age)	Blood glucose monitoring	Hypoglycemic events
Tsalikian [72]	Parallel-group, open-labeled, multicenter: Insulin aspart compared to regular insulin with basal NPH (12 weeks, n = 123, age range 7–17 y)	No comment in abstract	No difference in frequency of hypoglycemic episodes
Holcombe [73]	Cross-over, open-label, multicenter: Insulin lispro compared to regular insulin with basal NPH (4 months, n = 481, 9.1–18.9 y pubertal)	Significantly lower glucose levels after breakfast and supper (9.7 versus 10.6 and 8.6 versus 9.3 mmol/L, respectively), but higher levels at 3:00 AM (9.7 versus 8.8 mmol/L)	Significantly lower rate of hypoglycemic episodes in total (4.02 versus 4.37 episodes per month) and nocturnal (1.0 versus 1.7) with insulin lispro
Deeb [35]	Cross-over, open-label, multicenter: Regular insulin compared to insulin lispro given either 15 minutes before meal or immediately after meal (3 months, n = 61, 2.9–11.4 y prepubertal)	Significantly lower glucose levels 2 h after breakfast and dinner with preprandial insulin lispro, but regular insulin comparable to postprandial lispro	No difference in frequency of hypoglycemic episodes
Tupola [65]	Cross-over, open-label: Regular insulin compared to insulin lispro given postprandially with NPH as basal insulin (3 months, n = 22, 3.9 ± 9.9 y, prepubertal)	No differences in the glucose within 2 h after meal; higher fasting blood glucose with insulin lispro (11.5 ± 4.5 versus 8.4 ± 3.8 mmol/L)	No difference in frequency of hypoglycemic episodes
Ford-Adams [33]	Open-label, cross-over: Regular insulin compared with insulin lispro; NPH as basal insulin (4 months, n = 23, 7–11 y)	Lower postmeal blood glucose with insulin lispro; no difference in fasting blood glucose	No difference in frequency of symptomatic hypoglycemic episodes (1.6 versus 1.7 episodes/subject/week) Lower prevalence of lower blood sugar in early night hours 10:00 PM–4:00 AM (8% versus 13% of blood glucose was lower than 3.5) with insulin lispro.
Fairchild [74]	Open-label, cross-over: Insulin lispro compared to regular insulin, on a two-injection regimen (3 months, n = 35, 5–10 y)	No significant differences were found in blood glucose levels at all measurements, except higher blood glucose at 3:00 AM with lispro (10.5 ± 0.3 versus 9.02 ± 0.4 mmol/L)	No difference in frequency of hypoglycemic episodes with blood glucose lower than 3 mmol/L.

In none of these studies was there a significant difference in HbA1c levels with the different treatment regimens.

of severe hypoglycemic episodes in 676 children, teens, and young adults who have T1D who were switched from regular insulin to insulin lispro compared to 208 who remained on regular insulin. The subjects were divided into four age groups (< 5 years, 5–12 years, 12–18 years, and > 18 years) and the impact was assessed after 2 years of treatment with insulin lispro. They found a significant decrease in HbA1c levels among subjects > 18 years of age, with no corresponding increase in severe hypoglycemia. They also observed a decline in HbA1c levels in patients aged 5 to 12 years who received insulin lispro compared to patients who received regular insulin [12].

Very long-acting human insulin analogues

The clinical efficacy of these analogues has been studied predominantly in the adult population. In most of the studies, in children and adults, their most striking impact seems to be a significant reduction in nocturnal and severe hypoglycemic events, rather than a significant improvement in metabolic control.

Insulin glargine in adults who have type 1 diabetes

Several open-label multicenter RCTs and observational studies have assessed the efficacy of insulin glargine in adults who have T1D [20,41–43,53,55,75]. These studies compared once-daily insulin glargine with once- or twice-daily NPH or Ultralente insulin. All individuals recruited into these trials ($n = 22$-619) used a basal bolus insulin regimen. The total study periods ranged between 4 and 28 weeks. Most studies reported no statistically significant difference in HbA1c levels between groups that received insulin glargine and groups that received NPH [41,52,53]. A few studies reported significant HbA1c decreases of 0.1% to 0.5% when insulin glargine was compared to NPH [20,43,55] and decreases of 0.2% when compared to Ultralente [42]. Although the Diabetes Control and Complications Trial has reported that any decline in HbA1c is beneficial in reducing microvascular complications, decreases of < 0.5% in HbA1c should be interpreted with caution [2]. After 4 to 16 weeks of treatment, the mean decline in fasting blood glucose from baseline was significantly greater with insulin glargine (by 1.76–2.22 mmol/L) compared to NPH (0.33–0.72 mmol/L) [41,52,55]. This difference was not sustained after 28 weeks of treatment, however [53]. Some studies found no significant difference in the incidence of symptomatic hypoglycemia between insulin glargine, NPH, and Ultralente treatment groups [52,53], whereas others reported fewer patients experiencing nocturnal [43,55] and diurnal [20] hypoglycemia and less severe hypoglycemic events (blood glucose levels of < 2 mmol/L) in patients who received insulin glargine [42,53]. There was no difference in insulin requirements with transition from NPH to insulin glargine [43].

Table 3

Summary of studies of clinical effectiveness of insulin glargine and insulin detemir in children and adolescents with type 1 diabetes. (CSII = continuous subcutaneous insulin infusion; RCT = randomized controlled trial)

Study	Study design (duration, n, age)	Comparison groups	HbA1c	Blood glucose	Hypoglycemic events
Chase [39]	Retrospective analysis (9 mo, n = 114, age range 2–18 y)	Transition after 9 mo of NPH/Lente/Ultralente before glargine at bedtime with NPH in the morning with premeal boluses of insulin lispro	13–18 y: no difference <13 y: a significant decrease with insulin glargine (9.4% versus 9.1%).		<13 y: significant reduction in the mean weekly frequency of low (1.5 versus 2.2 /week), and a lower number of severe, mostly nocturnal hypoglycemic episodes, 14 versus 22 (NS)
Schiaffini [83]	Retrospective analysis (12 mo, n = 36, 6–17.8 y)	Transition from human regular insulin + NPH to CSII (n = 20) with fast-acting analogue or glargine at bedtime with premeal fasting analogue	Significant decrease with CSII (7.6% versus 8.5%) but not in insulin glargine group (8.2% versus 8.9%)		No difference in frequency of severe events
Alemzadeh [21]	Cohort (12 mo, n = 80, 10.3–17.8 y)	Transition from Ultralente twice daily to bedtime glargine or CSII	Significant decrease with CSII (7.8% versus 8.4%) but not with insulin glargine (8.5% versus 8.2%)		Significant lower rate of moderate and severe hypoglycemia events/100 patient years (from 56.3–30.4, and from 18.8–7.5, respectively)

Study	Design	Intervention	HbA1c outcome	BG outcome	Hypoglycemia outcome
Schober [56]	RCT, multicenter, open-label (6 mo, n = 349, 5–16 y)	Insulin glargine once daily versus NPH once or twice daily with premeal boluses of regular insulin	No difference in the HbA1c change from baseline to endpoint	Fasting BG levels decreased significantly with insulin glargine (-1.29 versus -0.68 mmol/L, $P < 0.02$).	No difference in symptomatic events; fewer severe diurnal and nocturnal episodes (23% versus 28.6% and 13% versus 18%, respectively) (NS)
Murphy [82]	RCT: two-way cross-over, open-label (16 wk, n = 25, 12–18 y)	Regular insulin + NPH at bedtime versus insulins lispro + glargine at bedtime	No significant decrease (9.1% versus 8.7%)	Significant decrease in pre- and postmeal BG; mean overnight BG significantly higher with insulin glargine (7.5 versus 5.6 mmol/L)	No severe episodes; fewer episodes of asymptomatic nocturnal hypoglycemia (8 versus 25, $P < 0.05$) with insulin glargine
Robertson [84]	RCT, open-label, multicenter (26 wk, n = 347, 11.9 ± 2.8 y)	NPH versus insulin detemir, with premeal boluses of insulin aspart	Similar decrease in both groups (8.8%–8.0%)	Lower levels of fasting BG (8.44 versus 9.58 mmol/L)	No difference in the risk of overall hypoglycemia, but lower risk (36%) for nocturnal hypoglycemia

Abbreviations: BG, blood glucose; NS, not significant.

Insulin detemir in adults who have type 1 diabetes

Several open-label multicenter RCTs also have assessed the efficacy of insulin determir in adults who have T1D, comparing once- or twice-daily dosages of insulin detemir with once- or twice-daily NPH [54,76–78]. All individuals recruited into these trials ($n = 250$ - 575) used a basal bolus regimen with insulin aspart, lispro, or regular insulin to manage their prandial blood glucose levels. The study periods ranged between 16 and 52 weeks. Most studies reported no statistically significant difference in HbA1c levels between the treatment groups [54,77,78]. Although the nocturnal blood glucose pattern was smoother and more stable with detemir compared to NPH, with less intrapatient variability, no significant difference was found in fasting plasma glucose between the treatment groups [54,76,79]. Results regarding the risk of hypoglycemic episodes varied. Some studies reported a significant reduction in the risk of overall and nocturnal hypoglycemia with insulin detemir compared with NPH [54,79], some reported a significant reduction only in nocturnal hypoglycemia [76,77], and others reported only a trend but with no significant difference in hypoglycemic events [80].

Of particular interest is that subjects who received insulin detemir had a significantly lower change in mean body weight compared to NPH after 16 to 52 weeks of treatment [54,77,79,80]. This change was attributed to the lower intrapatient variability of blood glucose and the lower risk for hypoglycemia resulting in less defensive snacking [81].

Very long-acting insulin analogues in children and adolescents who have type 1 diabetes

There is limited information on very long-acting insulin analogues in children and teens who have T1D. Most of this information is derived from six studies, two of them randomized (Table 3) [21,39,56,82–84]. The only randomized study that compared insulin glargine to NPH for 6 months failed to show any decrease in HbA1c levels or in the frequency of symptomatic hypoglycemic events. It did demonstrate a significant decrease in morning fasting blood glucose levels and in the frequency of severe diurnal and nocturnal hypoglycemic episodes, however [56]. The same conclusions were drawn from the randomized multicenter study with insulin detemir [84]. Similar to studies in adults, baseline-adjusted body mass index was lower with detemir compared to NPH (19.3 versus 19.8 kg/m^2, respectively) [84]. No change in body mass index or insulin daily dose was reported after 9 to 12 months' treatment with insulin glargine [21,39,83].

In general, the observational studies did not add more information, apart from the study by Chase and colleagues [39]. In a group of children younger than 13 years who have T1D, the study demonstrated a decrease of 0.3% in HbA1c in addition to a significant decrease in the mean weekly frequency of low blood glucose levels, including severe and nocturnal. Chase and colleagues [39] added an injection of NPH in the morning in addition to the bedtime insulin glargine.

There seems to be significant advantage to using very long-acting analogues to reduce hypoglycemic episodes in children and adolescents with suboptimal glucose control without jeopardizing glycemic control. This change may result in better awareness and improved counterregulation to severe hypoglycemia in the long-term.

Because CSII remains the reference standard against which any basal insulin candidate should be compared, two of the observational studies evaluated the metabolic effects of transition from NPH and regular to either multiple daily injections with insulins glargine and lispro or to CSII. There was a significant decrease in HbA1c after transition from NPH to CSII, whereas none was observed after transition to insulin glargine. The metabolic outcomes cannot be compared directly, however, because the study patients were not randomized to either treatment regimen [21,83].

Other approaches to insulin therapy

Premixed insulins

Attempts to simplify insulin therapy for people with diabetes have included the introduction of premixed (biphasic) insulins that originally contained a constant premixed preparation of regular insulin with a protamine component similar to NPH insulin at various ratios (eg, 10% to 50% regular insulin and 50% to 90% NPH). The same rationale also led to the formation of premixed insulin preparations that contained insulin aspart and insulin lispro with NPH. In a large cross-sectional study (Hvidore Study Group) there was less frequent usage of premixed insulins compared to other regimens [11]. We do not think premixes have a place in treatment of children and teens who have T1D, other than in the relatively rare circumstance in which simplification of the regimen is mandatory for a particular child or family. The major disadvantage of premixes is that they commit patients to a fixed dose and are not amenable to alteration with changes in ambient blood glucose level, variable carbohydrate intake, or planned exercise [16].

Continuous subcutaneous insulin infusion (pump therapy)

CSII uses an externally worn insulin pump with insulin delivered through an infusion catheter inserted into the subcutaneous tissue. CSII currently offers the best possibility of mimicking physiologic insulin secretion and reduces the variability of insulin absorption as compared to subcutaneous injections. When fastidiously implemented, CSII has the potential to improve glycemic control and reduce the occurrence of severe hypoglycemic events [62] with an added advantage of being able to accommodate more easily the habit of older children and teens to snack in the late afternoon. The need for a higher degree of sophistication, more frequent glucose monitoring, significantly higher treatment costs, and the risk of technical problems, site infections, and discomfort are some of the challenges of CSII.

Inhaled insulin

The concept of administering insulin via the respiratory tract, either nasally or into the lung, is not new. Only recently have adequate delivery devices been developed, however, with insulin administered via powder or aerosol. The Cochrane Metabolic and Endocrine Disorders Group reviewed three randomized controlled studies in which patients who have T1D were followed for at least 10 weeks of treatment with inhaled insulin as the bolus insulin in conjunction with injected basal insulin. They were compared to subjects who received an entirely subcutaneous insulin regimen. Results for HbA1c were similar for all trials with no difference in frequency of total hypoglycemic episodes. All trials that reported patient satisfaction and quality of life showed that they were significantly greater in the inhaled insulin group. One must note, however, that generally only subjects who were interested in trying this route of administration volunteered for these studies, No adverse pulmonary effects were observed in any of the studies [85]. A longer follow-up of 6 months (335 adults) did show a decrease in fasting and postprandial glucose, but mild to moderate cough was more frequent, as was increase in insulin antibody levels [86]. Current phase III studies are being conducted in preadolescents and adolescents with favorable preliminary results [87]. Longer follow-up is required to ensure that there are no adverse side effects involving lung parenchyma or the pulmonary vasculature.

Adjunctive therapies

In many individuals with T1D, currently available insulin regimens are inadequate for achieving and maintaining euglycemia. An emerging approach to management in these individuals is the addition of pharmacologic agents to the insulin therapy. Such adjunctive therapies were recently reviewed by Jefferies and colleagues [88] and grouped into three categories based on their mechanism of action: (1) insulin-sensitizing agents (eg, biguanides) aimed at decreasing the insulin resistance typical of the pubertal years; (2) agents that alter gastrointestinal nutrient delivery (eg, acarbose, amylin) aimed at decreasing the postprandial hyperglycemia, which is a risk factor for the development of macrovascular atherosclerotic changes; and (3) others (eg, pirenzepine, IGF-1, glucagon-like peptide 1).

Metformin (biguanide) acts essentially by decreasing hepatic glucose output and improving peripheral insulin sensitivity. Several recent studies have reported the use of metformin in dosages of 25 to 30 mg/kg/d to a maximum of 2000 mg/d in adolescents who have T1D in addition to their insulin regimen [89,90]. At least two such RCTs have demonstrated significant reductions in HbA1c (0.6% to 0.9%), with either no change or reduction in insulin dose and no significant increase in body mass index. Side effects were limited to gastrointestinal discomfort. A recent study failed to exhibit the same effects using pioglitazone, one of the thiazolidinediones [91].

Acarbose is an alpha glucosidase inhibitor that delays carbohydrate digestion in the small intestine. Studies in adults who have T1D demonstrated a 20% to 30% reduction in postprandial hyperglycemia [92,93] and a significant reduction in HbA1c (0.48% to 0.7%) [93,94]. This reduction occurred at the expense of frequent gastrointestinal symptoms, however, such as diarrhea and flatulence [92–95].

Pramlintide (human amylin analog). Amylin is a 37-amino acid peptide that is co-located and co-secreted with insulin from pancreatic beta cells that has been shown to be deficient in patients who have T1D. It regulates gastric emptying, slows glucose delivery to the small intestine, inhibits postprandial nutrient-stimulated glucagon secretion, and reduces glucose emergence from the liver [96]. Because human amylin self-aggregates, its analog, pramlintide, which is given by subcutaneous injections, was used in adult clinical trials. Those trials demonstrated reductions in HbA1c accompanied by a reduction in body weight without an increase in severe hypoglycemic events [97,98]. Heptulla and colleagues [99] reported reduced immediate postprandial hyperglycemia with suppressed glucagon levels after pramlintide administration in children who have T1D.

Glucagon-like peptide 1 is a hormone produced by enteroendocrine cells of the small and large intestine and is secreted in a nutrient-dependent manner. It regulates nutrient assimilation via inhibition of gastric emptying and food intake and controls blood glucose via stimulation of glucose-dependent insulin secretion, insulin biosynthesis, islet proliferation, and neogenesis and inhibition of glucagon secretion [100]. Long-acting GLP-1 agonist is a reptilian peptide that activates the mammalian receptor for glucagon-like peptide 1 with relatively prolonged actions [101]. Subcutaneous administration of glucagon-like peptide 1 and long-acting GLP-1 agonist in patients who have T1D and a range of residual endogenous insulin secretion normalized glycemic excursions after a meal when given in combination with insulin. This effect was associated with delayed gastric emptying and suppression of glucagon secretion without an increase in insulin blood levels [101–103].

The rationale for the use of IGF-1 and pirenzepine (an anticholinergic agent) is based on the dysregulation of the growth hormone (GH)/IGF-1 axis in T1D, with low serum IGF-1 levels and lack of negative feedback on GH secretion. Studies of both agents have demonstrated significant reduction in HbA1c after administration for short periods of time in adolescents who have T1D; however, longer duration RCTs are required to better assess their role and possible side effects [89].

Summary

Insulin analogues have been developed in response to the increasing demand for the achievement and maintenance of meticulous glycemic control starting at the onset of diabetes. Results of the Diabetes Control and Complications Trial in T1D demonstrate unequivocally the need for near normoglycemia as the best means of delaying the onset or slowing the progression of diabetes-related complications. The rapid-acting and very long-acting analogues provide the potential to meet the bolus (meal-related or prandial) and basal demands for physiologic insulin delivery. Data accumulated so far suggest that use of these analogues can decrease the risk of hypoglycemia significantly and may facilitate achievement of lower HbA1c levels. A word of caution is warranted, however. Although studies of these analogues have been somewhat disappointing with respect to glycemic outcomes (lower HbA1c levels in the range of 0.1%–0.2% may have limited clinical significance), one must remember that many of the studies were performed for safety purposes before clinicians and investigators had acquired any experience in their use. Longer term use of these analogues may allow better outcomes to be achieved.

With respect to analogue use, specifically in children and teens with diabetes, two issues are worthy of comment. First, there have been few clinical trials in these populations. The lack of adequate studies in the pediatric population is a common experience when new medications are introduced into clinical care. Second, regimens that aim to achieve and maintain meticulous glycemia with either the new analogues or even with traditional insulins make therapeutic demands that some children or teens who have T1D and their families may find difficult, if not impossible, to meet for various reasons, many of which are related to psychosocial or socioeconomic factors. The health care providers involved with these families must remain sensitive to these issues and not forget the multifaceted nature of diabetes management.

References

[1] Tisch R, McDevitt H. Insulin-dependent diabetes mellitus. Cell 1996;85(3):291–7.
[2] The Diabetes Control and Complication Trial Research Group. The effect of intensive treatment of diabetes on the development and progression of long-term complications in insulin-dependent diabetes mellitus. N Engl J Med 1993;329(14):977–86.
[3] Diabetes Control and Complications Trial Research Group. Effect of intensive diabetes treatment on the development and progression of long-term complications in adolescents with insulin-dependent diabetes mellitus: diabetes control and complications trial. J Pediatr 1994; 125(2):177–88.
[4] Diabetes Control and Complications Trial/Epidemiology of Diabetes Interventions and Complications Research Group. Beneficial effects of intensive therapy of diabetes during adolescence: outcomes after the conclusion of diabetes control and complications trial. J Pediatr 2001;139(6):804–12.
[5] The Diabetes Control and Complication Trial Research Group. Hypoglycemia in the diabetes control and complication trial research group. Diabetes 1997;46(2):271–86.

[6] Matyka K, Wigg L, Pramming S, et al. Cognitive function and mood after profound nocturnal hypoglycemia in children with conventional insulin treatment for diabetes. Arch Dis Child 1999;81(2):138–42.

[7] Porter PA, Byrne G, Stick S, et al. Nocturnal hypoglycemia and sleep disturbances in young teenagers with insulin dependent diabetes mellitus. Arch Dis Child 1996;75(2):120–3.

[8] Mortensen HB, Hougaard P. For the Hvidore study group on childhood diabetes: comparison of metabolic control in a cross sectional study of 2873 children and adolescents with insulin-dependent diabetes from 18 countries. Diabetes Care 1997;20(5):714–20.

[9] Bergszaszi M, Tubiana-Rufi N, Benali K, et al. Nocturnal hypoglycaemia in children and adolescents with insulin dependent diabetes mellitus: prevalence and risk-factors. J Pediatr 1997;131(1):27–33.

[10] Acerini CL, Cheetham TD, Edge JA, et al. Both insulin sensitivity and insulin clearance in children and young adults with type 1(insulin dependent) diabetes vary with growth hormone concentrations and with age. Diabetologia 2000;43(1):61–8.

[11] Mortensen HB, Robertson KJ, Aantoot HJ, et al. For the Hvidore study group on childhood diabetes: insulin management and metabolic control of type 1diabetes mellitus in children and adolescents in 18 countries. Diabet Med 1998;15(9):752–9.

[12] Chase P, Lockspeiser T, Peery B, et al. The impact of the diabetes control and complications trial and humalog insulin on glycohemoglobin levels and severe hypoglycemia in type 1 diabetes. Diabetes Care 2001;24(1):430–4.

[13] Kovacs M, Jyengar S, Goldston D, et al. Psychological functioning of children with insulin-dependent diabetes mellitus: a longitudinal study. J Pediatr Psychol 1990;15(5):619–32.

[14] Amiel SA, Sherwin RS, Simonson DC, et al. Impaired insulin action in puberty: a contributing factor to poor glycemic control in adolescents with diabetes. N Engl J Med 1986;315(4):215–9.

[15] Ruggles JA, Kelemen D, Baron A. Emerging therapies: controlling glucose homeostasis, immunotherapy, islet cell transplantation, gene therapy and islet cell neogenesis and regeneration. Endocrinol Metab Clin N Am 2004;33(1):239–52.

[16] International Society for Pediatric and Adolescent Diabetes. Consensus Guidelines. The Netherlands: Medical Forum International for the International Society for Pediatric and Adolescent Pediatrics; 2000. p. 1.

[17] Zinman B. The physiological replacement of insulin: an elusive goal. N Engl J Med 1989; 321(6):363–70.

[18] Bolli GB, Owens DR. Insulin glargine. Lancet 2000;356(9228):443–5.

[19] Owens DR, Zinman B, Bolli GB. Insulins today and beyond. Lancet 2001;358(9283):739–46.

[20] National Institute for Clinical Excellence. Guidance on the use of long acting insulin analogues for the treatment of diabetes-insulin glargine. Technology appraisal guidelines no. 53. London: National Institute for Clinical Excellence; 2002. p. 1–26.

[21] Almezadeh R, Ellis JN, Holzum MK, et al. Beneficial effects of continuous subcutaneous insulin infusion and flexible multiple daily insulin regimen using insulin glargin in type 1 diabetes. Pediatrics 2004;114(11):e91–5.

[22] Reynolds NA, Wagastaff AJ. Insulin aspart: a review of its use in the management of type1 and type 2 diabetes mellitus. Drugs 2004;64(17):1957–74.

[23] Gammeltoft S, Hansen BF, Dideriksen L. Insulin aspart: a novel rapid acting human insulin analogue. Expert Opin Investig Drugs 1999;8(9):1431–41.

[24] Bolli GB, Di Marchi RD, Park GD, et al. Insulin analogues and their potential in the management of diabetes mellitus. Diabetologia 1999;42(10):1151–67.

[25] Homko C, Deluzio A, Jimenez C, et al. Comparison of insulin aspart and lispro: pharmacokinetic and metabolic effects. Diabetes Care 2003;26(7):2027–31.

[26] Mudaliar SR, Lindberg FA, Joyce M, et al. Insulin aspart (B28 Asp-insulin): a fasting acting analog of human insulin. Absorption kinetics and action profile compared with regular human insulin in healthy nondiabetic subjects. Diabetes Care 1999;22(9):1501–6.

[27] Rami B, Schober E. Postprandial glycaemia after regular and lispro insulin in children and adolescents with diabetes. Eur J Pediatr 2000;156(11):838–40.

[28] Mortensen H, Lindholm A, Olsen B, et al. Rapid appearance and onset of action of insulin aspart in paediatric subjects with type 1 diabetes. Eur J Pediatr 2000;159(7):483–8.
[29] Howey DC, Bowsher RR, Brunelle RL, et al. [Lys(B28), Pro(B29)]-human insulin: a rapidly absorbed analogue of human insulin. Diabetes 1994;43(3):396–402.
[30] DeVries JH, Lindholm A, Jacobsen JL, et al. The Tri-Continental Insulin Aspart Study Group: a randomized trial of insulin aspart with intensified basal NPH insulin supplementation in people with type 1 diabetes. Diabet Med 2003;20(4):312–8.
[31] Home PD, Lindholm AL, Hylleberg B, et al for the UK Insulin Aspart Study Group. Improved glycemic control with insulin aspart: a multicenter randomized double blind crossover trial in type 1 diabetes patients. Diabetes Care 1998;21(11):1904–9.
[32] Mohn A, Matyka KA, Harris DA, et al. Lispro or regular insulin for multiple injection therapy in adolescence: difference in free insulin and glucose levels overnight. Diabetes Care 1999;22(1):27–32.
[33] Ford-Adams ME, Murphy NP, Moore EJ, et al. Insulin lispro: a potential role in preventing nocturnal hypoglycemia in young children with diabetes mellitus. Diabet Med 2003;20(8):656–60.
[34] Danne T, Aman J, Schober E, et al for the ANA 1200 study group. A comparison of postprandial and preprandial administration of insulin aspart in children and adolescents with type 1 diabetes. Diabetes Care 2003;26(8):2359–64.
[35] Deeb LC, Holcombe JH, Brunelle R, et al. Insulin lispro lowers postprandial glucose in prepubertal children with diabetes. Pediatrics 2001;108(5):1175–9.
[36] Rutledge KS, Chase HP, Klingensmith GL, et al. Effectiveness of postprandial humalog in toddlers with diabetes. Pediatrics 1997;100(6):968–72.
[37] Jehle PM, Micheler C, Jehle DR, et al. Inadequate suspension of neutral protamine Hagedorn (NPH) insulin in pens. Lancet 1999;354:1604–7.
[38] Lepore M, Pampanelli S, Fanelli C, et al. Pharmacokinetics and pharmacodynamics of subcutaneous injection of long acting human insulin analog glargine, NPH insulin, and Ultralente human insulin and continuous subcutaneous infusion of insulin lispro. Diabetes 2000;49(12):2142–8.
[39] Chase HP, Dixon B, Pearson J, et al. Reduced hypoglycemic episodes and improved glycemic control in children with type 1 diabetes using insulin glargine and neutral protamine hagedorn insulin. J Pediatr 2003;143(6):737–40.
[40] Chapman TM, Perry CM. Insulin detemir: a review of its use in the management of type 1 and 2 diabetes mellitus. Drugs 2004;64(22):2577–95.
[41] Rosenstock J, Park G, Zimmerman J. Basal insulin glargine (HOE 901) versus NPH insulin in patients with type 1 diabetes on multiple daily insulin regimens. Diabetes Care 2000;23(8):1137–42.
[42] Kudva YC, Basu A, Jenkins GD, et al. Randomized controlled clinical trial of glargine versus ultralente insulin in the treatment of type 1 diabetes. Diabetes Care 2005;28(1):10–4.
[43] Rossetti P, Pampanelli S, Fanelli C, et al. Intensive replacement of basal insulin in patients with type 1 diabetes given rapid-acting insulin analog at mealtime: a 3 month comparison between administration of NPH insulin four times daily and glargine insulin at dinner or bedtime. Diabetes Care 2003;26(5):1490–6.
[44] Mohn A, Strang S, Wernicke-Panten K, et al. Nocturnal glucose control and free insulin levels in children with type 1 diabetes by use of the long acting insulin HOE 901 as part of a three injection regimen. Diabetes Care 2000;23(4):557–9.
[45] Garg SK, Gottlieb PA, Hisatomi ME, et al. Improved glycemic control without an increase in severe hypoglycemic episodes in intensively treated patients with type 1 diabetes receiving morning, evening, or split dose insulin glargine. Diabetes Res Clin Pract 2004;66(1):49–56.
[46] Hamann A, Matthaei S, Rosek C, et al for HOE901/4007 study group. A randomized clinical trial comparing breakfast, dinner, or bedtime administration of insulin glargine in patients with type 1 diabetes. Diabetes Care 2003;26(6):1738–44.
[47] Doyle EA, Weinzimer SA, Steffen AT, et al. A randomized, prospective trial comparing the

efficacy of continuous subcutaneous insulin infusion with multiple daily injections using glargine. Diabetes Care 2004;27(7):1554–8.

[48] Heise T, Nosek L, Ronn BB, et al. Lower within-subject variability of insulin detemir in comparison to NPH insulin and insulin glargine in people with type 1 diabetes. Diabetes 2004; 53(6):1614–20.

[49] Danne T, Lupke K, Walte K, et al. Insulin detemir is characterized by a consistent pharmacokinetic profile across age-groups in children, adolescents, and adults with type 1 diabetes. Diabetes Care 2003;26(11):3087–92.

[50] Hermansen K, Madsbad S, Perrild H, et al. Comparison of the soluble basal insulin analog insulin detemir with NPH insulin. Diabetes Care 2001;24(2):296–301.

[51] Jhee SS, Lyness WH, Rojas B, et al. Similarity of insulin detemir pharmacokinetics, safety, and tolerability profiles in healthy caucasian and Japanese American subjects. J Clin Pharmacol 2004;44(3):258–64.

[52] Raskin P, Klaff L, Bergenstal R, et al. A 16 week comparison of the novel insulin analog insulin glargine (HOE 901) and NPH human insulin used with lispro in patients with type 1 diabetes. Diabetes Care 2000;23(11):1666–71.

[53] Ratner RE, Hirsh IB, Neifing JL, et al. Less hypoglycemia with insulin glargine in intensive insulin therapy for type 1 diabetes. Diabetes Care 2000;23(5):639–43.

[54] Vague P, Selam JL, Skeie S, et al. Insulin detemir is associated with more predictable glycemic control and reduced risk of hypoglycemia than NPH insulin in patients with type 1 diabetes on a basal-bolus regimen with premeal insulin aspart. Diabetes Care 2003;26(3):590–6.

[55] Pieber TR, Eugene-Jorchine I, Derobert E. Efficacy and safety of HOE 901 versus NPH insulin in patients with type 1 diabetes. Diabetes Care 2000;23(2):157–62.

[56] Schober E, Schoenle E, Van Dyk J, et al. The pediatric study group of insulin glargine: comparative trial between insulin glargine and NPH insulin in children and adolescents with type 1 diabetes mellitus. J Pediatr Endocrinol Metab 2002;15(4):369–76.

[57] Milazzo G, Sciacca L' Papa V, Goldfine ID, et al. AspB10 insulin induction of increased mitogenic responses and phenotypic changes in human breast epithelial cells: evidence for enhanced interactions with the insulin-like growth factor-I receptor. Mol Carcinogen 1997; 18(1):19–25.

[58] Kurtzhals P, Schaffer L, Sorensen A, et al. Correlations of receptor binding and metabolic and mitogenic potencies of insulin analogues designed for clinical use. Diabetes 2000;49(6): 999–1005.

[59] Berti L, Kellerer M, Bossenmaier B, et al. The long acting human insulin analogue HOE 901: characteristics of insulin signaling in comparison to Asp (B10) and regular insulin. Horm Metab Res 1998;30(3):123–9.

[60] Bahr M, Kolter T, Seipke G, et al. Growth promoting and metabolic activity of the human insulin analogue [Gli ^{A21}, Arg ^{B31}, Arg ^{B23}] insulin (HOE 901) in muscle cells. Eur J Pharmacol 1997;320(2):259–65.

[61] Siebenhofer A, Plank J, Berghold A, et al. Short acting insulin analogues versus regular insulin in patients with diabetes mellitus. Cochrane Database of Systemic Reviews 2004;3.

[62] Seibenhofer A, Plank J, Berghold A, et al. Meta-analysis of short-acting insulin analogues in adult patients with type 1 diabetes: continuous subcutaneous insulin infusion versus injection therapy. Diabetologia 2004;47(11):1895–905.

[63] Garg SK, Carmain JA, Braddy KC, et al. Pre-meal insulin analogue insulin lispro vs humulin R insulin treatment in youth subjects with type 1 diabetes. Diabet Med 1996;13(1):47–52.

[64] Lunt H, Kendali D, Moore MP, et al. Prospective audit of conversion from regular to lispro insulin during routine clinical care. Int Med J 2004;34:320–3.

[65] Tupola S, Komulainen J, Jaaskelainen J, et al. Post-prandial insulin lispro vs. human regular insulin in prepubertal children with type 1 diabetes mellitus. Diabet Med 2001;18:654–8.

[66] Home PD, Lindholm A, Riis A for the European Insulin Aspart Study Group. Insulin aspart vs. human insulin in the management of long term blood glucose control in type 1 diabetes mellitus: a randomized controlled trial. Diabet Med 2000;17(11):762–71.

[67] Schernthaner G, Wein W, Sanndholzer K, et al. Postprandial insulin lispro: a new therapeutic option for type 1 diabetic patients. Diabetes Care 1998;21(4):570–3.

[68] Pampanelli S, Torlone E, Lalli C, et al. Improved postprandial metabolic control after subcutaneous injection of a short-acting insulin analogue in IDDM of short duration with residual pancreatic β-cell function. Diabetes Care 1995;18(11):1452–9.

[69] Brunelle RL, Llewellyn J, Anderson Jr JH, et al. Meta-analysis of the effect of insulin lispro on severe hypoglycemia in patients with type 1 diabetes. Diabetes Care 1998;21(10):1726–31.

[70] Raskin P, Guthrie RA, Leiter L, et al. Use of insulin aspart, a fast acting insulin analogue, as the mealtime insulin in the management of patients with type 1 diabetes. Diabetes Care 2000; 23(5):105–14.

[71] Tamas G, Marre M, Astotga R, et al. Glycaemic control in type 1 diabetic patients using optimised insulin aspart or human insulin in a randomized multinational study. Diabetes Res Clin Pract 2001;54(2):105–14.

[72] Tsalikian E. Insulin aspart in pediatric and adolescent patients with type 1 diabetes [abstract 767]. Diabetologia 2000;43(1):200.

[73] Holcombe JH, Zalani S, Arora VK, et al for the Lispro in Adolescents Study Group. Comparison of insulin lispro with regular human insulin for the treatment of type 1 diabetes in adolescents. Clin Ther 2002;24(4):629–38.

[74] Fairchild JM, Ambler GR, Genoud-Lowton CH, et al. Insulin lispro versus regular insulin in children with type 1 diabetes on twice daily insulin. Pediatric Diabetes 2000;1(3):135–41.

[75] Porcellati F, Rossetti P, Pampanelli S, et al. Better long term glycemic control with the basal insulin glargine as compared with NPH in patients with type 1 diabetes mellitus given meal time lispro insulin. Diabet Med 2004;21(11):1213–20.

[76] Home P, Bartley P, Russel Jones D, et al for the Study to Evaluate the Administration of Detemir Insulin Efficacy, Safety and Suitability (STEADINESS) Study Group. Insulin detemir offers improved glycemic control compared with NPH insulin in people with type 1 diabetes. Diabetes Care 2004;27(5):1081–7.

[77] De Leeuw I, Vague P, Selam JL, et al. Diabetes, insulin detemir used in basal-bolus therapy in people with type 1 diabetes is associated with a lower risk of nocturnal hypoglycaemia and less weight gain over 12 months in comparison to NPH insulin. Diabetes Obes Metabolism 2005;7(1):73–82.

[78] Roberts A, Standl E, Bayer T, et al. Efficacy and safety of 6 months treatment with insulin detemir in type 1 diabetic patients on a basal-bolus regimen [abstract 795 plus poster]. Diabetologia 2001;44S1:207.

[79] Hermansen K, Fontaine P, Kukolja KK, et al. Insulin analogues (insulin detemir and insulin aspart) versus traditional human insulins (NPH insulin and regular human insulin) in basal-bolus therapy for patients with type 1 diabetes. Diabetologia 2004;47(4):622–9.

[80] Standl E, Lang H, Roberts A. The 12-month efficacy and safety of insulin detemir and NPH insulin in basal-bolus therapy for the treatment of type 1 diabetes. Diabetes Technol Ther 2004; 6(5):579–88.

[81] Fritsche A, Haring H. At last, a weight neutral insulin? Int J Obes Relat Metab Disord 2004;28(Suppl 2):S41–6.

[82] Murphy NP, Keane SM, Ong KK, et al. Randomized cross-over trial of insulin glargine plus lispro or NPH insulin plus regular human insulin in adolescents with type 1 diabetes on intensive insulin regimen. Diabetes Care 2003;26(3):799–804.

[83] Schiaffini R, Ciampalini P, Spera S, et al. An observational study comparing continuous subcutaneous insulin infusion (CSII) and insulin glargin in children with T1DM. Diabetes Metab Res Rev 2005;21:347–52.

[84] Robertson K, Schonle E, Gucev Z, et al. Benefits of insulin detemir over NPH insulin in children and adolescents with type 1 diabetes: lower and more predictable fasting plasma glucose and lower risk nocturnal hypoglycemia [abstract and poster]. Diabetes 2004; 53(Suppl 2):A144.

[85] Royle P, Waugh N, McAuley L, et al. Inhaled insulin in diabetes mellitus. Cochrane Database of Systematic Reviews 2004;3:CD003890.

[86] Quattrin T, Belanger A, Bohannon NJ, et al, Exubera Phase III Study Group. Efficacy and safety of inhaled insulin (Exubera) compared with subcutaneous insulin therapy in patients with type 1 diabetes: results of a 6-month, randomized, comparative trial. Diabetes Care 2004;27(11):2622–7.

[87] Tamborlane WV, Bonfig W, Boland E. Recent advances in treatment of youth with type 1 diabetes: better care through technology. Diabet Med 2001;18(11):864–70.

[88] Jefferies CA, Hamilton J, Daneman D. Potential adjunctive therapies in adolescents with type 1 diabetes mellitus. Treat Endocrinol 2004;3(5):337–43.

[89] Hamilton J, Cummings E, Zdravkovik V, et al. Metformin as an adjuvant therapy in adolescents with type 1 diabetes and insulin resistance: randomized controlled trial. Diabetes Care 2003; 26(1):138–43.

[90] Sarnblad B, Kroon M, Aman J. Metformin as additional therapy in adolescents with poorly controlled type 1 diabetes: randomized placebo-controlled trial with aspects on insulin sensitivity. Eur J Endocrinol 2003;149(4):323–9.

[91] Zdravkovic V, Hamilton J, Daneman D, et al. Pioglitazone as adjunctive therapy in adolescents with type 1 diabetes and insulin resistance. Diabetes 2005;54(Suppl):A452.

[92] Dimitriadis G, Karaiskos C, Raptis S. Effects of prolonged (6 months) alpha-glucosidase inhibition on blood glucose control and insulin requirements in patients with insulin-dependent diabetes mellitus. Horm Metab Res 1986;18(4):253–5.

[93] Riccardi G, Giacco R, Parillo M, et al. Efficacy and safety of acarbose in the treatment of type 1 diabetes mellitus: a placebo-controlled, double blind, multicenter study. Diabet Med 1999; 16(3):228–32.

[94] Hollander P, Pi-Sunyer X, Coniff RF. Acarbose in the treatment of type 1 diabetes. Diabet Care 1997;20(3):248–53.

[95] Sels JP, Verdonk HE, Wolffenbuttel BH. Effects of acarbose (Glucobay) in persons with type 1 diabetes: a multicenter study. Diab Res Clin Pract 1998;41(2):139–45.

[96] Efelman SV, Weyer C. Unresolved challenges with insulin therapy in type 1 and type 2 diabetes: potential benefit of replacing amylin, a second β cell hormone. Diabetes Technol Ther 2002;4(2):175–89.

[97] Whitehouse F, Kruger DF, Fineman M, et al. A randomized study and open-label extension evaluating the long term efficacy of pramlintide as an adjunct to insulin therapy in type 1 diabetes. Diabetes Care 2002;25(4):724–30.

[98] Gottlieb A, Velte M, Fineman M, et al. Pramlintide as an adjunct to insulin therapy improved glycemic and weight control in people with type 1 diabetes during treatment for 52 weeks. Diabetes 2000;49:A109.

[99] Heptulla RA, Rodriguez LM, Bomgaars L, et al. The role of amylin and glucagons in the dampening of glycemic excursions in children with type 1 diabetes. Diabetes 2005;54(4): 1100–7.

[100] Drucker DJ, Miniriview L. The glucagon-like peptides. Endocrinology 2001;142(2):521–7.

[101] Dupre J, Behme MT, McDonald TJ. Exendin-4 normalized postcibal glycemic excursions in type 1 diabetes. J Clin Endocrinol Metab 2004;89(7):3469–73.

[102] Dupre J, Behme MT, Hramiak IM, et al. Subcutaneous glucagon-like peptide 1 combined with insulin normalizes postcibal glycemic excursions in IDDM. Diabetes Care 1997;20(3):381–4.

[103] Dupre J, Behme MT, Hramiak IM, et al. Glucagon-like peptide I reduces postprandial glycemic excursions in IDDM. Diabetes 1995;44(6):626–30.

ELSEVIER
SAUNDERS

PEDIATRIC CLINICS
OF NORTH AMERICA

Pediatr Clin N Am 52 (2005) 1677–1688

Insulin Pump Treatment of Childhood Type 1 Diabetes

Stuart A. Weinzimer, MD[a],*, Kristin A. Sikes, MSN[b],
Amy T. Steffen, BS[b], William V. Tamborlane, MD[a,c]

[a]Department of Pediatrics, Yale University School of Medicine, PO Box 208064,
New Haven, CT 06520–8064, USA
[b]Yale Pediatric Diabetes Research Program, Yale School of Medicine, 2 Church Street South,
Suite 312, New Haven, CT 06519, USA
[c]General Clinical Research Center, Yale University School of Medicine, 333 Cedar Street,
New Haven, CT 06520-8064, USA

Continuous subcutaneous insulin infusion (CSII) pump therapy was introduced to treat patients with type 1 diabetes (T1DM) more than 25 years ago [1,2].
At that time, most children and adolescents were being treated with one or two
daily injections of mixtures of neutral protamine hagedorn (NPH) and regular
insulin of animal origin and treatment was adjusted based on urinary glucose
excretion. With these inadequate methods, it was unsafe to strive for strict metabolic control in young patients, glucose levels often averaged over 300 mg/dL,
and children were at high risk for the later development of the devastating complications of diabetes. With CSII, clinicians could more closely simulate the
patterns of plasma insulin levels seen in normal children. The more predictable
pharmacokinetics of fast-acting versus intermediate-acting insulin [3] and the
administration of bolus doses immediately before each meal were two obvious
advantages of this approach to insulin replacement. Although not fully recognized at the time, the basal-bolus regimen offered by CSII and subsequently
applied to multiple daily injection regimens fundamentally changed the diabetes
treatment paradigm from adjusting the patient's lifestyle to a fixed insulin
regimen to adjusting the insulin regimen to the patient's lifestyle.

Supported by grants from the National Institute of Health (K12 DK063709, RR 06022, U10
HD041906), the Juvenile Diabetes Research Foundation, and the Stephen J. Morse Pediatric Diabetes
Research Fund.

* Corresponding author.
E-mail address: stuart.weinzimer@yale.edu (S.A. Weinzimer).

pediatric.theclinics.com

The development of pump therapy in the late 1970s coincided with the introduction of self-monitoring of blood glucose, hemoglobin (Hb) A_{1c} assays, and more aggressive approaches to conventional insulin therapy, using multiple daily insulin injections (MDI). It was suggested that the improved metabolic control achieved with these intensive therapies might finally provide an answer to the question of the role of hyperglycemia in the development and progression of microvascular and neuropathic complications of diabetes [1]. This issue was finally resolved in 1993 with publication of the results of the Diabetes Control and Complications Trial (DCCT) [4]. Even in the relatively small subset of adolescents who were 13 to 17 years of age on entry in the DCCT, intensive treatment significantly reduced the risk of onset and progression of retinopathy and microalbuminuria [5]. Subsequent follow-up of adolescents in the DCCT has shown that the risk of these complications remained reduced many years after completion of the DCCT, even though HbA_{1c} levels no longer differed between former intensive and former conventional treatment group patients [6]. It has been recommended that the goals of treatment in children with diabetes should be to achieve glucose and HbA_{1c} levels as close to normal as possible and as early in the course of the disease as possible.

Despite the putative advantages of CSII over conventional insulin injection regimens, CSII was used in very small numbers of children before publication of the DCCT results. The advantages of pumped versus injected insulin include the following:

- Uses only rapid-acting insulin
- Bolus doses given before each meal and snack
- Variable basal infusion rate between meals and overnight
- Increased flexibility and improved lifestyle
- One injection every 2 to 3 days

Factors that limited more widespread use of this method of insulin delivery in children before the DCCT included the large size and difficulties in use of early pump models, psychologic issues about wearing an external device, and the extra costs of pump therapy [7]. The most important obstacle to use of these devices, however, was uncertainty regarding the long-term benefits of intensive treatment itself. Results of the DCCT removed this important obstacle to use of pumps in children and, as pediatric treatment teams were challenged to find more effective methods to achieve intensive treatment goals, insulin pump therapy was rediscovered. Consequently, the safety and efficacy of this "new" approach to treatment of childhood diabetes has been the subject of intense interest over the past few years.

The rediscovery of insulin pump treatment in children coincided with a number of important improvements in pump technology that have made the devices safer and easier to use. Advanced pump features include the following:

- Multiple variable basal rates and small increments
- Smaller pumps and better infusion sets

- Greater safety and reliability
- Wireless link to glucose meter
- Dose calculators that incorporate carbohydrate to insulin ratios and correction doses
- Bolus history and other memory functions

The development of pumps with variable basal rate profiles allowed for a closer match in insulin needs particularly overnight, offering the opportunity to reduce the risk of nocturnal hypoglycemia. Current devices are small in size, easy to program, and have a variety of alarms and variable basal rates that can be adjusted in very small increments. Catheters and infusion sets have also improved. The most recent advances in pump technology include software programming of bolus and correction doses based on insulin to carbohydrate ratios and wireless transmission from meter to pump of blood glucose levels.

The introduction of very rapid-acting insulin analogues has been of benefit to both CSII and multiple daily injection regimens. In comparison with regular insulin, rapid-acting insulin analogues have earlier and sharper peaks and less overshoot hyperinsulinemia, facilitating better control of meal-related hyperglycemia with less late postprandial and nocturnal hypoglycemia [8–10]. These advantages of rapid-acting insulin analogues are of particular importance in adolescents with diabetes who require relatively large premeal bolus doses to overcome the peripheral insulin resistance of puberty [11].

Safety and efficacy of continuous subcutaneous insulin infusion in youth: clinical outcome studies

When considering the relative benefits and risks of CSII and MDI in children and adults [12], most studies before 2000 can be disregarded because both treatments have changed so dramatically. The initial reports examining the safety and efficacy of CSII in youth with T1DM in the "new era" were clinical outcome studies where the patients served as their own controls [13]. Although the results of these nonrandomized investigations must be interpreted with caution, the DCCT provides a historical standard by which to judge the usefulness of CSII. During the course of the DCCT, intensively treated adolescents were able to lower HbA$_{1c}$ levels to a mean of 8.1% (normal $\leq$6%) versus 9.8% in the conventional treatment group [5]. Improved diabetes control was achieved at the cost of a threefold increase in the risk of hypoglycemia, however, compared with conventional treatment. During the first 12 months of intensive treatment in the DCCT, the frequency of severe hypoglycemic events requiring the assistance of another person in adolescents was approximately one event per patient per year and 39% of these episodes resulted in seizure or coma. Intensive treatment also increased the risk of excessive weight gain.

The authors' multidisciplinary treatment team began using CSII in earnest in 1997. Their initial report described clinical outcomes in the first 161 patients

(aged 18 months to 18 years) who were started on CSII in the Yale Children's
Diabetes Clinic between January, 1997, and March, 2000 [14]. Only patients with
T1DM who had been followed for at least 1 year before the start of pump therapy
were included in the study and clinical data were collected prospectively before
and during pump treatment using standardized case report forms and a database
developed for this purpose. As shown in Fig. 1, before the start of CSII, mean
HbA_{1c} level was 7.8%, whereas after 12 months of pump therapy it had fallen to
7.1%. This improvement in metabolic control was maintained at the patient's
end-of-study visit, 26 ± 9 months after the start of CSII. Lower HbA_{1c} levels
were achieved with CSII without increasing daily insulin doses or body mass
index (BMI)-z score. Although lower HbA_{1c} levels are expected to be accompanied by an increase in the rate of severe hypoglycemia [5], the frequency of
severe hypoglycemic events fell from 37 to 24 events per 100 patient years after
they switched to pump therapy (Fig. 2). Moreover, preschool children <7 years of
age had the greatest reduction in the risk of severe hypoglycemia. Because these
results were considerably better than the DCCT standards for intensive treatment
in children [5], it was concluded that CSII is an effective alternative to injection
therapy in a large pediatric diabetes clinic setting and that even very young
patients can use CSII safely to lower HbA_{1c} levels [14].

The number of children using pump therapy in the authors' clinic is now more
than 600 youngsters. All are using rapid-acting insulin analogues, and the quar-
terly mean HbA_{1c} levels for this cohort range between 7.2% and 7.4%.

Over the past 4 years, a number of centers have reported their experience in
youngsters who switched from injection to pump treatment [15–24]. As shown
by the representative studies listed in Table 1, most of these investigations involved fairly large cohorts of patients who covered the entire pediatric age range.
In comparison with glycemic control on injection therapy, these studies have
reported decreases in HbA_{1c} levels that ranged between 0.2% and 0.7%, reaching
values that were generally equal to or better than the DCCT standard [5].

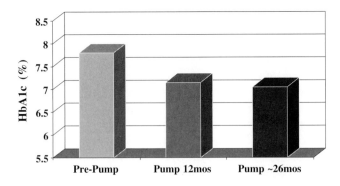

Fig. 1. Reduction in HbA_{1c} levels after switching from injection to pump therapy in the initial Yale
Children's Diabetes Clinic Study. (*Data from* Ahern JA, Boland EA, Doane R, et al. Insulin pump
therapy in pediatrics: a therapeutic alternative to safely lower therapy HbA1c levels across all age
groups. Pediatr Diabetes 2002;3:10–5.)

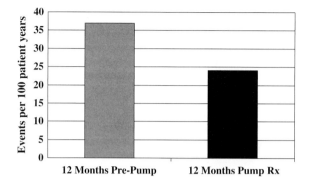

Fig. 2. Reduction in the rate of seizure and coma events during 12 months before and following switching to pump therapy in the initial Yale Children's Diabetes Clinic Study. (*Data from* Ahern JA, Boland EA, Doane R, et al. Insulin pump therapy in pediatrics: a therapeutic alternative to safely lower therapy HbA1c levels across all age groups. Pediatr Diabetes 2002;3:10–5.)

Although such decreases in HbA_{1c} levels might have been expected to increase the risk of hypoglycemia [5], a reduction in the frequency of severe hypogly-cemia has been consistently observed (see Table 1). Unlike the DCCT, excessive weight gain has not been a problem after switching from injection to pump therapy in children even in the face of better control. It should be noted, how-ever, that in many of these studies mean BMI was already 0.5 to 1 standard deviations above the mean for age before switching to pump therapy.

One of the last frontiers for pump therapy has been the use of this method of insulin delivery in infants, toddlers, and preschool children. Because treatment of very young patients with T1DM provides a special challenge, the authors recently analyzed long-term outcome data in this age group. Outcomes in 65 children who were less than 7 years of age at the start of insulin pump therapy were examined [21]. HbA_{1c} levels fell from 7.4% ± 1% to 6.9% ± 1%, and this level of control was sustained for up to 48 months. Even more important for children in this age group, the frequency of severe hypoglycemic events was reduced by more than

Table 1

Results of switching from injection to continuous subcutaneous insulin injection therapy in non-randomized pediatric studies

Author (ref)	N	Age (y)	Hemoglobin A_{1c} (%)	Hypoglycemia	BMI-z
Ahern et al [14]	161	1–18	7.8–7.1	Reduced	No change
Maniatis et al [15]	56	7–23	8.5–8.2	Reduced	No change
Plotnick et al [16]	95	4–18	8.1–7.7	Reduced	No change
Sulli and Shashaj [17]	40	4–25	9.5–8.8	Reduced	No change
Willi et al [18]	51	5–17	8.4–7.9	Reduced	No change
Mack-Fogg et al [20]	70	2–12	7.8–7.3	Reduced	Slight increase
Weinzimer et al [21]	65	1–6	7.4–6.8	Reduced	Slight decrease

Abbreviation: BMI-z, body mass index (z-score).

50%. Similar improvements in diabetes control were achieved in children with working mothers and mothers who stayed at home during the day.

Tubiana-Rufi and colleagues [22] also examined the usefulness of pump therapy in infants and toddlers. They studied youngsters who were experiencing recurrent episodes of hypoglycemia while on injection therapy. After switching to pump treatment, the frequency of severe hypoglycemic events was sharply reduced without sacrificing overall diabetes control. Similarly, positive results were reported in young children who were switched from injection to pump treatment by Litton and colleagues [23] and Shehadeh and colleagues [24].

Safety and efficacy of continuous subcutaneous insulin infusion in youth: results of randomized clinical trials

The first randomized study in pediatrics that compared the two therapies was undertaken in newly diagnosed patients. Although β-cell function was not prolonged, HbA_{1c} levels were significantly lower in the CSII group [25]. Weintrob and colleagues [26] used a randomized crossover design to compare the efficacy of CSII with a four shots per day regimen that used NPH insulin as basal insulin. Twenty-three children aged 9 to 13 years were studied for 3.5 months on each treatment. The changes in HbA_{1c} were similar with both treatments over time and there was a low rate of adverse events with each therapy.

The successful use of NPH insulin in the study by Weintrob and colleagues [26] is noteworthy, because it has been suggested that the clinical pharmacology of NPH insulin poses an important obstacle to safe and effective MDI therapy. Because NPH is a suspension, there is considerable dose-to-dose variability in the amount of insulin that is administered and absorbed [27] and the peaking action of this insulin makes it less than ideal for basal insulin replacement [28]. These limitations have been overcome to a great extent by the introduction of glargine insulin, the first soluble insulin analogue that has a flat and prolonged time-action profile [28]. Bolus-basal therapy that combines premeal aspart or lispro with glargine insulin has emerged as the gold standard for intensive MDI therapy in adults with T1DM.

A practical disadvantage of MDI with glargine in youth with T1DM is the large number of injections that are required daily. Unlike insulin suspensions, glargine cannot be mixed with rapid-acting insulin and must be injected separately. Because glargine does not peak, injections of rapid-acting insulin are also required for each meal and large snack to control postprandial hyperglycemia. Compliance problems with the frequent daily injections may, in part, explain why randomized pediatric trials have failed to show lower HbA_{1c} levels with glargine compared with NPH insulin [29,30].

The authors have recently completed a randomized, parallel group clinical trial comparing the effectiveness of CSII and MDI with glargine in lowering HbA_{1c} levels in children and adolescents with T1DM. Sixteen conventionally treated diabetic subjects who were naive to previous treatment with CSII and glargine

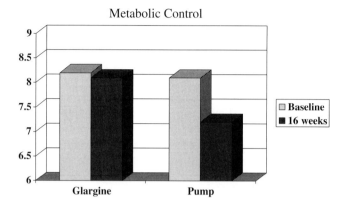

Fig. 3. Changes in HbA$_{1c}$ levels in the Yale randomized clinical trial comparing CSII with glargine-based MDI therapy. The difference in HbA$_{1c}$ levels between the CSII and glargine group at baseline was not significant. In contrast, at 16 weeks, HbA$_{1c}$ levels in the CSII group were significantly lower than baseline ($P < .02$) and versus glargine ($P < .05$). (*Data from* Doyle EA, Weinzimer SA, Steffen AT, et al. A randomized, prospective trial comparing the efficacy of continuous subcutaneous insulin infusion with multiple daily injections using insulin glargine. Diabetes Care 2004;27:1554–8.)

were randomized into each treatment group and changes in HbA$_{1c}$ levels assessed after 16 weeks of therapy. As shown in Fig. 3, subjects randomized to the glargine group were able to achieve as effective control of their diabetes as on conventional injection regimens. In contrast, patients randomized to CSII were able to significantly lower HbA$_{1c}$ values compared with their own baseline levels and versus the glargine group at 16 weeks [31]. It is noteworthy that 50% of patients in the CSII group were able to lower HbA$_{1c}$ to 7% or less versus only 12.5% in the MDI group. Two randomized clinical trials in preschool children with T1DM showed similar or slightly lower HbA$_{1c}$ levels with CSII versus injection therapy [32,33].

Subjective and other benefits of continuous subcutaneous insulin infusion

A qualitative approach with structured interviews has been used recently to examine the subjective response of patients and parents to pump treatment [34]. In that study, parents of very young patients consistently reported that CSII gave them their former lives back and that they were freed from the slavery of diabetes management that had previously affected the whole family. Shehadeh and colleagues [24] also reported improved diabetes quality of life and treatment satisfaction in parents of young children treated with CSII [24]. Low and colleagues [35] reported greater satisfaction with CSII in adolescents. Even though HbA$_{1c}$ levels did not differ, patients in the randomized cross-over study by Weintrob and colleagues [26] also reported higher treatment satisfaction with CSII than with MDI and 16 of the 23 patients elected to use pump rather than MDI therapy at the end of the study [26].

One of the less well-publicized advantages of insulin pump therapy is that the bolus history function of newer models allows clinicians and parents to track the child's compliance with administration of premeal bolus doses. Using this function, Burdick and colleagues [36] demonstrated that missing boluses is a common problem in youngsters with rising HbA_{1c} levels on CSII. There is no similar way to track bolus dose administration by patients on MDI therapy. In youth with T1DM, the risk of hypoglycemia is increased both during and on the night following prolonged aerobic exercise [37]. Children and adolescents on insulin pump therapy can decrease or suspend their rates of basal insulin infusion during exercise and use alternate overnight basal rates to reduce the risk of hypoglycemia. Acute reductions in the amount of basal insulin to prevent exercise-induced hypoglycemia are not readily achievable with long-acting insulins like glargine.

Importance of team management

The overriding conclusion from nonrandomized and randomized studies is that CSII provides an effective method of treatment of children and adolescents with T1DM across all age groups. It is also clear, however, that no single approach to treatment is ideal for every patient. The availability of multiple therapeutic options allows clinicians who care for children with T1DM to choose the best treatment for that individual patient at that particular time. Indeed, it can be effectively argued that the dedication, skill, and enthusiasm of the multidisciplinary team that cares for these youngsters play a primary role of the success of diabetes treatment. At the authors' center, diabetes nurse specialists (all advanced practice nurses) are the key members of the team who interact most frequently with the patients and parents [38]. These primary nurse managers remain in close contact with the families between office visits by telephone, email, and fax to adjust the treatment regimen and to maintain their commitment to treatment goals. Other members of the team, including the dietitian, psychologist, social worker, and pediatric endocrinologist, support the nurse managers. One of the major crises that pediatric diabetes care faces at the present time is that current insurance reimbursement rates cover only a small fraction of the actual costs of multidisciplinary care of children with this condition [39].

Toward a brighter future

Self-monitoring of blood glucose in combination with insulin pump therapy offers the possibility of controlling postprandial hyperglycemia and of reducing the risk of severe hypoglycemia. Most children and adolescents with T1DM only measure premeal blood glucose levels during the day, however, and they rarely measure glucose levels during the night, the time of greatest vulnerability to hypoglycemia [40]. Marked glycemic excursions from high to low values are undoubtedly missed by the brief glimpses into 24-hour glucose profiles provided by self-monitoring of blood glucose. Consequently, the recent development of methods for continuous monitoring of interstitial glucose concentrations has the potential to be one of the most important advances in the management of children and adolescents with T1DM in the past 20 years. Glucose sensor data regarding nocturnal glucose profiles should allow clinicians to exploit fully the variable basal rate capabilities of insulin pumps. Similarly, analysis of postprandial glycemic excursions can provide a more rational method of dividing daytime insulin replacement between basal and bolus doses in CSII-treated patients.

The Continuous Glucose Monitoring System (CGMS) developed by Medtronic MiniMed (Northridge, California) was the first continuous glucose-monitoring device approved by the US Food and Drug Administration. The CGMS sensor is inserted through a needle into the subcutaneous tissue of the anterior abdominal wall and measures interstitial glucose concentrations. The other Food and Drug Administration approved glucose sensing system is the GlucoWatch 2 Biographer (GW2B), developed by Cygnus (Redwood City, California). It looks like a watch and is worn on the forearm. Glucose is pulled from the interstitial fluid underneath the skin by reverse iontophoresis.

In comparison with the mature glucose meter technology that has benefited from 25 years of development, glucose sensor system technology is still in its infancy. Studies from the Diabetes Research in Children Network have demonstrated some of the limitations of the first-generation systems. As shown in Fig. 4, both the original CGMS and GW2B lack the accuracy and precision of current fingerstick blood-glucose meters, especially in the detection of hypoglycemia [41–43]. Moreover, in a recent randomized clinical trial involving

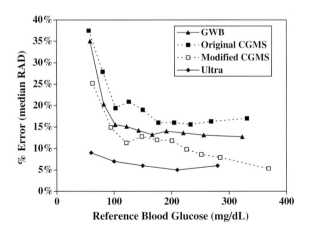

Fig. 4. Accuracy of the GlucoWatch G2 Biographer, original and modified CGMS, and One Touch Ultra meter in 89 children and adolescents with type 1 diabetes. % error (y-axis) represents the median relative absolute difference (RAD) of sensor and meter glucose levels compared with reference serum glucose values measured at a central laboratory for the DirecNet Study Group. (*Data from* references [41–43].)

200 children with T1DM, adding use of the GW2B to conventional glucose meter monitoring did not lower HbA$_{1c}$ levels or the frequency of hypoglycemia compared with conventional glucose monitoring alone [44]. By the end of the 6 months of that study, more than 25% of the GW2B group had stopped using the device altogether and the rest used it very infrequently. The modified CGMS sensor was shown to be more accurate than the original [45], however, and a real-time version of this system and others is on the verge of being introduced. Although much work still needs to be done, these breakthroughs in continuous glucose sensing suggest that clinicians may finally be at the threshold of the development of a practically applicable artificial endocrine pancreas, a prospect that has been anticipated for more than 30 years [46].

References

[1] Tamborlane WV, Sherwin RS, Genel M, et al. Reduction to normal of plasma glucose in juvenile diabetics by subcutaneous administration of insulin with a portable infusion pump. N Engl J Med 1979;300:573–8.
[2] Pickup JC, Keen H, Parsons JA, et al. Continuous subcutaneous insulin infusion: an approach to achieving normoglycemia. BMJ 1978;1:204–7.
[3] Lauritzen T, Pramming S, Deckert T, et al. Pharmacokinetics of continuous subcutaneous insulin infusion. Diabetologia 1983;24:326–9.
[4] DCCT Research Group. The effect of intensive treatment of diabetes on the development and progression of long-term complications in insulin-dependent diabetes mellitus. The Diabetes Control and Complications Trial. N Engl J Med 1993;329:977–86.
[5] The DCCT Research Group. The effect of intensive diabetes treatment on the development and progression of long-term complications in adolescents with insulin-dependent diabetes mellitus: the Diabetes Control and Complications Trial. J Pediatr 1994;125:177–88.
[6] DCCT/EDIC Research Group. Beneficial effects of intensive therapy of diabetes during adolescence: outcomes after the conclusion of the Diabetes Control and Complications Trial. J Pediatr 2001;139:804–12.
[7] DCCT Research Group. Resource utilization and costs of care in the Diabetes Control and Complications Trial. Diabetes Care 1995;18:1468–78.
[8] Howey DC, Bowsher RR, Brunelle RL, et al. [Lys(B28),Pro(B29)]-human insulin: a rapidly absorbed analogue of human insulin. Diabetes 1994;43:396–402.
[9] Zinman B, Tildesley H, Chiasson TJ, et al. Insulin lispro in CSII: results of a double-blind crossover study. Diabetes 1997;46:440–3.
[10] Mohn A, Matyka KA, Harris DA, et al. Lispro or regular insulin for multiple injection therapy in adolescence: differences in free insulin and glucose levels overnight. Diabetes Care 1999;22:27–32.
[11] Amiel SA, Caprio S, Sherwin RS, et al. Insulin resistance of puberty: a defect restricted to peripheral glucose metabolism. J Clin Endocrinol Metab 1991;72:277–82.
[12] Pickup J, Mattock M, Kerry S. Glycaemic control with continuous subcutaneous insulin infusion compared with intensive insulin injections in patients with type 1 diabetes: meta-analysis of randomised controlled trials. BMJ 2002;324:705–10.
[13] Boland EA, Grey M, Oesterle A, et al. Continuous subcutaneous insulin infusion: a new way to achieve strict metabolic control, decrease severe hypoglycemia and enhance coping in adolescents with type I diabetes. Diabetes Care 1999;22:1779–84.
[14] Ahern JA, Boland EA, Doane R, et al. Insulin pump therapy in pediatrics: a therapeutic alternative to safely lower therapy HbA1c levels across all age groups. Pediatr Diabetes 2002;3:10–5.

[15] Maniatis AK, Klingensmith GJ, Slover RH, et al. Continuous subcutaneous insulin infusion therapy for children and adolescents: an option for routine diabetes care. Pediatrics 2001; 107:351–6.

[16] Plotnick LP, Clark LM, Brancati FL, et al. Safety and effectiveness of insulin pump therapy in children and adolescents with type 1 diabetes. Diabetes Care 2003;26:1142–6.

[17] Sulli N, Shashaj B. Continuous subcutaneous insulin infusion in children and adolescents with diabetes mellitus: decreased HbA1c with low risk of hypoglycemia. J Pediatr Endocrinol 2003; 16:393–9.

[18] Willi SM, Planton J, Egede L, et al. Benefits of continuous subcutaneous insulin infusion in children with type 1 diabetes mellitus. J Pediatr 2003;143:796–801.

[19] Liberatore Jr R, Perlman K, Buccino J, et al. Continuous insulin infusion pump treatment in children with type 1 diabetes mellitus. J Pediatr Endocrinol 2004;17:223–6.

[20] Mack-Fogg JE, Orlowski CC, Jospe N. Continuous subcutaneous insulin infusion in toddlers and children with type 1 diabetes mellitus is safe and effective. Pediatr Diabetes 2005;6:17–21.

[21] Weinzimer SA, Ahern JA, Doyle EA, et al. Persistence of benefits of continuous subcutaneous insulin infusion in very young children with type 1 diabetes: a follow-up report. Pediatrics 2004; 114:1601–5.

[22] Tubiana-Rufi N, deLonlay P, Bloch J, et al. Remission of severe hypoglycemic incidents in young diabetic children treated with subcutaneous infusion. Arch Pediatr 1996;3:969–76.

[23] Litton J, Rice A, Friedman N, et al. Insulin pump therapy in toddlers and pre-school children with type 1 diabetes mellitus. J Pediatr 2002;141:490–5.

[24] Shehadeh N, Battelino T, Galatzer A, et al. Insulin pump therapy for 1–6 year old children with type 1 diabetes. Isr Med Assoc J 2004;6:284–6.

[25] de Beaufort CE, Houtzagers CM, Bruining GJ, et al. Continuous subcutaneous insulin infusion (CSII) versus conventional injection therapy in newly diagnosed diabetic children: two-year follow-up of a randomized, prospective trial. Diabet Med 1989;6:766–71.

[26] Weintrob N, Benzaquen H, Galatzar A, et al. Comparison of continuous subcutaneous insulin infusion and multiple daily injection regimens in children with type 1 diabetes: a randomized open crossover trial. Pediatrics 2003;112(3 Pt 1):559–64.

[27] Heise T, Nosek L, Ronn BB, et al. Lower within-subject variability of insulin detemir in comparison to NPH insulin and insulin glargine in people with type 1 diabetes. Diabetes 2004; 53:1614–20.

[28] Lepore M, Pampanelli S, Fanelli C, et al. Pharmacokinetics and pharmacodynamics of subcutaneous injection of long-acting human insulin analog glargine, NPH insulin, and ultralente human insulin and continuous subcutaneous infusion of insulin lispro. Diabetes 2000;49:2142–8.

[29] Schober E, Schoenle E, Van Dyk J, et al. Comparative trial between insulin glargine and NPH insulin in children and adolescents with type 1 diabetes mellitus. J Pediatr Endocrinol Metab 2002;15:369–76.

[30] Murphy NP, Keane SM, Ong KK, et al. Randomized cross-over trial of insulin glargine plus lispro or NPH insulin plus regular human insulin in adolescents with type 1 diabetes on intensive insulin regimens. Diabetes Care 2003;26:799–804.

[31] Doyle EA, Weinzimer SA, Steffen AT, et al. A randomized, prospective trial comparing the efficacy of continuous subcutaneous insulin infusion with multiple daily injections using insulin glargine. Diabetes Care 2004;27:1554–8.

[32] Wilson DM, Buckingham BA, Kunselman EL, et al. A two-center randomized controlled feasibility trial of insulin pump therapy in young children with diabetes. Diabetes Care 2005;28: 15–9.

[33] Di Meglio LA, Pottorff TM, Boyd SR, et al. A randomized, controlled study of insulin pump therapy in diabetic preschoolers. J Pediatr 2004;145:380–4.

[34] Sullivan-Bolyai S, Knafl K, Tamborlane W, et al. Parent's reflections on managing their children's diabetes with insulin pumps. J Nurs Scholarsh 2004;36:316–23.

[35] Low KG, Massa L, Lehman D, et al. Insulin pump use in young adolescents with type 1 diabetes: a descriptive study. Pediatr Diabetes 2005;6:22–31.

[36] Burdick J, Chase HP, Slover RH, et al. Missed insulin meal boluses and elevated hemoglobin A1c levels in children receiving insulin pump therapy. Pediatrics 2004;113(3 Pt 1):e221–4.

[37] The DirecNet Study Group. Impact of exercise on overnight glycemic control in children with type 1 diabetes. Diabetes 2005;54(Suppl 1):A64.

[38] Ahern JA, Ramchandani N, Cooper J, et al. Using a primary nurse manager to implement DCCT recommendations in a large pediatric program. Diabetes Educ 2000;26:990–4.

[39] Melzer SM, Richards GE, Covington ML. Reimbursement and costs of pediatric ambulatory diabetes care by using the resource-based relative value scale: is multidisciplinary care financially viable? Pediatr Diabetes 2004;5:133–42.

[40] Davis EA, Keating B, Byrne GC, et al. Hypoglycemia: incidence and clinical predictors in a large population based sample of children and adolescents with IDDM. Diabetes Care 1997; 20:22–5.

[41] Diabetes Research in Children Network (DirecNet) Study Group. The accuracy of the CGMS in children with type 1 diabetes: results of the Diabetes Research in Children Network (DirecNet) accuracy study. Diabetes Technol Ther 2003;5:781–9.

[42] Diabetes Research in Children Network (DirecNet) Study Group. The accuracy of the GlucoWatch G2 biographer in children with type 1 diabetes: results of the Diabetes Research in Children Network (DirecNet) accuracy study. Diabetes Technol Ther 2003;5:791–800.

[43] Diabetes Research in Children Network (DirecNet) Study Group. A multicenter study of the accuracy of the One Touch Ultra home glucose meter in children with type 1 diabetes. Diabetes Technol Ther 2003;5:933–41.

[44] The DirecNet Study Group. A randomized multicenter trial comparing the GlucoWatch Biographer with standard glucose monitoring in children with type 1 diabetes. Diabetes Care 2005;28:1101–6.

[45] The DirecNet Study Group. Accuracy of the modified Continuous Glucose Monitoring System (CGMS) sensor in an outpatient setting: results from a Diabetes Research in Children Network (DirecNet) study. Diabetes Technol Ther 2005;7:109–14.

[46] Albisser AM, Leibel BS, Ewart TG, et al. Clinical control of diabetes by the artificial pancreas. Diabetes 1974;23:397–404.

ELSEVIER
SAUNDERS

PEDIATRIC CLINICS
OF NORTH AMERICA

Pediatr Clin N Am 52 (2005) 1689–1703

Oral Agents in Managing Diabetes Mellitus in Children and Adolescents

Elka Jacobson-Dickman, MD[a,b], Lynne Levitsky, MD[a,b],*

[a]Department of Pediatrics, Massachusetts General Hospital for Children and
Harvard Medical School, 25 Shattuck Street, Boston, MA 02115, USA
[b]Pediatric Endocrine Unit, Massachusetts General Hospital, 55 Fruit Street, Boston, MA 02114, USA

Most cases of diabetes in childhood are immunologically mediated and eventually lead to complete insulin deficiency. Oral therapies for children with type 1 autoimmune diabetes mellitus (T1DM) are experimental and of unproven efficacy. Eight percent to 45% of children with newly diagnosed diabetes have non–immune-mediated diabetes [1]. Oral medication is often a feasible option for this group of children. The phenotype of type 2 diabetes mellitus (T2DM) is similar in adults and children and includes hyperglycemia, obesity, dyslipidemia, and insulin resistance. Patients who have T2DM are at risk for the same cluster of long-term complications as persons with T1DM, including nephropathy, retinopathy, and neuropathy [2]. Children and young people who have T2DM have a greater risk of early retinopathy and nephropathy than youth with T1DM and have a greater risk of macrovascular disease [3]. The United Kingdom Prospective Diabetes Study (UKPDS) showed that aggressive treatment of hyperglycemia can reduce complications in adults with T2DM [4]. The treatment of T2DM in adults can be intricate because the disorder is usually accompanied by other metabolic and cardiovascular disorders that also require therapy [2]. These therapies can complicate diabetes treatment. For example, thiazides and beta blockers worsen hyperglycemia. Therapy for T2DM in children and adolescents is usually less complicated by comorbidity. Because children may live many more years with diabetes and are diagnosed relatively early in the course of their disease, an argument for intensive treatment is easily made. Despite the

* Corresponding author. Pediatric Endocrine Unit, BHX 410, Massachusetts General Hospital, 55 Fruit Street, Boston, MA 02114.
E-mail address: llevitsky@partners.org (L. Levitsky).

0031-3955/05/$ – see front matter © 2005 Elsevier Inc. All rights reserved.
doi:10.1016/j.pcl.2005.07.008

wealth of experience and knowledge concerning the epidemiology, pathophysiology, and medical management of T2DM in adults, we know little about the disease in children [1]. It is possible that reversal of insulin resistance and restoration of euglycemia could lead to a remission of the disorder in a substantial number of young people.

Type 1 diabetes mellitus

Attempts to develop an insulin preparation that could be administered orally and would be absorbed either by the intestinal route or by the buccal mucosa continue. To date, all such preparations remain experimental and of unproved long-term efficacy [5]. Oral administration of large quantities of insulin in an attempt to prevent T1DM or progression of the disorder has not been successful, although small subgroups in these studies may have responded positively [6,7]. Other agents, such as nicotinamide and diazoxide, have been administered in short-term trials in an attempt to ameliorate the severity of T1DM and prolong the remission phase. None has been shown to be of significant long-term benefit [8,9]. Agents to reduce insulin resistance, such as biguanide, metformin, or the thiazolidinediones, pioglitazone, or rosiglitazone, theoretically could enhance diabetes control by ameliorating the insulin resistance of puberty or prolonging the remission phase of T1DM. Neither class of drug has been studied in a formal manner to prove efficacy in children with this disorder. Alpha glucosidase inhibitors (eg, acarbose, miglitol) have been suggested as useful agents for reducing postprandial hyperglycemia, but there are no careful prospective studies [10]. These agents are discussed in the section on T2DM.

Type 2 diabetes mellitus

Until recently, insulin was the only drug approved by the US Food and Drug Administration for the treatment of T2DM in children. However, most pediatric endocrinologists have used oral agents in this population. There is little evidence that insulin is superior to oral agents for initial therapy for mild T2DM [1]. Some experts assert that insulin remains the most effective drug in treating T2DM, which assumes that patients and caregivers are willing to use the large doses that are required to achieve euglycemia [11]. Aggressive and earlier treatment with insulin may increase remission rates and decrease HbA1c by approximately 2.5% [12]. However, T2DM is a disorder of both beta cell function and insulin sensitivity. Beta cell function worsens with duration of diabetes, which leads to eventual insulin dependence [13]. Some classes of oral agents theoretically could prevent or delay the gradual loss of beta cell function by reducing insulin resistance or the need for maximal islet insulin secretion.

General advantages of oral agents include potential greater adherence and convenience for the patient and family. Oral therapies available for the treatment of T2DM have expanded, providing greater flexibility for physicians and patients. Some agents may offer additional therapeutic advantage by reducing insulin resistance and its comorbidities, including hypertension, early cardiovascular disease, hyperlipidemia, and polycystic ovary disease. The goal of treatment is normalization of blood glucose values and HbA1c and control of such comorbidities [14]. The ultimate goal of treatment is to decrease the risk of acute and chronic complications associated with diabetes.

Currently, five categories of glucose-lowering oral agents are available in the United States for the treatment of T2DM [15,16]. Drugs used in T2DM include biguanides, thiazolidinediones, sulfonylureas, glitinides, and glycosidase inhibitors. It is useful to classify these medications based on their mechanism of action: drugs that decrease insulin resistance (ie, metformin, thiazolidinediones), drugs that stimulate insulin release (ie, sulfonylureas, glitinides), and drugs that decrease glucose absorption (ie, glucosidase inhibitors) (Table 1).

Drugs that decrease insulin resistance

Metformin

Metformin hydrochloride is an oral antihyperglycemic agent that has been marketed in the United States for the treatment of adult T2DM since 1995. Phenformin, the prototype biguanide, was withdrawn from the US market many years ago because of reports of lactic acidosis. It was associated with hypertension and tachycardia and with excess cardiovascular mortality in the University Group Diabetes Program. Metformin is rarely associated with serious side effects.

Metformin is the only oral agent currently approved by the US Food and Drug Administration for use in children. This drug improves glycemic control by reducing hepatic glucose production, increasing insulin sensitivity, and reducing intestinal glucose absorption without increasing insulin secretion [17]. It is effective in obese and nonobese patients. Its cellular mechanism of action is poorly understood. Many studies in humans and animal models have identified the liver as the primary target of metformin action [18]. One target for metformin is an AMP-activated protein kinase, which, when stimulated, inhibits lipogenesis and decreases hepatic steatosis [19]. In an uncontrolled study, metformin decreased transaminases in patients with nonalcoholic steatohepatitis [20]. Metformin has been shown to lower HbA1c by 1.5% to 2% [21]. Metformin is the most commonly prescribed oral antidiabetic agent in the United States for the treatment of T2DM. Before the publication of a multicenter trial in 2002, however, it had never been formally studied in children with T2DM. This pharmaceutical company–sponsored clinical trial evaluated the safety and efficacy of metformin at doses up to 1000 mg twice daily in 82 subjects aged 10 to 16 years with body mass index more than the fiftieth percentile, fasting plasma glucose levels ranging from 126 to 240 mg/dL (7.0 and 13.3 μmol/L), mean HbA1c of 7%, and stimulated C-peptide 1.5 ng/mL (0.5 nmol/L). Children were treated for up to 16 weeks in a randomized, double-blind, placebo-controlled trial. Met-

Table 1
Oral hypoglycemic agents

Drug	Mechanism of action	Duration of biologic effect (h)	Usual daily dose (mg)	Doses/day	Side effects	Caution
Biguanide	Insulin sensitizer				Gastrointestinal disturbance, lactic acidosis	
Metformin			1500–2500	2–3		Avoid in hepatic or renal impairment
Sulfonylureas						
First generation						
acetohexamide		12–18	500–750	1 or divided		
chlorpropamide		27–72	250–500	1		
tolbutamide		14–16	1000–2000	1 or divided		
Second generation						
glipizide		14–16	2.5–10 XL:5–10	1 or divided 1		
gliburide		20–24+	2.5–10	1 or divided		
glimepride		24+	2–4	1		
Glitinides	Promote insulin secretion					
repaglinide		≤24	2–16	3		Titrate carefully in renal or hepatic dysfunction
nateglinide		4	360	3		
α-Glucosidase inhibitors	Slow hydrolysis and absorption of complex carbohydrates				Transient gastrointestinal disturbances	
acarbose			150–300	3 (with meals)		
miglitol			150–300	3 (with meals)		
Thiazolidinedione	Peripheral insulin sensitizer				Upper respiratory tract infection, headache, edema, weight gain	
rosiglitazone			4–8	1 or divided		
pioglitazone			15–45	1		

formin significantly improved glycemic control and HbA1c values. It did not have a negative impact on body weight or lipid profile. Adverse events were similar to those reported in adults treated with metformin and included abdominal pain, diarrhea, nausea, vomiting, and headache. No cases of clinical hypoglycemia, lactic acidosis, or clinically significant changes in physical examinations occurred during this study. The study concluded that metformin was a safe and effective for treatment of T2DM in children and adolescents [22].

Metformin reduces HbA1c and blood glucose with little risk of hypoglycemia. Body weight remains stable or decreases slightly, hypertension is improved, and low-density lipoprotein (LDL) cholesterol and triglyceride levels decrease [1]. It is commonly recommended that patients be started on a low dose of metformin (500 mg once daily) and titrated up as tolerated to 1000 mg twice daily. Treatment with metformin may normalize ovulatory abnormalities in patients with polycystic ovarian syndrome and increase fertility and risk of unplanned pregnancies. Preconception and contraception counseling should be part of the treatment regimen with initiation of this drug. No oral hypoglycemic agents are approved for use during pregnancy, which further emphasizes the importance of such counseling [1].

Metformin is contraindicated in patients with impaired renal function because of concerns about induction of lactic acidosis. For the same reason, metformin should be discontinued temporarily before administration of parenteral radiocontrast material. Metformin also should not be used in patients with known hepatic disease, hypoxemic conditions, severe infections, or alcohol abuse, although nonalcoholic steatohepatitis may improve with metformin therapy. The drug should be discontinued temporarily with any acute illness associated with dehydration or hypoxemia, and insulin should be used for acute glycemic control. The most common side effects are gastrointestinal upset, including loss of appetite, nausea, flatulence, and diarrhea [1,16]. Side effects are diminished by administering metformin with food—but not with milk alone—and by slow titration of dose. Patients should be warned that initial gastrointestinal discomfort may be noted for 3 to 7 days but does not usually persist.

Thiazolidinediones

Thiazolidinediones are the newest class of approved antidiabetic agents. Thiazolidinediones originally were identified while screening for potential hypolipidemic agents. These agents act as peripheral insulin sensitizers. They bind to one receptor in a family of nuclear receptors known as peroxisomal proliferative activated receptors (PPAR-γ), which have a range of ligands, including fibric acids. Among other actions, they affect the differentiation of preadipocytes to adipocytes. The precise mechanism of glycemic reduction is unknown [23]. The nuclear receptor PPAR-γ is predominantly expressed in adipose tissue and, to a lesser extent, in liver and muscle [24]. A proposed mechanism of PPAR-γ effects in muscle and liver is indirect and results from modification of gene expression in adipose tissue by increasing adiponectin expression, which in mice has insulin-sensitizing effects, especially in the liver [25]. This group of drugs seems to enhance insulin action in peripheral tissues and the liver. Direct comparison of troglitazone and metformin suggested that the primary mechanism of troglitazone action is stimulation of peripheral glucose disposal [26].

Studies in animals and more than 5000 people with T2DM demonstrated troglitazone to be without significant side effects, except at high doses. In postmarketing retrospective examination, rare episodes of liver failure leading to transplantation and death were reported. The occurrence of mild liver dysfunction was rare and reversible. After these findings, the US Food and Drug Administration required frequent monitoring of liver function tests during the first year of this drug's use. After two new thiazolidinediones (ie, pioglitazone and rosiglitazone) were approved, troglitazone was taken off the market. It is believed that a side chain of the troglitazone molecule not found in the newer agents likely was responsible for liver dysfunction. Liver function testing is still required, but not as frequently. Current recommendations are that liver enzymes should be checked before the initiation of therapy in all patients and periodically thereafter based on the clinical judgment of the medical provider. Therapy should not be initiated if baseline liver function tests are more than double the upper limit of normal. If at any time during treatment liver enzymes increase to levels triple the upper limit of normal or symptoms of liver failure ensue, the medication should be discontinued while the problem is investigated. Rosiglitazone and pioglitazone were compared with troglitazone in a prospective, randomized conversion study. There were similar effects of rosiglitazone and pioglitazone with respect to weight gain and glycemic control after conversion from troglitazone. The lipid profile of patients receiving these newer agents improved [27].

Rosiglitazone and pioglitazone are indicated either as monotherapy or in combination with a sulfonylurea, metformin, or insulin when diet, exercise, and a single agent do not result in adequate glycemic control. They are considered relatively weak hypoglycemic drugs and lower HbA1c by only 0.5% to 1%. When used in monotherapy, weight gain and hypoglycemia do not seem to be a major problem. Both drugs may improve lipids, blood pressure, inflammatory biomarkers, endothelial function, and fibrinolytic status. These beneficial effects of thiazolidinediones on glycemia and cardiovascular risk factors have made them potentially useful agents for patients with T2DM who are at high risk for coronary vascular disease. Edema can occur in patients treated with either drug and could precipitate congestive heart failure. Although the safety profile of thiazolidinediones in patients without underlying heart disease is favorable, the risk must be considered in patients with underlying heart disease. [28].

A large-scale pharmaceutical company–sponsored multicenter trial demonstrated that pioglitazone was a well-tolerated and efficacious monotherapy for patients with T2DM. At maximal doses tested, the HbA1c reduction observed was between 0.5% and 1%, but dyslipidemia was ameliorated as an additional benefit [29].

Drugs that stimulate insulin release

Sulfonylureas

Sulfonylureas are the oldest class of drugs and were first developed 50 years ago. For more than two decades, second-generation drugs that have fewer side effects and drug interactions and are more potent have been available for use [30]. Sulfonylureas act by stimulating insulin secretion, likely by binding to a specific (SUR1) beta cell receptor. They are ineffective in patients who have T1DM and T2DM who do not have the capacity for adequate insulin release. Sulfonylureas lower blood glucose in 80% to 90% of newly treated type 2 patients and decrease HbA1c by 1% to 1.5%. However, the secondary failure rate is approximately 10% per year [31]. Within 5 years of beginning sulfonylurea therapy, most patients require a second drug to achieve near normoglycemia. The University Group Diabetes Program and UKPDS studies are the longest interventional studies with sulfonylureas. They demonstrated that after initial response to sulfonylureas, glycemic control drifted upward, and within approximately 5 years, glycemia returned to baseline [32,33].

Hypoglycemia and weight gain are the major side effects of sulfonylureas. The University Group Diabetes Program study suggested that tolbutamide, a first-generation sulfonylurea, was associated with excess cardiovascular mortality. These results have been debated, however, and the UKPDS results did not support this contention.

Tolbutamide is no longer commercially available. Chlorpropamide, an early, long-acting sulfonylurea (hypoglycemic effects may persist for up to 5 days), is used rarely because of its duration of action and risk of hypoglycemia. Glyburide, glipizide, and glimepiride are the most commonly used drugs in this class currently. Usage indications are described in Table 1. Glipizide and glimepiride should be used in individuals with renal disease because metabolism is largely hepatic. Glyburide may cause more hypoglycemia and may interfere with myocardial preconditioning in ischemic heart disease. It might not be considered the first drug of choice in adults. Data in children and adolescents are not available.

Glitinides

Glitinides (eg, repaglinide and nateglinide) stimulate endogenous insulin secretion by activating the voltage-dependent calcium channel of the beta cell. Because they have a more rapid on-and-off effect than the sulfonylureas, the expectation was that there would be less unpredictable hypoglycemia. This benefit, however, has not yet been demonstrated, although they have been available in the United States since 1998. These drugs are administered immediately before meals and enhance postprandial insulin release. They may be particularly suitable early in T2DM in adolescents and children when postprandial hyperglycemia is a major manifestation of the disorder. An ongoing clinical trial is also evaluating their use in cystic fibrosis–related diabetes in which postprandial hyperglycemia is a major concern. The glitinides have rapid clearance and action and can be used safely in patients who have renal failure.

There are limited data regarding efficacy. One study compared 24-week outcome in 701 patients who had T2DM who were randomly assigned to metformin, nateglinide, both agents, or placebo. In the study, nateglinide was less potent than metformin as monotherapy [34]. The mean decrease in HbA1c during monotherapy with these agents is 1.5% to 2% [16].

Drugs that interfere with carbohydrate absorption

Alpha-glucosidase inhibitors were approved in the United States in 1996. These drugs inhibit luminal enzymes involved in the digestion of carbohydrate in the small intestine and must be taken before meals. Inhibition of carbohydrate digestion decreases postprandial glycemia and may affect release of some gut hormones that potentiate altered blood glucose responses. This effect has been used to advantage to treat the metabolic component of dumping syndrome. Unabsorbed carbohydrate is delivered to the large intestine, where bacterial fermentation produces increased gas formation. Approximately 30% of patients suffer gastrointestinal side effects of borborygmi, abdominal discomfort, and flatulence. Otherwise, because the drugs are not absorbed, they have no systemic side effects. They are relatively weak hypoglycemic agents and lower HbA1c by 0.5% to 1% [35], and they may be used as a single agent in patients with mild T2DM or in combination with other oral agents or insulin.

Treatment plan for management of type 2 diabetes mellitus

A suggested treatment plan is summarized in Fig. 1. The first "oral therapy" for the treatment of mild T2DM arguably should be the reduction of caloric intake. Exercise promotion and advice from a pediatric dietician should complement medical management. Successful treatment with diet and exercise in children has been defined by an American Diabetes Association consensus committee as cessation of weight gain with normal linear growth, near-normal fasting blood glucose values, (<126 mg/dL), and near-normal HbA1c (<7% in most laboratories) [1]. There is some rationale for a more stringent standard in children and adolescents so that when possible, return to true normoglycemia with an HbA1c less than 6%, a fasting blood glucose less than 100 mg/dL, and a normal 2-hour postglucose response of less than 140 mg/dL should be an aim.

Diet modification and exercise regimen implementation are effective first-line interventions for T2DM but are often difficult to implement. If desired control is not achieved or if at diagnosis hyperglycemia is severe, pharmacologic therapy is necessary. Only 8% of adults who had newly diagnosed T2DM were able to maintain glycemic control through diet, exercise, and weight reduction [36].

The initial treatment of T2DM varies depending on the clinical presentation. The management of a well child with new-onset T2DM depends on the degree of

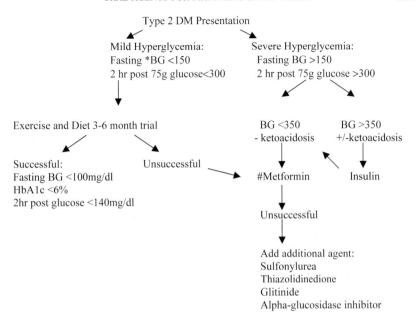

Fig. 1. Type 2 diabetes mellitus management.

hyperglycemia and insulin resistance. Diet modification and regular exercise implementation may appropriate initial steps for a patient with milder T2DM, whereas one may add a first-line oral hypoglycemic agent in a patient who has more severe and progressed disease. Metformin, which is the only oral agent approved by the US Food and Drug Administration for use in children, is a reasonable first-line agent.

The unwell patient with ketosis or ketoacidosis or blood glucose more than 300 mg/dL should be treated with insulin on presentation. The diagnosis and management can be reviewed subsequently if there are clinical features suggesting T2DM, including a strong family history, obesity, presence of skin findings of acanthosis nigricans, and slow historic onset of disease. High C-peptide levels and negative anti-islet autoantibodies offer laboratory confirmation of T2DM [13]. A minority of children with apparent T2DM have islet autoantibodies. These patients may not require insulin within the first several years of diagnosis and seem to have a slowly progressive latent autoimmune form of diabetes [37]. The absence of beta cell autoimmune markers (islet cell antibodies, glutamic acid decarboxylase antibodies, and insulin autoantibodies without previous insulin therapy) has been a diagnostic prerequisite for T2DM. Although the incidence of diabetes antibody markers was significantly lower in T2DM versus T1DM, in one study, 8.1% of patients with T2DM had positive islet cell antibodies, 30.3% had positive glutamic acid decarboxylase antibodies, and 34.8% had positive insulin autoantibodies without ever being treated with insulin.

In the T2DM group, none of the Hispanic patients had islet cell antibodies. These data suggest that islet cell antibody positivity at diagnosis could be a predictor of future insulin need [38].

The pathophysiology of T2DM in the pediatric population seems to be similar to that in adults, so it is reasonable to assume that oral agents other than metformin will be effective in children. Efficacy and safety data currently are not available for this population, however.

Almost all combinations of therapies have been attempted in the treatment of T2DM. Substitution of one drug for another has not been as successful as addition of other agents to the antidiabetic regimen. It is reasonable to personalize such therapies based on the particular needs of the individual with the understanding that each child must be treated to a close to euglycemic target and, if such treatment fails, must receive insulin therapy. Continued adherence to a healthy nutrition and exercise regimen contributes to the success of the oral therapies. The principle in using several drugs should be to combine medications with varied mechanisms of action. For example, combining a sulfonylurea with metformin has been shown to improve glycemic control in patients who fail to improve on sulfonylurea therapy alone [21,39]. Likewise, combining acarbose with insulin, sulfonylurea, or diet lowers the HbA1c further by 0.5% to 1% [35]. Metformin and a thiazolinedione in combination also have enhanced the effect of metformin alone [16].

If single-drug therapy with metformin is not successful over a period of 3 to 6 months, several alternatives can be considered. One can add a sulfonylurea, other insulin secretagogues, and glucosidase inhibitors, although they have been less frequently chosen alternatives in children and adolescents [1]. Effectiveness of these agents can be assessed within days by examining blood glucose and within 1 or 2 months by examining HbA1c. Addition of a thiazolidinedione has the theoretic advantage of further reducing insulin resistance, but these drugs lead to weight gain and redistribution of fat from intra-abdominal to peripheral sites, which may be cosmetically difficult for adolescents. Edema, although not usually severe enough to cause cardiac compromise in children, also may become a cosmetic problem. Thiazolidinediones take several months to reach full effect.

The ultimate goal of treatment of T2DM is to reduce long-term cardiovascular and other morbidities associated with hyperglycemia and perhaps insulin resistance. Endothelial dysfunction in T2DM tends to be progressive and is strongly associated with cardiovascular disease risk. Studies of children and adolescents with long-term follow-up into adulthood are not available, but adult studies using surrogate markers suggest potential effectiveness of some of these drugs. For example, 16 weeks of metformin treatment in patients with T2DM treated with insulin was associated with significant improvement of endothelial function markers but not of chronic, low-grade inflammation. Changes in the plasma levels of these markers were independent of metformin-associated favorable changes in body weight, glycemic control, insulin dose, and LDL cholesterol concentration. No effect of short-term treatment with metformin on markers of low-grade inflammation (ie, soluble intercellular adhesion molecule and C-reactive protein) was found [40].

Adult studies demonstrate that treatment of euglycemia using oral agents and insulin reduces long-term morbidity and mortality. The Diabetes Control and Complications Trial demonstrated the importance of intensive therapy in decreasing the risk of development and progression of all diabetes-specific complications in T1DM [41]. The UKPDS Group studied the effect of intensive blood glucose control with either sulfonylureas or insulin compared with conventional treatment and risk of complications in patients who have T2DM [32,33]. This study originally was planned and initiated in 1977, and results were published in 1998. The UKPDS results demonstrated a benefit of intensive therapy, which lowered HbA1c by 1%, with a reduction of risk of poor diabetic outcomes by 12%. The benefits were looked at separately. Metformin therapy resulted in less weight gain and hypoglycemic episodes than other intensive therapies. Aggregate diabetes mortality, but not diabetes-related outcomes, was significantly reduced by metformin. Early addition of metformin to sulfonylureas resulted in a large and statistically significant increase in cardiovascular mortality, however. Although the validity of some of the analysis strategies and the UKPDS's complex design have been called into question, the essential observation that intensive diabetes management improves outcome was largely seen by reduction in retinopathy and cataracts. There was no significant benefit with regard to cardiovascular disease [42].

Monitoring and treatment of T2DM comorbid conditions are crucial to the care of these patients. Careful control of hypertension in these children is critical. Angiotensin-converting enzyme inhibitors are the agents of choice in children with microalbuminuria. This group of antihypertensive agents has the added benefit of preventing diabetic nephropathy and is considered first-line therapy by most pediatric endocrinologists. The Joint National Committee VI report also recommends beta blockers, calcium antagonists (long acting), and low-dose diuretics [43]. There has been concern that use of beta blockers may worsen hypoglycemia and mask hypoglycemic symptoms. In select patients, however, the risks may be outweighed by the benefits. Dyslipidemia outweighs other risk factors for cardiovascular disease in adults who have T2DM. Children and adolescents who have T2DM may have hyperlipidemia and should be screened as soon as initial glycemic control is achieved. If normal lipid values are obtained, screening should be repeated every 2 years. Optimal lipid levels for persons with diabetes are defined as LDL < 100 mg/dL, high density lipoprotein > 35 mg/dL, and triglycerides < 150 mg/dL. In the absence of improvement with weight loss, increased activity, and improvement of glycemic control, medications could be used for children with the following profile[40]: older than 10 years, LDL ≥ 160 mg/dL, or LDL 130–159 mg/dL depending on the child's cardiovascular risk profile. The HMG CoA reductase inhibitors (statins) may be used first line with or without the addition of resins (bile acid sequestrants). Resins continue to be generally recommended as first-choice treatments in this age group; however, compliance rates with this class of medications are so low that therapeutic efficacy is lacking. Statin drugs also should be considered as a first-line agent. Fibric acid derivatives are recommended if triglycerides > 1000 mg/dL. It is important to note that the statins are contraindicated in pregnancy and should not be used in girls of childbearing age in the absence of extensive counseling and use of effective contraception. When statins are used, treatment should begin at the lowest available dose and dose increases should be based on LDL levels and side effects. Liver function tests should be monitored and medication should be discontinued if liver function tests are more than triple the upper limit of normal. If there is any persistent complaint of significant muscle pain or muscle soreness, the medication should be discontinued with observation for symptoms resolution [44].

Ongoing studies that may influence future management

Important ongoing trials that should broaden our knowledge and likely influence our therapeutic decisions in youth who have T2DM include the Treatment Options for T2DM in Adolescents and Youth (TODAY) study and A Diabetes Outcome Progression Trial (ADOPT) study. The TODAY study is an ongoing trial that compares three treatments of T2DM in children and teens, which is currently being conducted in 12 medical centers and affiliated sites in the United States. Patients are being randomly assigned to one of three treatment groups: metformin alone, metformin plus rosiglitazone, and metformin plus intensive lifestyle change aimed at diet and exercise intervention. Participating researchers plan to enroll 750 children and adolescents between 10 and 17 years of age, and the trial is expected to have a 5-year duration. The TODAY study's investigative goals include treatment safety, influence on individual and family behaviors, cost-effectiveness, and efficacy with outcome measures of insulin production and resistance, body composition, nutrition, fitness, diabetes-associated morbidity, quality of life, and psychological outcomes. ADOPT is a double-blinded, prospective, randomized, controlled trial that was developed to compare three mechanistically distinct antidiabetic agents currently available for the first-line pharmacologic treatment of T2DM (ie, metformin, rosiglitazone, and glyburide) in terms of their effects on glycemic control, beta cell function, and cardiovascular risk factors in adults. The study began in March 2000 and approximately 500 centers in North America, Canada, and Europe are participating in the study. Eligible patients are aged 30 to 75 years and have been diagnosed with T2DM within 3 years from study screening and have been previously managed only with diet and exercise [36].

Summary

T2DM is a chronic disease with potentially devastating long-term complications. Despite the tremendous body of research and experience concerning T2DM in adults, little is known about this condition and its optimal treatment in children. The pediatric community still must await further safety and efficacy studies of oral hypoglycemic agents in children and adolescents and continue to use efficacy data gathered in adult populations.

References

[1] American Diabetes Association. Type 2 diabetes in children and adolescents. Pediatrics 2000; 105(3 Pt 1):671–80.

[2] Nathan D. Long-term complications of diabetes mellitus. N Engl J Med 1993;328(23):1676–85.

[3] Henricsson M, Nystrom L, Blohme G, et al. The incidence of retinopathy 10 years after diagnosis in young adult people with diabetes: results from the nationwide population-based Diabetes Incidence Study in Sweden (DISS). Diabetes Care 2003;26(2):349–54.

[4] Adler AI, Stratton IM, Neil HA, et al. Association of systolic blood pressure with macrovascular and microvascular complications of type 2 diabetes (UKPDS 36): prospective observational study. BMJ 2000;321(7258):412–9.

[5] Uwaifo G, Ratner R. Novel pharmacologic agents for type 2 diabetes. Endocrinol Metab Clin N Am 2005;34:155–97.

[6] Skyler J, Krischer J, Wolfsdorf J, et al. Effects of oral insulin in relatives of patients with type 1 diabetes: the Diabetes Prevention Trial-Type 1. Diabetes Care 2005;28:1068–76.

[7] Ergun-Longmire B, Marker J, Zeidler A, et al. Oral insulin therapy to prevent progression of immune-mediated (type 1) diabetes. Ann N Y Acad Sci 2004;1029:260–77.

[8] Crino A, Schiaffini R, Manfrini S, et al. A randomized trial of nicotinamide and vitamin E in children with recent onset type 1 diabetes (IMDIAB IX). Eur J Endocrinol 2004;150:719–24.

[9] Ortqvist E, Bjork E, Wallensteen M, et al. Temporary preservation of beta-cell function by diazoxide treatment in childhood type 1 diabetes. Diabetes Care 2004;27:2191–7.

[10] Rios M. Acarbose and insulin therapy in type 1 diabetes mellitus. Eur J Clin Invest 1994; 24(Suppl 3):36–9.

[11] Nathan D. Clinical practice: initial management of glycemia in type 2 diabetes mellitus. N Engl J Med 2002;347(17):1342–9.

[12] Ilkova H, Glaser B, Tunckale A, et al. Induction of long-term glycemic control in newly diagnosed type 2 diabetic patients by transient intensive insulin treatment. Diabetes Care 1997; 20(9):1353–6.

[13] Porter J, Barrett T. Acquired non-type 1 diabetes in childhood: subtypes, diagnosis, and management. Arch Dis Child 2004;89(12):1138–44.

[14] American Diabetes Association. Standards of medical care for patients with diabetes mellitus: position statement. Diabetes Care 1999;22(1S):32S–41S.

[15] De Fronzo R. Pharmacologic therapy for type 2 diabetes mellitus. Ann Intern Med 1999; 131(4):281–303.

[16] Riddle M. Glycemic management of type 2 diabetes: an emerging strategy with oral agents, insulin, and combinations. Enocrinol Metab Clin N Am 2005;34:77–98.

[17] Baily CJ. Biguanides and NIDDM. Diabetes Care 1992;15(6):755–72.

[18] Tiikkainen M, Hakkinen A, Korshennikova E, et al. Effects of rosiglitazone and metformin on liver fat content, hepatic insulin resistance, insulin clearance, and gene expression in adipose tissue in patients with type 2 diabetes. Diabetes 2004;53:2169–76.

[19] Zhou G, Myers R, Li Y, et al. Role of AMP-activated protein kinase in mechanism of metformin action. J Clin Invest 2001;108:1167–74.

[20] Caballero A, Arora S, Saouaf R, et al. Micro and macro-vascular reactivity is reduced in subjects at risk for type 2 diabetes. Diabetes 1999;48:1856–62.

[21] De Fronzo R, Goodman A. Efficacy of metformin in patients with non-insulin-dependent diabetes mellitus: the Multicenter Metformin Study Group. N Engl J Med 1995;333(9):541–9.

[22] Jones K, Arslanian S, Peterokova V, et al. Effect of metformin in pediatric patients with type 2 diabetes: a randomized controlled trial. Diabetes Care 2002;25(1):89–94.

[23] Spiegelman B. PPAR-gamma: adipogenic regulator and thiazolidinedione receptor. Diabetes 1998;47(4):507–14.

[24] Vidal-Puig A, Considine R, Jimenez-Linan M, et al. Peroxisome-proliferator activated receptor gene expression in human tissues: effects of obesity, weight loss, and regulation by insulin and glucocorticoids. J Clin Invest 1997;99:2416–22.

[25] Combs T, Berg A, Obici S, et al. Endogenous glucose production is inhibited by adipose-derived protein Acrp30. J Clin Invest 2001;2001:1875–81.

[26] Inzucchi S, Maggs D, Spollett G, et al. Efficacy and metabolic effects of metformin and troglitazone in type II diabetes mellitus. N Engl J Med 1998;338(13):867–72.

[27] Khan M, St Peter J, Xue J. A prospective, randomized comparison of the metabolic effects of pioglitazone or rosiglitazone in patients with type 2 diabetes who were previously treated with troglitazone. Diabetes Care 2002;25(4):708–11.

[28] Nesto R, Bell D, Bonow R, et al. Thiazolidinedione use, fluid retention, and congestive heart failure: a consensus statement from the American Heart Association and American Diabetes Association. Diabetes Care 2004;27(1):256–63.

[29] Aronoff S, Rosenblatt S, Braithwaite S, et al. Pioglitazone hydrochloride monotherapy improves glycemic control in the treatment of patients with type 2 diabetes: a 6-month randomized placebo-controlled dose-response study. The Pioglitazone 001 Study Group. Diabetes Care 2000;23(11):1605–11.

[30] Groop L. Sulfonylureas in NIDDM. Diabetes Care 1992;15(6):737–54.

[31] Haupt E, Laube F, Loy H, et al. Secondary failures in modern therapy of diabetes mellitus with blood glucose lowering sulfonamides. Med Klin 1977;72(38):1529–36.

[32] Group UKPDS. Effect of intensive blood-glucose control with metformin on complications in overweight patients with type 2 diabetes (UKPDS 34). Lancet 1998;352(9131):854–65.

[33] Group UKPDS. Intensive blood-glucose control with sulphonylureas or insulin compared with conventional treatment and risk of complications in patients with type 2 diabetes (UKPDS 33). Lancet 1998;352(9131):837–53.

[34] Horton E, Clinkingbeard C, Gatlin M, et al. Nateglinide alone and in combination with metformin improves glycemic control by reducing mealtime glucose levels in type 2 diabetes. Diabetes Care 2000;23(11):1660–5.

[35] Chiasson J, Josse R, Hunt JA, et al. The efficacy of acarbose in the treatment of patients with non-insulin-dependent diabetes mellitus: a multicenter controlled clinical trial. Ann Intern Med 1994;121(12):928–35.

[36] Viberti G, Kahn S, Greene D, et al. A diabetes outcome progression trial (ADOPT): an international multicenter study of the comparative efficacy of rosiglitazone, glyburide, and metformin in recently diagnosed type 2 diabetes. Diabetes Care 2002;25(10):1737–43.

[37] Torn C, Landin-Olsson M, Ostman J, et al. Glutamic acid decarboxylase antibodies (GADA) is the most important factor for prediction of insulin therapy within 3 years in young adult diabetic patients not classified as Type 1 diabetes on clinical grounds. Diabetes Metab Res Rev 2000;16(6):442–7.

[38] Hathout E, Thomas W, El-Shahawy M, et al. Diabetic autoimmune markers in children and adolescents with type 2 diabetes. Pediatrics 2001;107:E102.

[39] Hermann L, Schersten B, Bitzen P, et al. Therapeutic comparison of metformin and sulfonylurea, alone and in various combinations: a double-blind controlled study. Diabetes Care 1994;17(10):1100–9.

[40] De Jager J, Kooy A, Lehert P, et al. Effects of short-term treatment with metformin on markers of endothelial function and inflammatory activity in type 2 diabetes mellitus: a randomized placebo-controlled trial. J Intern Med 2005;257:100–9.

[41] DCCT Research Group. The effect of intensive treatment of diabetes on the development and progression of long-term complications in insulin-dependent diabetes mellitus. N Engl J Med 1993;329(14):977–86.

[42] Nathan D. Some answers, more controversy, from UKPDS: United Kingdom Prospective Diabetes Study. Lancet 1998;352(9131):832–3.

[43] National Institutes of Health, National Heart, Lung, and Blood Institute (NHLBI). The sixth report of the joint national committee on prevention, detection, evaluation, and treatment of high blood pressure. NIH Publication 98–4080. Bethesda (MD): National Institutes of Health; 1998.

[44] American Diabetes Association. Management of dyslipidemia in children and adolescents with diabetes. Diabetes Care 2003;26:2194–7.

ELSEVIER
SAUNDERS

PEDIATRIC CLINICS
OF NORTH AMERICA

Pediatr Clin N Am 52 (2005) 1705–1733

Hypoglycemia: A Complication of Diabetes Therapy in Children

Christopher Ryan, PhD[a], Nursen Gurtunca, MD, FCP[b], Dorothy Becker, MBBCh[b],*

[a]Department of Psychiatry, University of Pittsburgh,
Western Pennsylvania Psychiatric Institute and Clinic, Pittsburgh, PA 15213, USA
[b]Division of Endocrinology, Department of Pediatrics, Children's Hospital of Pittsburgh,
University of Pittsburgh, 3705 Fifth Avenue, 4A 400, Pittsburgh, PA 15213, USA

Hypoglycemia is the most common acute complication associated with the treatment of type 1 diabetes. At the very least, it can be an unpleasant experience for many children, because they begin to experience symptoms such as shakiness and emotional lability when their blood glucose levels fall. Many children and their parents find that hypoglycemia can be a terrifying event because under certain circumstances, more severe hypoglycemia leads to seizures or loss of consciousness and the possible development of permanent brain dysfunction, an uncertain area currently under intense investigation. For these reasons, iatrogenic hypoglycemia remains the major limiting factor in attempts to achieve the glycemic level required to prevent chronic micro- and macrovascular complications.

Since the publication in 1993 of the results of the Diabetes Control and Complications Trial (DCCT) [1], there has been widespread acceptance of intensive insulin therapy for adults and children with diabetes. Early results from that study demonstrated a greatly increased risk of moderate to severe hypoglycemia in individuals (adolescents and adults) randomized to the intensive therapy intervention [2,3], but as confirmed by more recent data, intensive therapy is also associated with a marked decline or delay in the incidence of microvas-

This article is supported by grant R01HD-29487 RO1 DK-069472 JDRF.
* Corresponding author.
E-mail address: Dorothy.Becker@chp.edu (D. Becker).

cular complications, such as retinopathy [4], renal insufficiency [5], and periph-eral neuropathy [6]. Advances in diabetes treatment regimens also have led to a dramatic decrease in mortality rates [7]. Despite these positive treatment out-comes, the frequency of hypoglycemic events seems to be unchanged in adults and children [8]. Results from the DCCT showed that hypoglycemia was more frequent and more severe in adolescents than in adults in the intensive and con-ventional treatment group [2]. Whether these differences between adolescents and adults are related to a greater metabolic vulnerability of the younger group or to compliance and lifestyle issues remains undetermined.

This article reviews the causes and consequences (or correlates) of hypo-glycemia in childhood and adolescence and discusses prevention strategies.

Defining hypoglycemia

Over the past 50 years, investigators have used different operational defi-nitions of hypoglycemia that have varied according to the age of the individual and the application of biochemical or clinical criteria [9,10]. It is important to define hypoglycemia objectively to establish its prevalence, assess its causes, and identify the glycemic level that induces deleterious metabolic or cognitive effects. Standardized criteria also permit researchers to evaluate the effectiveness of new drugs, devices, or management strategies in reducing the occurrence and severity of hypoglycemic events.

Conventional definitions have been based largely on symptomatology. For example, hypoglycemia has been characterized as mild when minimal symptoms are present, as moderate when assistance is required, and as severe when an individual experiences a seizure or loss of consciousness. The DCCT definition, which was used to ascertain the incidence of severe hypoglycemia during that clinical trial, defined an episode of severe hypoglycemia as any episode that re-quired assistance, did or did not involve a loss of consciousness, and was asso-ciated with either a blood glucose level of ≤ 50 mg/dL or an immediate response to treatment with oral or intravenous carbohydrate or glucagon injection [11]. Unfortunately, this definition has not been helpful in documenting hypoglycemia in young children because they always require treatment assistance during an even mild episode of hypoglycemia. In the pediatric population, it may be more useful to focus on a child's actual blood glucose value, regardless of the pres-ence of symptoms. This focus is particularly important not only because symp-tomatology is idiosyncratic from one individual to another but also because it is likely to be diminished by prior hypoglycemia (hypoglycemia unawareness syndrome) and during sleep [12].

We propose an arbitrary biochemical classification of mild or moderate hypo-glycemia, whether symptomatic or asymptomatic, with mild hypoglycemia being capillary blood glucose values between 70 and 55 mg/dL and moderate hypo-glycemia being <55 mg/dL without loss of consciousness. Any episode asso-ciated with a blood glucose value <70 mg/dL and either a loss of consciousness or a seizure should be considered to be severe. Although we previously recommended 65 mg/dL as the glycemic level defining hypoglycemia because cognitive function and counterregulatory responses are typically altered at this level in individuals with and without diabetes [13,14], the American Diabetes Association Working Group on Hypoglycemia recently adopted a value of < 70 mg/dL as its definition of biochemical hypoglycemia [15].

Prevalence of hypoglycemia

It has been difficult to establish the prevalence of hypoglycemia in children with diabetes because of the application of different criteria to define hypoglycemia, the absence of standardized conventions for reporting the frequency of hypoglycemia in clinical studies, and the use of small, highly selected populations [16]. Limitations in current glucose monitoring technology also have prevented the accurate ascertainment of the prevalence of asymptomatic hypoglycemia in the naturalistic setting. Recent refinements of glucose sensors may allow future detailed determination of the prevalence of hypoglycemia, its causes, and correlates.

In their recent review, Jones and Davis [17] noted that the reported rates of severe hypoglycemia in prospective studies vary considerably around the world, and they emphasize the likelihood that it may reflect, at least in part, the use of different definitions of hypoglycemia and the application of different data analytic strategies [18]. The highest rates were found among the adolescent subjects who participated in the intensive therapy arm (mean HbA1c = 8.3%) of the DCCT, in which 64% of the pediatric sample experienced at least one episode during the study. This rate corresponds to a rate of 26.7 events per 100 patient years [2]. Adolescents in the conventional therapy arm (mean HbA1c = 9.3%) of the DCCT experienced 9.7 events per 100 patient years. Rates intermediate between these two extremes (15.6–22 events per 100 patients years) have been reported from several recent prospective epidemiologic studies [19–23], in which the mean HbA1c value ranged between 8.6% and 9.1% and typically used a more stringent definition of severe hypoglycemia. A frequently overlooked fact from the DCCT is adolescents' greatly elevated vulnerability to hypoglycemia. Compared with their adult counterparts, rates of severe hypoglycemia were three times greater in the intensively and conventionally treated adolescent groups.

Severe hypoglycemic events occur most frequently at night [24]. In the few studies that have measured adequately the blood glucose levels at night, the prevalence of biochemical hypoglycemia, defined as levels between 55 and 70 mg/dL, indicated rates ranging between 10% [25] and 55% [26] in children, with no relationship to the number of daily insulin injections [27]. One small, carefully monitored study measured nocturnal blood glucose levels in the home and found values as low as 34 mg/dL in children treated with conventional insulin therapy [28].

Physiologic defenses and adaptation to hypoglycemia

Glucose is the primary fuel that generates the chemical energy required for normal brain metabolism [29]. Because the brain is unable to store glucose for an extended period of time, any reduction in circulating peripheral glucose levels may affect brain activity adversely. This may be particularly true during childhood, when brain energy consumption is highest [30]. For example, rates of glucose use increase dramatically from birth to 4 years, when they reach a value that is more than twice the glucose use rate of adults. This rate is maintained up until approximately 10 years of age, when use rates begin to decline until the age of 16 to 18, at which point they are comparable to that of adults [30]. These higher rates of glucose use during development may place younger children at an increased risk of brain dysfunction secondary to neuroglycopenia when peripheral blood glucose values fall into the hypoglycemic range.

Glucose counterregulation

Falling blood glucose levels ordinarily trigger glucose counterregulation, a process that normally prevents or rapidly corrects hypoglycemia. Declines in blood and interstitial glucose levels are detected by the glucokinase sensing mechanism in islet cells and in the hypothalamus [31], which induces a series of events that include a reduction in endogenous insulin secretion together with an increase in glucagon, epinephrine, cortisol, and growth hormone [32]. In patients who have diabetes, the normal physiologic counterregulatory process is disrupted because exogenously administered insulin levels cannot be suppressed accurately. Patients who have diabetes also manifest impairment in the normal glucagon response and a significant attenuation of the normal surge in epinephrine release during a fall in blood glucose levels. The imbalance between circulating insulin levels and insulin requirements that is associated with the absent glucagon and the impaired epinephrine response results in inadequate glycogenolysis and gluconeogenesis and in the presence of defective glucose counterregulation, leads to greater or persisting hypoglycemia [32]. Of clinical importance is the fact that the deficient glucagon response to hypoglycemia occurs despite normal or excessive glucagon secretion stimulated by amino acids and protein (eg, during a meal) [33].

In the absence of sufficient glucose supplies, ketone bodies (beta-hydroxybutyrate and acetoacetate) and lactate may provide an alternate fuel for brain energy metabolism and thereby preserve cognitive function [34,35]. When hypoglycemia is associated with fasting or glycogen storage disease, insulinopenia allows lipolysis and ketogenesis to occur. Although muscle metabolizes ketones and lactate rapidly, there is a time delay for the required metabolic adaptation and upregulation of enzyme required for ketone body transport and use in the brain. During states of relative or absolute insulin excess, the generation of ketones is suppressed, although it is possible that locally stored or metabolized lactate may provide a short-term alternate energy supply [36].

Glucose transporters

The primary method for transferring glucose from the peripheral circulation into the central nervous system (CNS) is by facilitated diffusion, a process mediated by specific cell membrane transporters at the level of the blood-brain barrier. Because the brain is unable to store glucose for any extended period of time, its normal function and energy metabolism depend almost entirely on this process. Several specific glucose transporters (GLUTs) with different affinities for glucose have been described [37]. GLUT1 and GLUT3 mediate basal glucose uptake in most tissues and are the primary glucose transporters in the brain, nerves, and red blood cells. Their high affinities for glucose ensure adequate brain levels of glucose even during periods of relative hypoglycemia. At normal glucose concentrations, GLUT1 and GLUT3 have maximum affinities for glucose and are believed to be insulin independent, unlike GLUT4 in adipose tissue and muscle.

Our knowledge of the up- and downregulation of GLUT transporters in the CNS is based almost entirely on animal studies [38–40], although its potential importance in preserving brain function during hypoglycemia has been deduced from cerebral glucose uptake studies in humans [41,42]. Chronic hyperglycemia has been shown, although not consistently, to result in downregulation of GLUT 1 and GLUT 3 in rodents. This finding could explain why children and adults in poorer metabolic control also tend to experience more hypoglycemic events and manifest mild cognitive impairments [43,44]. Because it takes time to reverse this phenomenon, an episode of acute hypoglycemia would result in suboptimal glucose transport into the brain, compared with the normal individual, resulting in relative neuroglycopenia in a patient who has poorly controlled diabetes. This would account for the clinical experience of more severe hypoglycemic symptoms associated with exaggerated counterregulatory responses in those patients [45]. Upregulation of GLUT 1 during chronic hypoglycemia is well established in animal models [38,46] and presumably occurs after recurrent hypoglycemic episodes. This putatively adaptive phenomenon would allow increased glucose transport into the brain during periods of decreased circulating glucose, which accounts for apparent neurocognitive protection seen in patients who have experienced repeated episodes of hypoglycemia [47].

Another potential adaptive phenomenon to decreasing energy supplies is an increase in cerebral blood flow, as demonstrated in studies with adults who do not have diabetes [48,49], adults who do have diabetes [50–52], and children [53], and numerous animal studies [54,55]. This phenomenon is presumably a compensatory mechanism that maintains adequate delivery of glucose to the brain [56], although for reasons not well understood, these cerebral blood flow changes seem to be asymmetrical, insofar as increases are greater in the right than in the left cerebral hemisphere [48,52,53]. This asymmetry is a plausible explanation for the frequent transient hemiparalysis (Todd's paralysis) experienced by patients who have diabetes after a severe episode of acute hypoglycemia [53].

Pathophysiology of hypoglycemia

Neurochemical manifestations

Profound experimentally induced hypoglycemia has been found to induce neurochemical changes throughout the CNS. At the cellular level, low blood glucose levels will—over an extended period of time—alter ion pump activity and disrupt cellular homeostasis by permitting an influx of calcium into the cells and intracellular alkalosis [57,58]. The resulting release of excitatory amino acids, particularly aspartate and glutamate, into the interstitial space triggers neuronal necrosis [57], which may be accompanied by an isoelectric electroencephalogram (EEG). Animal studies have indicated that the hippocampus is the brain region that seems to be especially vulnerable to hypoglycemia [59–61], whereas data clinical case reports suggest in addition to inducing hippocampal damage, profound hypoglycemia can cause lesions in the basal ganglia as well as in the cerebral cortex [62–65].

The multiple neurochemical changes that occur during acute hypoglycemia can have marked effects on brain tissue. As summarized by Auer and Siesjö in their excellent review [57,66], cerebral oxygen consumption declines due to substrate deficiency, and there is depletion of high energy phosphate compounds (ATP and creatine phosphate). With profound hypoglycemia, loss of ionic homeostasis occurs: brain extracellular potassium rises [67] while extracellular calcium falls [68]. Increasing intracellular calcium is thought to activate a number of enzymes including proteases, nucleases and lipases whose action may lead to mitochondrial damage and eventually cell death [69].

Protein markers of neuronal injury have been found to be elevated in adults following an episode of profound hypoglycemia. For example, Strachan and associates [70] measured serum levels of neuron-specific enolase (NSE) and protein S-100 approximately 36 hours and 8.5 days following an episode of profound hypoglycemia in 3 diabetic adults who subsequently expired, and found greatly elevated levels of both proteins, as compared with diabetic adults who had no recent hypoglycemic episodes. On the other hand, no significant differences were evident when diabetic adults with a mild to moderately severe episode of hypoglycemia were compared with diabetic subjects without such a history. These results are consistent with animal studies that suggest that significant neuronal necrosis appears only following an episode of profound, and extended, hypoglycemia.

Physiologic consequences

The deficient counterregulatory hormone responses to hypoglycemia in type 1 diabetes is known as the 'syndrome of hypoglycemia-associated autonomic failure' (HAAF) [71], which is a functional disorder [32] that occurs irrespective of the presence or absence of diabetic autonomic neuropathy [32]. Epinephrine and cortisol release, which remain the major defenses against hypoglycemia, are decreased as part of the HAAF syndrome. This syndrome is apparently a consequence of prior episodes of hypoglycemia or exercise, and thus forms part of a vicious cycle allowing further episodes of hypoglycemia to occur [32,72]. The reduced epinephrine response to hypoglycemia is typically induced by up to 3 recent episodes of hypoglycemia [32] and is reversed by meticulous avoidance of even mild acute hypoglycemia [73]. The exact mechanisms underlying HAAF are currently under investigation, but appear to involve, at least in part, the up-regulation of glucose transport into the brain [38,42], particularly the hypothalamus, which mediates the normal counterregulatory response [74]. It has also been suggested that cortisol release plays an important role in the suppression of the adreno-sympathetic response insofar as cortisol is normally, but variably, increased during even mild hypoglycemia and the prevention of its release preserves epinephrine secretion [75,76]. However, this concept is controversial because no effect on counterregulation was seen during infusions of cortisol to achieve blood levels which were lower than those achieved in the above studies but more consistent with usual patient responses [77].

Hypoglycemia associated autonomic failure is almost always associated with the concomitant occurrence of 'hypoglycemic unawareness' because of the absence of normal sympathoadrenal responses to hypoglycemia [32,78]. The failure of patients to recognize hypoglycemia, together with impaired glucose counterregulation, places the patient at a marked risk for experiencing a severe and prolonged hypoglycemic episode. Like HAAF, hypoglycemia unawareness is reversible by as little as 2-3 weeks of avoidance of hypoglycemia [79]. It is not only the low glucose concentration and the duration of hypoglycemia, but also frequent asymptomatic hypoglycemia that can lead to defective glucose counterregulation and hypoglycemia unawareness. Therefore, since all hypoglycemic episodes can harm the diabetic child in the short or long term, they should be detected and avoided. Because warning symptoms of hypoglycemia are difficult to recognize and verbalize by the young diabetic child and may be absent in the older child who has HAAF, glucose measurements rather than symptom reports are needed to ascertain the presence of hypoglycemia to avoid hypoglycemic unawareness.

In patients with type 1 diabetes, particularly in younger children [26,28,80], severe hypoglycemia occurs most frequently during sleep [3,24]. Sleep reduces awareness of symptoms and also decreases epinephrine responses to hypoglycemia [12,27]. The consequences of this unawareness and failure of counterregulation are compounded by the fact that nocturnal hypoglycemia occurs at the time when glucose monitoring is infrequent or absent. Because episodes of nocturnal hypoglycemia are usually asymptomatic, they may be prolonged and potentially result in a "dead in bed" scenario [81,82]. These nocturnal hypoglycemic episodes are likely to be a major cause of the HAAF syndrome [32],and thus should be of greater concern than daytime hypoglycemia as a potential factor for future severe episodes [15,27]. Surprisingly, asymptomatic nocturnal hypoglycemia values, even those lower than 40 mg/dl, do not affect subsequent daytime mood or cognitive performance [28].

Exercise, without hypoglycemia, has been described as an additional cause of HAAF [32,83,84]. Antecedent hypoglycemia can decrease counterregulatory response to exercise [84], and antecedent exercise can decrease the counterregulatory response to hypoglycemia [85]. This failure of counterregulation, which in adults is more profound in men than women [86], compounds the glucose-lowering effect of the increased energy use by the exercising muscle [87]. This increased glucose use is mediated by the translocation of the most important glucose transporters in muscle (ie, GLUT4) [88,89].

Acute consequence of hypoglycemia

Symptoms

Hypoglycemic symptoms are typically classified as either 'autonomic' or 'neuroglycopenic.' Sympathoadrenal and parasympathetic responses result in the typical autonomic symptoms which include shakiness, hunger, anxiety, palpitations, and sweatiness. Neuroglycopenia results in dizziness, irritability, crying, sleepiness, headache and mental confusion. One study of children indicated that the most frequently experienced symptoms included hunger and emotional lability, as well as parents' report that their child appeared pale [90]. Neuroglycopenic symptoms, or fear of their occurrence, are obviously detrimental to the well-being of these children and may result not only in significant emotional distress, but may also interfere with children's daily activities and their management of diabetes.

It is important to keep in mind that hypoglycemia-associated symptoms tend to be idiosyncratic from one child to another, and may be difficult for the younger child to recognize and verbalize, leaving the parents to distinguish hypoglycemia from other transient physical conditions and behavioral states. The difficulty parents have in readily identifying hypoglycemia accurately may result in longer delays in treatment, and correspondingly, an increase in both the depth and the duration of the hypoglycemic event. Alternately, parents may become so concerned about missing an episode of hypoglycemia that they become obsessed with blood glucose testing, especially at night – a situation that is likely to adversely affect the child/parent relationship [91].

Symptom detection

Adolescents are not very accurate in identifying falling blood glucose levels. During our controlled hypoglycemic clamp studies in which mild hypoglycemia (60 mg/dl) was experimentally induced and maintained for a period of time, only 42% of adolescents reported autonomic symptoms, and 29% reported neuroglycopenic symptoms [92]. Although their symptom reports were not correlated with epinephrine or pancreatic polypeptide secretion, they were more frequent in those individuals who had higher anxiety scores during the eugly-cemic baseline. Elevated levels of anxiety are often considered to be an indicator of the personality trait known as 'negative affectivity' or 'neuroticism' [93,94]; individuals with this trait tend to be introspective, apprehensive, vigilant and negativistic. In this study, those higher on this trait were the most likely to detect hypoglycemic symptoms and accurately estimate their blood glucose values [92]. This finding underscores the importance of variables other than glycemic level, in influencing individuals' ability to detect and report symptoms indicative of mild to moderate hypoglycemia. Interestingly, 60% of subjects reported that they were experiencing symptoms in anticipation of acute hypoglycemia; indeed, during those reports, their glucose values were well within the euglycemic range. Throughout the hypoglycemic period of the study, only 28% were able to accu-rately estimate their blood glucose. Despite the very high level of hypoglycemia unawareness within this study, our subjects were more accurate in estimating their blood glucose values than those previously evaluated in more naturalistic settings (ie, at home; at diabetes camp) [95–97].

Fear of hypoglycemia

Although the 'fear of hypoglycemia' syndrome is usually thought of as the fear of experiencing an episode of unconsciousness or a seizure [91,98], in practical terms many patients fear the occurrence of autonomic symptoms despite the fact that these signify the protective counterregulatory hormone responses. Fear of hypoglycemia syndrome is a real entity and is a major impediment to adequate glycemic control in many patients. It most commonly, but not neces-sarily, follows an episode of moderate or severe hypoglycemia. Children (and more often their parents) who are extremely concerned about hypoglycemic events tend to keep blood glucose values above recommended targets in an effort to avoid a hypoglycemic episode [91,98,99]. This leads to poorer glycemic control which may be significantly more detrimental to the individual's health than an episode of even moderately severe hypoglycemia. In studies of adult patients, fear of hypoglycemia is especially prominent in those who have higher levels of anxiety and neuroticism [100]. It is likely that the development of accurate, continuous monitoring blood glucose systems with alarms would al-leviate or prevent this syndrome, but such systems are not yet available.

Acute neurologic sequelae

A severe hypoglycemic episode with loss of consciousness is usually not recalled by the child, but is often followed by physical discomfort, including headache and vomiting, for a several hours. Hemiparesis (Todd's paralysis) is not uncommon and appears to occur after period of prolonged, usually nocturnal, hypoglycemia [101]. This usually resolves after several hours and is not an indication for diagnostic brain imaging.

Transient changes in mood

Laboratory studies of diabetic and nondiabetic adults have demonstrated that changes in mood state are common as blood glucose levels fall and autonomic symptoms begin to appear. Hypoglycemic adults report a constellation of feelings that has been characterized as 'tense tiredness': feeling less happy, less energetic, and more tense [102–104]. In addition, many of these individuals describe themselves as feeling more angry than normal [105]. To date, there has been no formal assessment of mood in children and adolescents during acute hypoglycemia but based on our clinical experience, we would expect to find a similar pattern of results. One study has examined mood state in children following an episode of nocturnal hypoglycemia in the home, and contrary to expectations, no significant mood changes were reported [28], suggesting that if hypoglycemia does alter mood, the effects are very short-lived.

Transient cognitive deterioration

Since the introduction of insulin therapy, diabetic patients have frequently complained that their ability to think clearly is disrupted during a hypoglycemic episode, but it has only been since the development of two similar experimental techniques – the hyperinsulinemic glucose clamp paradigm [106] and the automated glucose-controlled insulin infusion system (Biostator) [107] – that researchers have been able to evaluate the extent to which hypoglycemia affects cognitive function. In their early research, Holmes and associates administered a variety of mental efficiency tests to young adults during periods of experimentally-controlled euglycemia and moderate hypoglycemia (55–60 mg/dl) and noted that performance was markedly slowed, but accuracy was unaffected [107–111]. Performance decrements were most apparent on tasks that required rapid decision-making (Choice Reaction Time), and these decrements became greater as the cognitive demands of the task increased. On the other hand, tasks which relied on highly overlearned or automated skills (eg, reading) or which did not have a significant speed component (eg, learning) were relatively unaffected.

This overall pattern of results has subsequently been replicated by numerous investigators using a variety of cognitive tasks and varying the degree and duration of the hypoglycemia. Attention, decision-making speed, psychomotor efficiency, and 'mental flexibility' are the cognitive processes that seem to be particularly vulnerable to acute hypoglycemia in adults [112–118] as well as in adolescents [13,119]. Our work with adolescents demonstrates that these changes may occur during even mild hypoglycemia (between 65 and 55 mg/dl), whereas adults rarely show evidence of cognitive change unless blood glucose values fall below 54 mg/dl. Learning and memory skills may also become increasingly impaired as blood glucose levels drop. Although this has not been studied in children or adolescents, the few studies of diabetic adults have demonstrated that the ability to learn lists of words or strings of numbers, to recall recently studied stories or designs after a brief delay, or to use 'working memory' processes may be disrupted during moderately severe hypoglycemia [117,120].

The severity of acute cognitive dysfunction is related to variables that include the depth and duration of hypoglycemia [14], recent episodes of prior hypoglycemia [121], as well as the complexity of the cognitive task [109]. In addition, it appears to be influenced to some extent by as yet unknown characteristics of the individual. For example, a number of studies have demonstrated very dramatic individual differences in susceptibility to hypoglycemia such that some subjects show a marked deterioration in cognitive function shortly after blood glucose values begin to fall below 70 mg/dl, whereas others show absolutely no cognitive change despite blood glucose values below 55–60 mg/dl in children [119] and below 45–50 mg/dl in adults [113,122]. There may also be marked differences across individuals (and cognitive tasks) in the rate at which cognitive function returns to normal following restoration of euglycemia. Although it is clear that the cognitive changes associated with mild to moderately severe hypoglycemia are completely reversible, there may be a delay of 30 minutes or more before performance has returned to normal, particularly on those tasks that require rapid decision-making [119,123].

The clinical relevance of hypoglycemia-induced cognitive dysfunction has been estimated by determining the proportion of individuals who, during acute hypoglycemia, perform in the 'brain damaged' range, as defined by published norms for impairment [124], or by defining performance as 'impaired' if it exceeds normative values by more than 2 standard deviation units [117,119,122]. Depending on the type of task as well as on the degree of hypoglycemia, as many as 25 to 65% of subjects studied met criteria for clinically significant impairment on at least one cognitive task. Whether those impairments actually affect the individual's ability to perform in the classroom or in the workplace has not been formally measured. It is certainly plausible to expect that children who are experiencing an episode of hypoglycemia that persists for an extended period of time and interferes with their ability to pay attention and learn new information, would ultimately perform more poorly on measures of academic achievement and verbal intelligence. As a group, diabetic children often [125–128], but not invariably [129], perform more poorly on such tasks as compared with their nondiabetic peers, but because of the difficulty in measuring blood glucose levels continuously over the course of the day, it has been impossible to attribute the poorer academic achievement of diabetic children to episodes of acute hypoglycemia.

Performance on 'ecologically valid' tests, like measures of driving, have also been used to assess the adverse effects of acute hypoglycemia on activities that are cognitively and metabolically demanding [130]. Using a sophisticated driving simulator, Cox and his associates have found that even mild hypoglycemia (72–54 mg/dl) was associated with more high speed driving and higher scores on a composite driving impairment score in adults [131]. As blood glucose levels fell further, there were significant decrements on most measures of driving skill, and these were accompanied by marked changes in EEG indices. As seen on other measures of cognitive function, these hypoglycemia-associated driving decrements were limited to a subset of subjects. Whether the subjects who made driving errors during experimentally induced hypoglycemia in the laboratory would have higher rates of accidents on the road remains to be determined, although a recent survey demonstrated that as a group, adults who have type 1 diabetes have higher rates of driving mishaps (eg, moving violations, crashes) than adults who have type 2 diabetes or persons who do not have diabetes. The three strongest predictors of serious traffic mishaps were previous episodes of hypoglycemic stupor during driving, less frequent blood glucose monitoring before driving, and taking insulin by subcutaneous injection rather than using an insulin pump. No studies have examined driving skills in adolescents who have diabetes, but we would expect an even stronger relationship between hypoglycemic events and driving mishaps in this group because driving skills are less likely to be highly overlearned and automatic in a relatively inexperienced driver.

Acute electroencephalographic changes

An enormous body of literature has demonstrated that experimentally induced hypoglycemia triggers dramatic changes in the resting EEG. Initially, there is a decrease in alpha activity; as blood glucose levels continue to drop, there is a corresponding increase in slow wave delta activity and theta activity [132–138]. In adults who have diabetes, this level recovers shortly after the restoration of euglycemia [134], but the EEGs of children who have diabetes are much slower to recover. Evidence suggests that children who have diabetes may more vulnerable to the CNS effects of acute hypoglycemia compared with either adults or children who do not have diabetes [132]. Not only do abnormalities in delta and theta activity tend to appear at glycemic levels that are higher than levels reported for adults who have diabetes (54 mg/dL versus 36 mg/dL) [132,134] but children who have diabetes are also more likely to manifest clinically significant EEG abnormalities. In one study, nearly half of the children who had diabetes showed epileptiform spikes during the hypoglycemic nadir (47 mg/dL), compared with only 9% of the children who did not have diabetes [132].

Electrophysiologic abnormalities during experimentally induced hypoglycemia are also apparent in studies that activate the brain by having subjects complete a demanding cognitive task. These so-called "event-related potential" paradigms measure brain wave activity while individuals perform tasks that require focused attention. When individuals are presented with a series of tones and required to count the number of infrequently occurring tones, the latency and amplitude of the resulting brain wave (P300 wave) provide an index of neural processing efficiency. Moderate hypoglycemia (<50 mg/dL) slows neural processing significantly in adults who have diabetes [112,139] and do not have diabetes [140], as evidenced by an increase in the P300 latency and the corresponding increase in response time on decision-making tasks. These changes were more likely to be seen during mild hypoglycemia (63 mg/dL) in conventionally treated patients who received twice-daily insulin injections; patients who received intensive insulin therapy were protected to some extent insofar as P300 abnormalities did not appear until blood glucose values fell to 40 mg/dL, and even then, the magnitude of the slowing was small [141]. To date, only a single study has recorded P300 waves in children during experimentally induced hypoglycemia, and none of those children had diabetes. Increased P300 latencies were apparent at modest hypoglycemic levels (75 mg/dL), and latencies continued to increase as blood glucose levels dropped further [142]. A comparison group of adults who did not have diabetes did not manifest any changes in latency until blood glucose values fell to 54 mg/dL. These results reinforced the view that the CNS of children is particularly vulnerable to mild hypoglycemia. Given the resting EEG findings reported by Bjørgaas and colleagues [132], we would expect to see even longer latencies in P300 studies in children with diabetes during hypoglycemia.

Chronic consequences of recurrent hypoglycemia

Permanent cognitive sequelae of severe or recurrent hypoglycemia

Although pediatricians are aware of the potential neurocognitive damage caused by profound or repeated hypoglycemic episodes in childhood, there is a dearth of published information about the long-term cognitive effects of profound hypoglycemia in children who have diabetes, perhaps because these cases are sporadic and infrequent. Nearly all case reports have been limited to adults, and few have assessed cognitive function formally using standard neuropsychological measures [64]. Conversely, continued research has produced a large body of literature on the effects of one or recurrent episodes of less severe hypoglycemia with or without seizures on neuropsychological function in children and adults. These data suggest that in general, contrary to expectations, permanent cognitive sequelae, although measurable, are relatively minor.

Early cross-sectional studies of adults who have diabetes suggested that persons who experienced five or more episodes of severe hypoglycemia (defined as requiring external assistance or triggering a seizure or coma) tended to perform more poorly on various cognitive tests than persons without prior hypoglycemia [143–145]. These deficits appeared most prominently on measures that required rapid decision-making and problem-solving skills ("fluid intelligence") [146–148]. Recent cross-sectional research from the same group failed to find any link between recurrent hypoglycemia and cognitive function [149]. Similarly, analyses of the neuropsychological test results from the DCCT failed to support the view that recurrent severe hypoglycemia induces detectable cognitive dysfunction. Despite 6.5 years of follow-up and high rates of severe hypoglycemia in the intensive therapy treatment group (61 severe hypoglycemic episodes per 100 patient-years, as compared with 19 episodes per 100 patient years in the conventionally treated group), neither the treatment arm nor the number of episodes of severe hypoglycemia had any effect on a wide variety of cognitive outcome measures [150,151]. This is not to say that adults who have diabetes do not develop cognitive dysfunction over time. A growing body of research suggests that chronic hyperglycemia, as indexed by the development of microvascular complications (eg, retinopathy), is more closely associated with reductions in mental efficiency than measurable (thus incompletely documented) episodes of recurrent hypoglycemia [149,152,153].

The possibility that recurrent hypoglycemia induces cognitive sequelae in children is more controversial. Studies of children who were diagnosed with diabetes after 5 or 6 years of age reported relatively mild cognitive impairments, but usually there is little evidence that these impairments reflect the development of brain damage secondary to recurrent hypoglycemia. The most common findings in these studies of later onset diabetes are somewhat lower scores on measures of verbal intelligence and academic achievement [125,127,128,154–157]. Because performance on these tasks may depend on adequate exposure to information presented in the classroom setting, it is also possible that poorer performance of children who have diabetes may be a consequence of their higher rates of school absence [158–160] and transient inattention secondary to acute mild hypoglycemic events. Studies also have demonstrated evidence of psychomotor slowing [125,161] (which is also frequent in adults who have type 1 and type 2 diabetes), but the growing body of literature has not been able to determine whether this common cognitive finding correlates with the degree of hyperglycemia or frequency of hypoglycemia or both. There is no convincing evidence that episodes of moderately severe hypoglycemia alone influence the neuropsychological test performance of children and adolescents who have a later onset of diabetes [44,162].

There is, however, a subgroup of children who have diabetes who have a greatly elevated risk of manifesting hypoglycemia-associated cognitive dysfunction: children who have an early onset of diabetes within the first 5 or 6 years of life. In younger children, tasks that require visuospatial information processing (eg, copying complex geometric designs, solving jigsaw puzzles, reproducing patterns with blocks) seem to be most compromised [163]. In adolescents, deficits are evident on virtually all types of cognitive tasks, including measures of intelligence, learning, memory, and problem solving [164]. Our work has demonstrated that approximately 25% of adolescents diagnosed before 6 years of age manifested clinically significant cognitive impairment; in contrast, only 6% of patients with a later onset of diabetes met criteria for clinically significant impairment, as did 6% of a sample of subjects drawn from the community who did not have diabetes [164]. Children and adolescents who have an early onset of diabetes also have more difficulty with tasks that require them to pay attention [128,156]. These cross-sectional findings have been confirmed in prospective studies in which children who have newly diagnosed diabetes have been followed for up to 6 years [126,165,166]. Children diagnosed before 4 years of age showed the greatest impairments, with deficits most prominent on cognitive tests that required attention, rapid information processing, and executive skills [126].

Cognitive deficits associated with an early onset of diabetes persist into adulthood and are associated with structural changes in the CNS. Ferguson and colleagues [167] demonstrated that adults diagnosed before 7 years of age performed more poorly on measures of intelligence and information-processing efficiency compared with persons diagnosed after that age. Brain imaging data showed evidence of cortical atrophy, as indexed by lateral ventricle volumes that were 37% greater in the subjects who had early-onset diabetes. Because subjects with less brain volume performed worse on most of the cognitive tests, the authors concluded that the diagnosis of diabetes early in life may affect normal brain development and influence cognition.

Hypoglycemia has been implicated in the development of these deficits because rates of severe hypoglycemia are far higher (45% versus 13%) during the first 5 to 6 years of life [168], perhaps because younger children who have diabetes have an increased sensitivity to insulin [169]. Because the developing nervous system is vulnerable to virtually any type of brain insult [170–172], a reduction in the brain availability of glucose may cause significant structural damage [173,174]. Cross-sectional and longitudinal studies repeatedly have demonstrated statistical associations among early onset of diabetes, episodes of moderately severe hypoglycemia, and cognitive dysfunction [126,156,161,163, 164,175,176], although growing evidence suggests that chronic hyperglycemia also may play an important role in the cognitive decline of children with an early onset of diabetes [126,177].

Chronic electroencephalographic abnormalities

An extensive body of literature has indicated that children who have diabetes manifest significant EEG abnormalities. In most of those studies, recurrent severe hypoglycemia is confounded with age at onset, insofar as individuals with more episodes of severe hypoglycemia tend to have an earlier age at onset [178] and tend to be in poorer metabolic control [179]. Individuals with one or more previous episodes of severe hypoglycemia are two [180] to five times [181] as likely to have an abnormal EEG, compared with individuals without a history of prior hypoglycemia. As a group, children and adolescents who have diabetes show an increase in slow activity (delta and theta) and a reduction in alpha frequency, which is most prominent in frontal regions [178,179]. A history of severe hypoglycemia predicts increased theta slowing [178,179], whereas poor metabolic control is associated with increases in delta activity and decreases in alpha frequency. Peripheral nerve conduction velocities are also correlated with increases in slow wave activity (delta and theta). That finding is consistent with the possibility of a link between peripheral neuropathy and what is known as central neuropathy [182], both of which may be induced by the microvascular or metabolic changes associated with chronic hyperglycemia. Because cognitive function has not been measured in any study examining EEG abnormalities in children and adolescents, it is impossible to determine whether these electrophysiologic abnormalities have a significant impact on neuropsychological abilities.

Permanent structural damage

To date, no neuroimaging studies of children or adolescents who have diabetes have been published. Some evidence exists in adults to suggest that as few as three or more episodes of severe hypoglycemia may be associated with a reduction in brain gray matter, as measured using MRI. This reduction is especially prominent in regions responsible for language processing and verbal memory, but the magnitude of this effect is small [183]. Other studies that used various neuroimaging procedures have been equivocal, with some—but not all—showing mild abnormalities in adults who have diabetes who experienced recurrent episodes of moderately severe hypoglycemia. For example, one MRI study reported cortical atrophy in 45% of the subjects who had diabetes with recurrent hypoglycemia, compared with none of 11 subjects with no past history of hypoglycemia [184]. On the other hand, more recent studies failed to find a relationship between brain structure and hypoglycemia [149]. Individuals who experienced hypoglycemic comas did not show abnormalities either in the cerebral metabolic rate of oxygen use, as measured with positron emission tomography [185], or in neural processing efficiency, as measured by event-related potential (P300) studies [186]. In some instances [185], these null results may reflect the small samples of subjects or the relative insensitivity of the techniques, but there is a growing consensus that even if structural changes are present, they are small and may not be attributable solely to recurrent hypoglycemia.

Risk factors for hypoglycemia

Adolescents are much more likely to experience severe hypoglycemia than adults, regardless of the intensity of therapy [2], and within the pediatric group, younger age has been a consistently reported risk factor for hypoglycemia [168,187]. Children with a history of prior hypoglycemia, lower glycohemoglobin levels, absence of residual C-peptide, and male gender are at the greatest risk [2,19,188–190], as are children treated in centers with the least experience [188]. The use of human insulins was initially a risk factor for hypoglycemia when used in regimens of two injections per day [191]. Surprisingly, no study reported a relationship between the frequency of hypoglycemia and the number of daily insulin injections administered [188].

Illnesses commonly seen in patients who have type 1 diabetes, such as hypothyroidism and celiac disease, are associated with frequent hypoglycemia [192,193]. The less common occurrence of autoimmune Addison's disease also can cause severe hypoglycemia [193]. These conditions should be excluded in any patient with recurrent, unexplained hypoglycemic episodes.

The reason that younger children are at greatest risk is partially explained by their highly variable eating habits, increased sensitivity to insulin [169], and high exercise-associated energy expenditure. Prolonged or intense exercise is probably the most frequent risk factor for diurnal and nocturnal hypoglycemia.

Exercise, although desirable, can cause hypoglycemia during activity [194] and several hours later. The physiologic basis for this postexercise, late-onset hypoglycemia remains unknown, but it typically occurs at night. In one large study, it accounted for more than half of the episodes of severe hypoglycemia [195].

Intervention strategies

The development and successful implementation of effective prevention interventions have been hampered by the lack of sensitive and accurate techniques to detect and document asymptomatic hypoglycemic episodes. These techniques are currently under intense investigation, and one can be optimistic that they will lead to appropriate future interventions. Currently, the evaluation of frequent blood glucose monitoring, using accurate meters, allows each individual patient—at least hypothetically—to detect patterns of glycemia that might predict a severe hypoglycemic episode that can be prevented by changes in meal planning or insulin doses [196,197]. The challenge is to teach families to test frequently and use this information to implement prevention strategies. One group has attempted to use a handheld computer to teach subjects more effectively to be proactive [198]. This strategy was believed to be useful in adults but has yet to be tested in children who have diabetes. Prevention of hypoglycemia can be accomplished with regular intake of well-balanced meals with increased caloric density and decreasing insulin dosing to compensate for the increased energy expenditure associated with exercise. These approaches are the mainstay of diabetes teaching by an experienced diabetes team. In patients treated with intermediate-acting insulins, the ingestion of an adequate nighttime snack is essential. This snack, by clinical experience, must contain a significant amount of protein/fat (eg, peanut butter) in addition to carbohydrate.

The recognition that most hypoglycemic episodes occur at night, especially after exercise, demands arduous nighttime glucose monitoring, which is difficult for more families to implement. Some parents' sleep is disrupted each night because their fear of hypoglycemia results in frequent testing, however, particularly if a severe episode has been experienced previously. Similar to reports in adults, pediatric studies have documented decreased frequency of nocturnal hypoglycemia by substituting short- and long-acting insulin analogs for regular- and intermediate-acting insulins, respectively (ie, insulins with prolonged peak) [8,199–202]. The use of subcutaneous insulin infusion with the recent development of improved pumps is theoretically the most effective way of rapidly altering insulin delivery to prevent hypoglycemia. Studies of patients before and after the institution of insulin pump therapy suggested that continuous insulin infusion may be an effective means of decreasing the frequency of nocturnal hypoglycemia, particularly in younger children [202,203]. Adolescents who chose pump therapy also had fewer episodes of hypoglycemia than their counterparts who chose treatment with multiple daily injections [204], although small randomized studies have not confirmed this difference between pump therapy and multiple daily injections [205,206]. Large randomized studies in children to evaluate the efficacy of insulin delivered by pump versus injections are needed.

Exercise-induced hypoglycemia should be anticipated and prevented by feeding carbohydrate-containing food while exercising [207] or decreasing short-acting insulin by 30% to 50% [208]. Prevention of nocturnal, postexercise hypoglycemia is less well studied. The usual practice is to decrease the evening insulin dose after strenuous exercise or provide a larger evening snack. In that situation, we usually recommend that the snack contain an increased portion of carbohydrate and protein.

It is generally believed that intensive insulin therapy by any of the previously mentioned regimens is most successful in experienced hands. Vigilance, frequent glucose monitoring, and education of the family are key for successful prevention of severe hypoglycemic episodes. Pediatric research has documented that most severe hypoglycemic episodes can be explained by errors in implementing such a plan [209]. Current continuous glucose monitoring techniques, although improving, still lack the ability to detect hypoglycemic episodes accurately because they still produce false-positive and false-negative results [210–212]. Ultimately, individualized patient therapy is required to meet the variable needs of each patient, taking into account age, activity level, family habits, knowledge, motivation, and ability to follow a complex medical regimen. The dangers and fears of hypoglycemia must be balanced with the documented need to maintain the best glycemic control possible.

Treatment of acute episodes

It has been recognized that posthypoglycemia hyperglycemia (ie, the Somogyi phenomenon) is most likely to represent the overtreatment of hypoglycemic episodes, compounded by the effect of hormonal counterregulation in individuals without the HAAF syndrome [213,214]. It is important to deliver only the amount of glucose and calories sufficient to counteract an episode of hypoglycemia. The amount of glucose required varies with the degree of hypoglycemia; an example of one set of treatment guidelines is presented in Box 1. The blood glucose level should be checked after an episode of hypoglycemia to ensure the adequacy of treatment.

Severe hypoglycemia must be counteracted immediately with intravenous glucose in a hospital setting or the delivery of subcutaneous glucagon (ideally, 0.03 mg/kg). For practical reasons, the glucagon dose is delivered as either 0.5- or 1-mg aliquots in the field to raise blood glucose levels immediately. Glucagon treatment should be followed by the administration of concentrated oral glucose as soon as possible to maintain euglycemia. Large volumes of fluid should be avoided under these circumstances because hypoglycemia per se and glucagon therapy often cause nausea and vomiting for several hours after the

---

Box 1. Hypoglycemia treatment guidelines

If patient is symptomatic and blood glucose is ≤ 70, provide prompt treatment

If patient is asymptomatic and blood glucose is ≤ 70, verify glucose level by rechecking it

Recheck glucose meter 30 minutes after treatment to verify that hypoglycemia has been reversed, regardless of whether symptoms continue

Treatment of mild or moderate hypoglycemia

If blood glucose is 55–70 mg/dL, provide three glucose tablets (5 g glucose each) or 4 oz orange juice and follow with six crackers

If blood glucose is less than 55 mg/dL, provide four glucose tablets or 6–8 oz of orange juice and follow with six crackers

If blood glucose level is described as previously and it is at mealtime, give only the juice or glucose tablets as directed, give insulin, and give the meal; do not change the portions of the meal

Treatment of severe hypoglycemia

If the child is unresponsive, seizing, or cannot swallow, test blood glucose and either

- administer 0.1 mg/kg of 25% dextrose solution intravenously if there is intravenous access and if medical staff are readily available to administer the dextrose *or*
- administer 0.5 mg (small child) or 1 mg of glucagon subcutaneously

An alternative involves the administration of cake icing or glucose gel into the cheek pouch, although this is not optimal because of the risk of inhalation

---

event. It is our contention that every patient with type 1 diabetes should have an emergency supply of glucagon at home and in the school setting.

Summary

The experience of hypoglycemia is probably the most feared and hated consequence of life with type 1 diabetes among pediatric patients and their parents. Although transient detrimental effects are clearly disturbing and may have severe results, there is surprisingly little evidence of long-term CNS damage, even after multiple hypoglycemic episodes, except in rare instances. Despite the latter evidence, we advocate that every treatment regimen be designed to prevent hypoglycemia without inducing unacceptable hyperglycemia and increasing the risk of micro- and macrovascular complications.

References

[1] Diabetes Control and Complications Trial Research Group. The effect of intensive treatment on the development and progression of long-term complications in insulin-dependent diabetes mellitus. N Engl J Med 1993;329:977–86.
[2] Diabetes Control and Complications Trial Research Group. Effect of intensive diabetes treatment on the development and progression of long-term complications in adolescents with insulin-dependent diabetes mellitus: Diabetes Control and Complications Trial. J Pediatr 1994; 125:177–88.
[3] Diabetes Control and Complications Trial Research Group. Epidemiology of severe hypoglycemia in the Diabetes Control and Complications Trial. Am J Med 1991;90:450–9.
[4] Diabetes Control and Complications Trial Research Group. The relationship of glycemic exposure (HbA_{1c}) to the risk of development and progression of retinopathy in the Diabetes Control and Complications Trial. Diabetes 1995;44:968–83.
[5] Writing Team for the Diabetes Control and Complications Trial/Epidemiology of Diabetes Interventions and Complications Research Group. Sustained effect of intensive treatment of type 1 diabetes mellitus on development and progression of diabetic nephropathy: the Epidemiology of Diabetes Interventions and Complications (EDIC) Study. JAMA 2003;290: 2159–67.
[6] Diabetes Control and Complications Trial Research Group. The effect of intensive diabetes therapy on the development and progression of neuropathy. Ann Intern Med 1995;122:561–8.
[7] Nishimura R, LaPorte RE, Dorman JS, et al. Mortality trends in type 1 diabetes: the Allegheny County (Pennsylvania) Registry 1965–1999. Diabetes Care 2001;24:823–7.
[8] Chase HP, Lockspeiser T, Perry B, et al. The impact of the Diabetes Control and Complications Trial and Humalog insulin on glycohemoglobin levels and severe hypoglycemia in type 1 diabetes. Diabetes Care 2001;24:430–4.
[9] Marks V. Hypoglycaemia: real and unreal, lawful and unlawful. The 1994 Banting Lecture. Diabet Med 1995;12:850–64.
[10] Schwartz RP. Neonatal hypoglycemia: how low is too low? J Pediatr 1997;131:171–3.
[11] DCCT Research Group. Hypoglycemia in the Diabetes Control and Complications Trial. Diabetes 1997;46:271–86.
[12] Jones TW, Porter P, Sherwin RS, et al. Decreased epinephrine responses to hypoglycemia during sleep. N Engl J Med 1998;338:1657–62.
[13] Gschwend S, Ryan C, Atchinson J, et al. Effects of acute hyperglycemia on mental efficiency and counterregulatory hormones in adolescents with insulin-dependent diabetes mellitus. J Pediatr 1995;126:178–84.
[14] Mokan M, Mitrakou A, Veneman T, et al. Hypoglycemia unawareness in insulin-dependent diabetes mellitus. Diabetes Care 1994;17:1397–403.
[15] American Diabetes Association Workgroup on Hypoglycemia. Defining and reporting hypoglycemia in diabetes: a report from the American Diabetes Association Workgroup on Hypoglycemia. Diabetes Care 2005;28:1245–9.
[16] Clarke WL, Gonder-Frederick L, Cox DJ. The frequency of severe hypoglycaemia in children with insulin-dependent diabetes mellitus. Horm Res 1996;45:48–52.
[17] Jones TW, Davis EA. Hypoglycemia in children with type 1 diabetes: current issues and controversies. Pediatr Diabetes 2003;4:143–50.

[18] Bulsara MK, Holman GDJ, Davis EA, et al. Evaluating risk factors associated with severe hypoglycaemia in epidemiology studies: what method should we use? Diabet Med 2004; 21:914–9.

[19] Davis EA, Keating B, Byrne GC, et al. Hypoglycemia: incidence and clinical predictors in a large population-based sample of children and adolescents with IDDM. Diabetes Care 1997; 20:22–5.

[20] Davis EA, Keating B, Byrne GC, et al. Impact of improved glycaemic control on rates of hypoglycaemia in insulin dependent diabetes mellitus. Arch Dis Child 1998;78:111–5.

[21] Danne T, Mortensen HB, Hougaard P, et al for the Hvidøre Study Group on Childhood Diabetes. Persistent differences among centers over 3 years in glycemic control and hypoglycemia in a study of 3,805 children and adolescents with type 1 diabetes from the Hvidøre Study Group. Diabetes Care 2001;24:1342–7.

[22] Norfeldt S, Ludvigsson J. Adverse events in intensively treated children and adolescents with type 1 diabetes. Acta Paediatr 1999;88:1184–93.

[23] Rewers A, Chase HP, Mackenzie TA, et al. Predictors of acute complications in children with type 1 diabetes. JAMA 2002;287:2511–8.

[24] Diabetes Control and Complications Trial Research Group. Hypoglycemia in the Diabetes Control and Complications Trial. Diabetes 1997;46:271–86.

[25] Whincup G, Milner RDG. Prediction and management of nocturnal hypoglycemia in diabetes. Arch Dis Child 1987;62:333–7.

[26] Beregszaszi M, Tubiana-Rufi N, Benali K, et al. Nocturnal hypoglycemia in children and adolescents with insulin-dependent diabetes mellitus: prevalence and risk factors. J Pediatr 1997;131:27–33.

[27] Matyka KA. Sweet dreams? Nocturnal hypoglycemia in children with type 1 diabetes. Pediatr Diabetes 2002;3:74–81.

[28] Matyka KA, Wigg L, Pramming S, et al. Cognitive function and mood after profound nocturnal hypoglycaemia in prepubertal children with conventional insulin treatment for diabetes. Arch Dis Child 1999;81:138–42.

[29] Clarke DD, Sokoloff LL. Circulation and energy metabolism of the brain. In: Siegel GJ, Agranoff BW, Albers RW, et al, editors. Basic neurochemistry. Philadelphia: Lippincott-Raven; 1999. p. 637–69.

[30] Chugani HT. A critical period of brain development: studies of cerebral glucose utilization with PET. Prev Med 1998;27:184–8.

[31] Dunn-Meynell AA, Routh VH, Kang L, et al. Glucokinase is the likely mediator of glucose sensing in both glucose-excited and glucose-inhibited central neurons. Diabetes 2002;51: 2056–65.

[32] Cryer PE. Diverse causes of hypoglycemia-associated autonomic failure in diabetes. N Engl J Med 2004;350:2272–9.

[33] Hoffman RP, Singer-Granick C, Drash AL, et al. Abnormal alpha cell hypoglycemia recognition in children with insulin-dependent diabetes. J Pediatr Endocrinol Metab 1994;7:225–34.

[34] Maran A, Cranston I, Lomas J, et al. Protection by lactate of cerebral function during hypoglycaemia. Lancet 1994;343:16–20.

[35] Amiel SA, Archibald HR, Chusney G, et al. Ketone infusion lowers hormonal responses to hypoglycaemia: evidence for acute cerebral utilization of a non-glucose fuel. Clin Sci 1991; 81:189–94.

[36] Abi-Saab WM, Maggs DG, Jones T, et al. Striking differences in glucose and lactate levels between brain extracellular fluid and plasma in conscious human subjects: effects of hyperglycemia and hypoglycemia. J Cereb Blood Flow Metab 2002;22:271–9.

[37] Duelli R, Kuschinsky W. Brain glucose transporters: relationship to local energy demand. News Physiol Sci 2001;16:71–6.

[38] Simpson IA, Appel NM, Hokari M, et al. Blood-brain barrier glucose transporter: effects of hypo- and hyperglycemia revisited. J Neurochem 1999;72:238–47.

[39] McCall AL, Moss JM. Cerebral glucose metabolism in diabetes mellitus. Eur J Pharmacol 2004;490:147–58.

[40] McEwen BS, Reagan LP. Glucose transporter expression in the central nervous system: relationship to synaptic function. Eur J Pharmacol 2004;490:13–24.

[41] Boyle PJ. Alteration in brain glucose metabolism induced by hypoglycemia in man. Diabetologia 1997;40:S69–74.

[42] Criego AB, Tkac I, Kumar A, et al. Brain glucose concentrations in patients with type 1 diabetes and hypoglycemia unawareness. J Neurosci Res 2005;79:42–7.

[43] Hershey T, Lillie R, Sadler M, et al. A prospective study of severe hypoglycemia and long-term spatial memory in children with type 1 diabetes. Pediatr Diabetes 2004;5:63–71.

[44] Ryan CM. Does moderately severe hypoglycemia cause cognitive dysfunction in children? Pediatr Diabetes 2004;5:59–62.

[45] Jones TW, Boulware SD, Kraemer DT, et al. Independent effects of youth and poor diabetes control on responses to hypoglycemia in children. Diabetes 1991;40:358–63.

[46] McCall AL, Fixman LB, Fleming N, et al. Chronic hypoglycemia increases brain glucose transport. Am J Physiol 1986;251:E442–7.

[47] Fanelli CG, Pampanelli S, Porcellati F, et al. Shift of glycaemic thresholds for cognitive function in hypoglycaemia unawareness in humans. Diabetologia 1998;41:720–3.

[48] Tallroth G, Ryding E, Agardh C-D. Regional cerebral blood flow in normal man during insulin-induced hypoglycemia and in the recovery period following glucose infusion. Metabolism 1992;41:717–21.

[49] Kerr D, Stanley JC, Barron M, et al. Symmetry of cerebral blood flow and cognitive responses to hypoglycemia in humans. Diabetologia 1993;36:73–8.

[50] Eckert B, Ryding E, Agardh C-D. The cerebral vascular response to a rapid decrease in blood glucose to values above normal in poorly controlled type 1 (insulin-dependent) diabetes mellitus. Diabetes Res Clin Pract 1995;27:221–7.

[51] MacLeod KM, Gold AE, Ebmeier KP, et al. The effects of acute hypoglycemia on relative cerebral blood flow distribution in patients with type 1 (insulin dependent) diabetes and impaired hypoglycemia awareness. Metabolism 1996;45:974–80.

[52] Tallroth G, Ryding E, Agardh C-D. The influence of hypoglycaemia on regional cerebral blood flow and cerebral volume in type 1 (insulin-dependent) diabetes mellitus. Diabetologia 1993;36:530–5.

[53] Jarjour IT, Ryan CM, Becker DJ. Regional cerebral blood flow during hypoglycaemia in children with IDDM. Diabetologia 1995;38:1090–5.

[54] Bryan RM, Pelligrino DA. Cerebral blood flow during chronic hypoglycemia in the rat. Brain Res 1988;475:397–400.

[55] Pelligrino DA, Segil LJ, Albrecht RF. Brain glucose utilization and transport and cortical function in chronic vs. acute hypoglycemia. Am J Physiol 1990;259:E729–35.

[56] Pelligrino DA, Lipa MD, Albrecht RF. Regional blood-brain glucose transfer and glucose utilization in chronically hyperglycemic, diabetic rats following acute glycemic normalization. J Cereb Blood Flow Metab 1990;10:774–80.

[57] Auer RN, Siesjö BK. Hypoglycaemia: brain neurochemistry and neuropathology. Baillieres Clin Endocrinol Metab 1993;7:611–25.

[58] Siesjö BK, Bengtsson F. Calcium fluxes, calcium antagonists, and calcium-related pathology in brain ischemia, hypoglycemia, and spreading depression: a unifying hypothesis. J Cereb Blood Flow Metab 1989;9:127–40.

[59] Auer RN, Olsson Y, Siesjo BK. Hypoglycemic brain injury in the rat: correlation of density of brain damage with the EEG isoelectric timed. A quantitative study. Diabetes 1984;33:1090–8.

[60] Auer RN, Wieloch T, Olsson Y, et al. The distribution of hypoglycemic brain damage. Acta Neuropathol (Berl) 1984;64:177–91.

[61] Brierley JB, Brown AW, Meldrum BS. The nature and time course of the neuronal alterations resulting from oligaemia and hypoglycaemia in the brain of Macaca mulatta. Brain Res 1971;25:483–99.

[62] Auer RN, Hugh J, Cosgrove E, et al. Neuropathologic findings in three cases of profound hypoglycemia. Clin Neuropathol 1989;8:63–8.

[63] Boeve BF, Bell DG, Noseworthy JH. Bilateral temporal lobe MRI changes in uncomplicated hypoglycemic coma. Can J Neurol Sci 1995;22:56–8.

[64] Chalmers J, Risk MTA, Kean DM, et al. Severe amnesia after hypoglycemia. Diabetes Care 1991;14:922–5.

[65] Fujioka M, Okuchi K, Hiramatsu K, et al. Specific changes in human brain after hypoglycemic injury. Stroke 1997;28:584–7.

[66] Auer RN. Progress review: hypoglycemic brain damage. Stroke 1986;17:699–708.

[67] Wieloch T, Harris RJ, Symon L, et al. Influences of severe hypoglycemia on brain extracellular calcium and potassium activities, energy and phospholipid metabolism. J Neurochem 1984; 43:160–8.

[68] Harris RJ, Wieloch T, Symon L, et al. Cerebral extracellular calcium activity in severe hypoglycemia: relation to extracellular potassium and energy state. J Cereb Blood Flow Metab 1984;4:187–93.

[69] Auer RN, Kalimo H, Olsson Y, et al. The temporal evolution of hypoglycemic brain damage. Acta Neuropathol (Berl) 1985;67:13–24.

[70] Strachan MWJ, Abraha HD, Sherwood RA, et al. Evaluation of serum markers of neuronal damage following severe hypoglycaemia in adults with insulin-treated diabetes mellitus. Diabetes Metab Res Rev 1999;15:5–12.

[71] Dagogo-Jack SE, Craft S, Cryer PE. Hypoglycemia-associated autonomic failure in insulin-dependent diabetes mellitus. J Clin Invest 1993;91:819–28.

[72] Cryer PE. Iatrogenic hypoglycemia as a cause of hypoglycemia-associated autonomic failure in IDDM: a vicious cycle. Diabetes 1992;41:255–60.

[73] Fanelli CG, Pampanelli S, Epifano L, et al. Long term recovery from awareness, deficient counterregulation and lack of cognitive dysfunction during hypoglycemia following institution of rational intensive therapy in IDDM. Diabetologia 1994;37:1265–76.

[74] Borg WP, Sherwin RS, During MJ, et al. Local ventromedial hypothalamus glucopenia triggers counterregulatory hormone release. Diabetes 1995;44:180–4.

[75] Davis SN, Shavers C, Costa F, et al. Role of cortisol in the pathogenesis of deficient counter-regulation after antecedent hypoglycemia in normal humans. J Clin Invest 1996;98:680–91.

[76] Davis SN, Shavers C, Davis B, et al. Prevention of an increase in plasma cortisol during hypoglycemia preserves subsequent counterregulatory responses. J Clin Invest 1997;100: 429–38.

[77] Raju B, McGregor VP, Cryer PE. Cortisol elevations comparable to those that occur during hypoglycemia do not cause hypoglycemia-associated autonomic failure. Diabetes 2003;52: 2083–9.

[78] Cryer PE, Davis SN, Shamoon H. Hypoglycemia in diabetes. Diabetes Care 2003;26:1902–12.

[79] Dagogo-Jack SE, Rattarasarn C, Cryer PE. Reversal of hypoglycemia unawareness, but not defective glucose-counter-regulation in IDDM. Diabetes 1994;43:1426–34.

[80] Puczynski S, Becker D, Dorn L, et al. An intervention protocol for parental management of nocturnal hypoglycemia in young children with IDDM. Diabetes 1997;46:98A.

[81] Thordarson H, Søvik O. Dead in bed syndrome in young diabetic patients in Norway. Diabet Med 1995;12:782–7.

[82] Edge JA, Ford-Adams ME, Dunger DB. Causes of death in children with insulin dependent diabetes 1990–96. Arch Dis Child 1999;81:318–23.

[83] Banarer S, Cryer PE. Sleep-related hypoglycemia-associated autonomic failure in type 1 diabetes: reduced awakening from sleep during hypoglycemia. Diabetes 2003;52:1195–203.

[84] Davis SN, Galassetti P, Wasserman DH, et al. Effects of antecedent hypoglycemia on subsequent counterregulatory responses to exercise. Diabetes 2000;49:73–81.

[85] McGregor VP, Greiwe JS, Banarer S, et al. Limited impact of vigorous exercise on defenses against hypoglycemia: relevance to hypoglycemia-associated autonomic failure. Diabetes 2002; 51:1485–92.

[86] Galassetti P, Neill A, Tate D, et al. Sexual dimorphism in counterregulatory responses to hypoglycemia after antecedent exercise. J Clin Endocrinol Metab 2001;86:3516–24.

[87] Koyama Y, Galassetti P, Coker R, et al. Prior exercise and the response to insulin-induced hypoglycemia in the dog. Am J Physiol Endocrinol Metab 2002;282:E1128–38.

[88] Rose AJ, Richter EA. Skeletal muscle glucose uptake during exercise: how is it regulated? Physiology 2005;20:260–70.

[89] Holloszy JO. Exercise-induced increase in muscle insulin sensitivity. J Appl Physiol 2005; 99:338–43.

[90] McCrimmon RJ, Gold AE, Deary IJ, et al. Symptoms of hypoglycemia in children with IDDM. Diabetes Care 1995;18:858–61.

[91] Marrero DG, Guare JC, Vandagriff JL, et al. Fear of hypoglycemia in the parents of children and adolescents with diabetes: maladaptive or healthy response? Diabetes Educ 1997;23: 281–6.

[92] Ryan CM, Dulay D, Suprasongsin C, et al. Detection of symptoms by adolescents and young adults with type 1 diabetes during experimental induction of mild hypoglycemia: role of hormonal and psychological variables. Diabetes Care 2002;25:852–8.

[93] Watson D, Clark LA. Negative affectivity: the disposition to experience aversive emotional states. Psychol Bull 1984;96:465–90.

[94] Watson D, Pennebaker JW. Health complaints, stress, and distress: exploring the central role of negative affectivity. Psychol Rev 1989;96:234–54.

[95] Nurick MA, Johnson SB. Enhancing blood glucose awareness in adolescents and young adults with IDDM. Diabetes Care 1991;14:1–7.

[96] Freund A, Johnson SB, Rosenbloom A, et al. Subjective symptoms, blood glucose estimation, and blood glucose concentrations in adolescents with diabetes. Diabetes Care 1986;9:236–43.

[97] Gonder-Frederick LA, Snyder AL, Clarke WL. Accuracy of blood glucose estimation by children with IDDM and their parents. Diabetes Care 1991;14:565–70.

[98] Green LB, Wysocki T, Reineck B. Fear of hypoglycemia in children and adolescents with diabetes. J Pediatr Psychol 1990;15:633–41.

[99] Clarke WL, Gonder-Frederick LA, Snyder AL, et al. Maternal fear of hypoglycemia in their children with insulin dependent diabetes mellitus. J Pediatr Endocrinol Metab 1998;11:189–94.

[100] Hepburn DA, Deary IJ, MacLeod KM, et al. Structural equation modeling of symptoms, awareness and fear of hypoglycemia, and personality in patients with insulin-treated diabetes. Diabetes Care 1994;17:1273–80.

[101] Pocecco M, Ronfani L. Transient focal neurologic deficits associated with hypoglycemia in children with insulin-dependent diabetes mellitus: Italian Collaborative Paediatric Diabetologic Group. Acta Paediatr 1998;87:542–4.

[102] Gold AE, Deary IJ, Frier BM. Hypoglycaemia and non-cognitive aspects of psychological function in insulin-dependent (type 1) diabetes mellitus (IDDM). Diabet Med 1997;14:111–8.

[103] Gold AE, MacLeod KM, Deary IJ. Changes in mood during acute hypoglycemia in healthy participants. J Pers Soc Psychol 1995;68:498–504.

[104] Hepburn DA, MacLeod KM, Frier BM. Physiological, symptomatic and hormonal responses to acute hypoglycaemia in type 1 diabetic patients with autonomic neuropathy. Diabet Med 1993; 10:940–9.

[105] McCrimmon RJ, Ewing FME, Frier BM, et al. Anger state during acute insulin-induced hypoglycaemia. Physiol Behav 1999;67:35–9.

[106] DeFronzo RA, Tobin JD, Andres R. Glucose clamp technique: a method for quantifying insulin secretion and resistance. Am J Physiol 1979;237:E214–23.

[107] Holmes CS, Hayford JT, Gonzalez JL, et al. A survey of cognitive functioning at different glucose levels in diabetic persons. Diabetes Care 1983;6:180–5.

[108] Holmes CS, Koepke KM, Thompson RG, et al. Verbal fluency and naming performance in type I diabetes at different blood glucose concentrations. Diabetes Care 1984;7:454–9.

[109] Holmes CS, Koepke KM, Thompson RG. Simple versus complex performance impairments at three blood glucose levels. Psychoneuroendocrinology 1986;11:353–7.

[110] Holmes CS. Metabolic control and auditory information processing at altered glucose levels in insulin-dependent diabetes. Brain Cogn 1987;6:161–74.

[111] Holmes CS. Neuropsychological sequelae of acute and chronic blood glucose disruption in

adults with insulin-dependent diabetes. In: Holmes CS, editor. Neuropsychological and behavioral aspects of diabetes. New York: Springer-Verlag; 1989. p. 122–54.

[112] Blackman JD, Towle VL, Sturis J, et al. Hypoglycemic thresholds for cognitive dysfunction in IDDM. Diabetes 1992;41:392–9.

[113] Driesen NR, Cox DJ, Gonder-Frederick L, et al. Reaction time impairment in insulin-dependent diabetes: task complexity, blood glucose levels, and individual differences. Neuropsychology 1995;9:246–54.

[114] Heller SR, Macdonald IA, Herbert M, et al. Influence of sympathetic nervous system on hypoglycaemic warning symptoms. Lancet 1987;2:359–63.

[115] Herold KC, Polonsky KS, Cohen RM, et al. Variable deterioration in cortical function during insulin-induced hypoglycemia. Diabetes 1985;34:677–85.

[116] Wirsén A, Tallroth G, Lindgren M, et al. Neuropsychological performance differs between type 1 diabetic and normal men during insulin-induced hypoglycaemia. Diabet Med 1992;9: 156–65.

[117] Draelos MT, Jacobson AM, Weinger K, et al. Cognitive function in patients with insulin-dependent diabetes mellitus during hyperglycemia and hypoglycemia. Am J Med 1995;98: 135–44.

[118] McAulay V, Deary IJ, Ferguson SC, et al. Acute hypoglycemia in humans causes attentional dysfunction while nonverbal intelligence is preserved. Diabetes Care 2001;24:1745–50.

[119] Ryan CM, Atchison J, Puczynski S, et al. Mild hypoglycemia associated with deterioration of mental efficiency in children with insulin-dependent diabetes mellitus. J Pediatr 1990;117: 32–8.

[120] Sommerfield AJ, Deary IJ, McAulay V, et al. Short-term delayed, and working memory are impaired during hypoglycemia in individuals with type 1 diabetes. Diabetes Care 2003;26: 390–6.

[121] Ovalle F, Fanelli CG, Paramore DS, et al. Brief twice-weekly episodes of hypoglycemia reduce detection of clinical hypoglycemia in type 1 diabetes mellitus. Diabetes 1998;47:1472–9.

[122] Gonder-Frederick LA, Cox DJ, Driesen NR, et al. Individual differences in neurobehavioral disruption during mild and moderate hypoglycemia in adults with IDDM. Diabetes 1994; 43:1407–12.

[123] Evans ML, Pernet A, Lomas J, et al. Delay in onset of awareness of acute hypoglycemia and of restoration of cognitive performance during recovery. Diabetes Care 2000;23:893–7.

[124] Hoffman RG, Speelman DJ, Hinnen DA, et al. Changes in cortical functioning with acute hypoglycemia and hyperglycemia in type 1 diabetes. Diabetes Care 1989;12:193–7.

[125] Ryan C, Vega A, Longstreet C, et al. Neuropsychological changes in adolescents with insulin-dependent diabetes mellitus. J Consult Clin Psychol 1984;52:335–42.

[126] Northam EA, Anderson PJ, Jacobs R, et al. Neuropsychological profiles of children with type 1 diabetes 6 years after disease onset. Diabetes Care 2001;24:1541–6.

[127] Kaufman FR, Epport K, Engilman R, et al. Neurocognitive functioning in children diagnosed with diabetes before age 10 years. J Diabetes Complications 1999;13:31–8.

[128] Hagen JW, Barclay CR, Anderson BJ, et al. Intellective functioning and strategy use in children with insulin-dependent diabetes mellitus. Child Dev 1990;61:1714–27.

[129] McCarthy AM, Lindgren S, Mengeling MA, et al. Effects of diabetes on learning in children. Pediatrics 2002;109:1–10.

[130] Cox DJ, Gonder-Frederick LA, Kovatchev BP, et al. The metabolic demands of driving for drivers with type 1 diabetes mellitus. Diabetes Metab Res Rev 2002;18:381–5.

[131] Cox DJ, Gonder-Frederick LA, Kovatchev BP, et al. Progressive hypoglycemia's impact on driving simulation performance. Diabetes Care 2000;23:163–70.

[132] Bjørgaas M, Sand T, Vik T, et al. Quantitative EEG during controlled hypoglycemia in diabetic and non-diabetic children. Diabet Med 1998;15:30–7.

[133] Bendtson I, Gade J, Rosenfalck AM, et al. Nocturnal electroencephalogram registrations in type 1 (insulin-dependent) diabetic patients with hypoglycaemia. Diabetologia 1991;34: 750–6.

[134] Pramming S, Thorsteinsson B, Stigsby B, et al. Glycaemic threshold for changes in

electroencephalograms during hypoglycaemia in patients with insulin dependent diabetes. BMJ 1988;296:665–7.

[135] Tallroth G, Lindgren M, Stenberg G, et al. Neurophysiological changes during insulin-induced hypoglycaemia and in the recovery period following glucose infusion in type 1 (insulin-dependent) diabetes mellitus and in normal man. Diabetologia 1990;33:319–23.

[136] Tribl G, Howorka K, Heger G, et al. EEG topography during insulin-induced hypoglycemia in patients with insulin-dependent diabetes mellitus. Eur Neurol 1996;36:303–9.

[137] Howorka K, Heger G, Schabmann A, et al. Severe hypoglycaemia unawareness is associated with an early decrease in vigilance during hypoglycaemia. Psychoneuroendocrinology 1996; 21:295–312.

[138] Amiel SA, Pottinger RC, Archibald HR, et al. Effect of antecedent glucose control on cerebral function during hypoglycemia. Diabetes Care 1991;14:109–18.

[139] Ziegler D, Hübinger A, Mühlen H, et al. Effects of previous glycaemic control on the onset and magnitude of cognitive dysfunction during hypoglycaemia in type 1 (insulin-dependent) diabetic patients. Diabetologia 1992;35:828–34.

[140] Fruehwald-Schultes B, Born J, Kern W, et al. Adaptation of cognitive function to hypoglycemia in healthy men. Diabetes Care 2000;23:1059–66.

[141] Jones TW, Borg WP, Borg MA, et al. Resistance to neuroglycopenia: an adaptive response during intensive insulin treatment of diabetes. J Clin Endocrinol Metab 1997;82:1713–8.

[142] Jones TW, Borg WP, Boulware SD, et al. Enhanced adrenomedullary response and increased susceptibility to neuroglycopenia: mechanisms underlying the adverse effects of sugar ingestion in healthy children. J Pediatr 1995;126:171–7.

[143] Gold AE, Deary IJ, Frier BM. Recurrent severe hypoglycaemia and cognitive function in type 1 diabetes. Diabet Med 1993;10:503–8.

[144] Perros P, Deary IJ. Long-term effects of hypoglycaemia on cognitive function and the brain in diabetes. In: Frier BM, Fisher BM, editors. Hypoglycaemia in clinical diabetes. Chichester (UK): John Wiley & Sons, Ltd; 1999. p. 187–210.

[145] Ryan CM. Effects of diabetes mellitus on neuropsychological functioning: a lifespan perspective. Semin Clin Neuropsychiatry 1997;2:4–14.

[146] Langan S, Deary I, Hepburn D, et al. Cumulative cognitive impairment following recurrent severe hypoglycaemia in adult patients with insulin-treated diabetes mellitus. Diabetologia 1991;34:337–44.

[147] Deary IJ, Langan SJ, Graham KS, et al. Recurrent severe hypoglycemia, intelligence, and speed of information processing. Intelligence 1992;16:337–59.

[148] Lincoln NB, Faleiro RM, Kelly C, et al. Effect of long-term glycemic control on cognitive function. Diabetes Care 1996;19:656–8.

[149] Ferguson SC, Blane A, Perros P, et al. Cognitive ability and brain structure in type 1 diabetes: relation to microangiopathy and preceding severe hypoglycemia. Diabetes 2003;52:149–56.

[150] Austin EJ, Deary IJ. Effects of repeated hypoglycemia on cognitive function. Diabetes Care 1999;22:1273–7.

[151] Diabetes Control and Complications Trial Research Group. Effects of intensive diabetes therapy on neuropsychological function in adults in the Diabetes Control and Complications Trial. Ann Intern Med 1996;124:379–88.

[152] Ryan CM, Geckle MO, Orchard TJ. Cognitive efficiency declines over time in adults with type 1 diabetes: effects of micro- and macrovascular complications. Diabetologia 2003;46: 940–8.

[153] Brand AMA, Biessels G-J, De Haan EHF, et al. The effects of type 1 diabetes on cognitive performance: a meta-analysis. Diabetes Care 2005;28:726–35.

[154] Holmes CS, Richman L. Cognitive profiles of children with insulin-dependent diabetes. J Dev Behav Pediatr 1985;6:323–6.

[155] Holmes CS, Dunlap WP, Chen RS, et al. Gender differences in the learning status of diabetic children. J Consult Clin Psychol 1992;60:698–704.

[156] Rovet J, Alverez M. Attentional functioning in children and adolescents with IDDM. Diabetes Care 1997;20:803–10.

[157] Rovet JF, Ehrlich RM, Czuchta D, et al. Psychoeducational characteristics of children and adolescents with insulin-dependent diabetes mellitus. J Learn Disabil 1993;26:7–22.

[158] Ryan C, Longstreet C, Morrow LA. The effects of diabetes mellitus on the school attendance and school achievement of adolescents. Child Care Health Dev 1985;11:229–40.

[159] Vetiska J, Glaab L, Perlman K, et al. School attendance of children with type 1 diabetes. Diabetes Care 2000;23:1706–7.

[160] Kovacs M, Goldston D, Iyengar S. Intellectual development and academic performance of children with insulin-dependent diabetes mellitus: a longitudinal study. Dev Psychol 1992; 28:676–84.

[161] Hershey T, Bhargava N, Sadler M, et al. Conventional vs. intensive diabetes therapy in children with type 1 diabetes: effects on memory and motor speed. Diabetes Care 1999;22: 1318–24.

[162] Wysocki T, Harris MA, Mauras N, et al. Absence of adverse effects of severe hypoglycemia on cognitive function in school-aged children with diabetes over 18 months. Diabetes Care 2003;26:1100–5.

[163] Rovet J, Ehrlich R, Hoppe M. Specific intellectual deficits associated with the early onset of insulin-dependent diabetes mellitus in children. Child Dev 1988;59:226–34.

[164] Ryan C, Vega A, Drash A. Cognitive deficits in adolescents who developed diabetes early in life. Pediatrics 1985;75:921–7.

[165] Northam EA, Anderson PJ, Werther GA, et al. Neuropsychological complications of IDDM in children 2 years after disease onset. Diabetes Care 1998;21:379–84.

[166] Northam EA, Anderson PJ, Werther GA, et al. Predictors of change in the neuropsychological profiles of children with insulin dependent diabetes mellitus two years after disease onset. Diabetes Care 1999;22:1438–44.

[167] Ferguson SC, Blane A, Wardlaw JM, et al. Influence of an early-onset age of type 1 diabetes on cerebral structure and cognitive function. Diabetes Care 2005;28:1431–7.

[168] Lteif AN, Schwenk WF. Type 1 diabetes mellitus in early childhood: glycemic control and associated risk of hypoglycemic reactions. Mayo Clin Proc 1999;74:211–6.

[169] Ternand C, Go VLW, Gerich JE, et al. Endocrine pancreatic response of children with onset of insulin-requiring diabetes before age 3 and after age 5. J Pediatr 1982;101:36–9.

[170] Caviness VS, Kennedy DN, Bates JF, et al. The developing human brain: a morphometric profile. In: Thatcher RW, Lyon GR, Rumsey J, et al, editors. Developmental neuroimaging: mapping the development of brain and behavior. San Diego (CA): Academic Press; 1997. p. 3–14.

[171] Huttenlocher PR. Morphometric study of human cerebral cortex development. Neuropsychologia 1990;28:517–27.

[172] Taylor HG, Alden J. Age-related differences in outcomes following childhood brain insults: an introduction and overview. J Intern Neuropsychol Soc 1997;3:555–67.

[173] Stenninger E, Flink R, Eriksson B, et al. Long term neurological dysfunction and neonatal hypoglycaemia after diabetic pregnancy. Arch Dis Child 1998;79:174F–9F.

[174] Murakami Y, Yamashita Y, Matsuishi T, et al. Cranial MRI of neurologically impaired children suffering from neonatal hypoglycaemia. Pediatr Radiol 1999;29:23–7.

[175] Bjørgaas M, Gimse R, Vik T, et al. Cognitive function in type 1 diabetic children with and without episodes of hypoglycaemia. Acta Paediatr 1997;86:148–53.

[176] Hershey T, Perantie DC, Warren SL, et al. Frequency and timing of severe hypoglycemia affects spatial memory in children with type 1 diabetes mellitus. Diabetes Care 2005;28:2372–7.

[177] Schoenle EJ, Schoenle D, Molinari L, et al. Impaired intellectual development in children with type 1 diabetes: association with HbA$_{1c}$, age at diagnosis, and sex. Diabetologia 2002;45: 108–14.

[178] Bjørgaas M, Sand T, Gimse R. Quantitative EEG in type 1 diabetic children with and without episodes of severe hypoglycemia: a controlled, blind study. Acta Neurol Scand 1996;93: 398–402.

[179] Hyllienmark L, Maltez J, Dandenell A, et al. EEG abnormalities with and without relation to severe hypoglycaemia in adolescents with type 1 diabetes. Diabetologia 2005;48:412–9.

[180] Gilhaus KH, Daweke H, Lülsdorf HG, et al. EEG veränderungen bei diabetischen kindern. Dtsch Med Wochenschr 1973;98:1449–54.

[181] Soltész G, Acsádi G. Association between diabetes, severe hypoglycemia, and electro-encephalographic abnormalities. Arch Dis Child 1989;64:992–6.

[182] Dejgaard A, Gade A, Larsson H, et al. Evidence for diabetic encephalopathy. Diabet Med 1991;8:162–7.

[183] Musen G, Lyoo IK, Sparks CR, et al. Effects of type 1 diabetes on gram matter density as measured by voxel-based morphometry. Diabetes, in press.

[184] Perros P, Deary IJ, Sellar RJ, et al. Brain abnormalities demonstrated by magnetic resonance imaging in adult IDDM patients with and without a history of recurrent severe hypoglycemia. Diabetes Care 1997;20:1013–8.

[185] Chabriat H, Sachon C, Levasseur M, et al. Brain metabolism after recurrent insulin-induced hypoglycemic episodes: a PET study. J Neurol Neurosurg Psychiatry 1994;57:1360–5.

[186] Kramer L, Fasching P, Madl C, et al. Previous episodes of hypoglycemic coma are not associated with permanent cognitive brain dysfunction in IDDM patients on intensive insulin treatment. Diabetes 1998;47:1909–14.

[187] Barkai L, Vámosi I, Lukács K. Prospective assessment of severe hypoglycaemia in diabetic children and adolescents with impaired and normal awareness of hypoglycaemia. Diabetologia 1998;41:898–903.

[188] Wagner VM, Grabert M, Holl RW. Severe hypoglycaemia, metabolic control and diabetes management in children with type 1 diabetes in the decade after the Diabetes Control and Complications Trial: a large scale multicentre study. Eur J Pediatr 2005;164:73–9.

[189] Porter PA, Keating B, Byrne G, et al. Incidence and predictive criteria of nocturnal hypoglycemia in young children with insulin-dependent diabetes mellitus. J Pediatr 1997;130:366–72.

[190] Mortensen HB, Hougaard P. Comparison of metabolic control in a cross-sectional study in 2,873 children and adolescents with IDDM from 18 countries: the Hvidore Study Group on Childhood Diabetes. Diabetes Care 1997;20:714–20.

[191] Egger M, Smith GD, Teuscher AU, et al. Influence of human insulin on symptoms and awareness of hypoglycaemia: a randomized double blind crossover trial. BMJ 1991;303:622–6.

[192] Mohn A, Cerruto M, Lafusco D, et al. Celiac disease in children and adolescents with type 1 diabetes: importance of hypoglycemia. J Pediatr Gastroenterol Nutr 2001;32:37–40.

[193] Mohn A, Di Michele S, Di Luzio R, et al. The effect of subclinical hypothyroidism on metabolic control in children and adolescents with type 1 diabetes mellitus. Diabet Med 2002;19:70–3.

[194] Temple MY, Bar-Or O, Riddell MC. The reliability repeatability of the blood glucose response to prolonged exercise in adolescent boys with IDDM. Diabetes Care 1995;18:326–32.

[195] MacDonald MJ. Postexercise late-onset hypoglycemia in insulin-dependent diabetic patients. Diabetes Care 1987;10:584–8.

[196] Cox DJ, Gonder-Frederick L, Polonsky W, et al. Blood glucose awareness training (BGAT-2): long-term benefits. Diabetes Care 2001;24:637–42.

[197] Clarke WL, Cox DJ, Gonder-Frederick L, et al. Biopsychobehavioral model of risk of severe hypoglycemia: self-management behaviors. Diabetes Care 1999;22:580–4.

[198] Cox D, Gonder-Frederick L, Polonsky W, et al. A multicenter evaluation of blood glucose awareness training: II. Diabetes Care 1995;18:523–8.

[199] Mohn A, Matyka KA, Harris DA, et al. Lispro or regular insulin for multiple injection therapy in adolescence: differences in free insulin and glucose levels overnight. Diabetes Care 1999;22:27–32.

[200] Chase HP, Dixon B, Pearson JS, et al. Reduced hypoglycemic episodes and improved glycemic control in children with type 1 diabetes using insulin glargine and neutral protamine hagedorn insulin. J Pediatr 2003;143:737–40.

[201] Danne T, Deisst D, Hopfenmuller W, et al. Experience with insulin analogs in children. Horm Res 2002;57:46–53.

[202] Weinzimer SA, Doyle EA, Tamborlane WV. Disease management in the young diabetic patients: glucose monitoring, coping skills, and treatment strategies. Clin Pediatr 2005;44: 393–403.

[203] Weinzimer SA, Ahern JH, Doyle EA, et al. Persistence of benefits of continuous subcutaneous insulin infusion in very young children with type 1 diabetes: a follow-up report. Pediatrics 2004;114:1601–5.

[204] Boland EA, Grey M, Oesterle A, et al. Continuous subcutaneous insulin infusion: a new way to lower risk of severe hypoglycemia, improve metabolic control, and enhance coping in adolescents with type 1 diabetes. Diabetes Care 1999;22:1779–84.

[205] Weintrob N, Schechter A, Benzaquen H, et al. Glycemic patterns detected by continuous subcutaneous glucose sensing in children and adolescents with type 1 diabetes mellitus treated by multiple daily injections vs. continuous subcutaneous insulin infusion. Arch Pediatr Adolesc Med 2004;158:677–84.

[206] Wilson DM, Buckingham BA, Kunselman EL, et al. A two-center randomized controlled feasibility trial of insulin pump therapy in young children with diabetes. Diabetes Care 2005; 28:15–9.

[207] Riddell MC, Bar-Or O, Ayub BB, et al. Glucose ingestion matched with total carbohydrate utilization attenuates hypoglycemia during exercise in adolescents with IDDM. Int J Sport Nutr 1999;9:24–34.

[208] Shiffrin A, Parikh S. Accommodating planned exercise in type 1 diabetic patients on intensive treatment. Diabetes Care 1985;8:337–42.

[209] Daneman D, Frank M, Perlman K, et al. Severe hypoglycemia in children with insulin dependent diabetes mellitus: frequency and predisposing factors. J Pediatr 1989;115:681–5.

[210] Diabetes Research in Children Network (DirecNet) Study Group. The accuracy of the CGMS in children with type 1 diabetes: results of the Diabetes Research in Children Network (DirecNet) Accuracy Study. Diabetes Technol Ther 2003;5:781–9.

[211] Diabetes Research in Children Network (DirecNet) Study Group. Accuracy of the GlucoWatch G2 Biographer and the Continuous Glucose Monitoring System during hypoglycemia. Diabetes Care 2004;27:722–6.

[212] Diabetes Research in Children Network (DirecNet) Study Group. Accuracy of the modified Continuous Glucose Monitoring System (CGMS) sensor in an outpatient setting: results from a Diabetes Research in Children Network (DirecNet) Study. Diabetes Technol Ther 2005;7: 109–14.

[213] De Feo P, Perriello G, Bolli GB. Somogyi and dawn phenomena: mechanisms. Diabetes Metab Rev 1988;4:31–49.

[214] Raskin P. The Somogyi phenomenon: sacred cow or bull? Arch Intern Med 1984;144:781–7.

ELSEVIER
SAUNDERS

PEDIATRIC CLINICS
OF NORTH AMERICA

Pediatr Clin N Am 52 (2005) 1735–1753

Complications of Diabetes Mellitus in Childhood

Sarah J. Glastras, MBBS (Hons), BSc Psychol (Hons)[a],
Fauzia Mohsin, MBBS, FCPS[a],
Kim C. Donaghue, MBBS, PhD, FRACP[a,b,*]

[a]Institute of Endocrinology and Diabetes, The Children's Hospital at Westmead, Locked Bag 4001, Westmead NSW 2145, Sydney, Australia
[b]Department of Medicine, University of Sydney, NSW 2006, Sydney, Australia

Microvascular complications of diabetes include retinopathy, nephropathy, and neuropathy. Such complications can have devastating long-term effects, including blindness caused by diabetic retinopathy, renal failure caused by diabetic nephropathy, and disabling pain caused by diabetic neuropathy. Although they uncommonly affect children and adolescents with diabetes, subclinical microvascular changes may be detected by sensitive testing methods during these early periods. Macrovascular complications that predispose to ischemic and peripheral vascular disease are rare under the age of 30 years. Childhood and adolescence are periods during which intensive education and treatment may prevent or delay the onset of complications.

Pathogenesis

Hyperglycemia is the primary pathogenic factor in the development of complications [1]. Several biochemical pathways may be activated in the presence of hyperglycemia, including polyol accumulation, formation of advanced glycation end products, oxidative stress, and activation of protein kinase C [2,3]. The combined effect of these mechanisms results in further cellular, functional, and structural changes. Vascular changes of diabetes result in hyperperfusion of or-

---

* Corresponding author. Institute of Endocrinology and Diabetes, The Children's Hospital at Westmead, Locked Bag 4001, Westmead NSW 2145, Sydney, Australia.
  E-mail address: kimd@chw.edu.au (K.C. Donaghue).

gans causing basement membrane and mesangial thickening and subsequent vascular permeability.

The importance of glycemic control

The Diabetes Control and Complications Trial (DCCT) was a large, multi-center, clinical trial that involved 1441 patients with type 1 diabetes (T1D). It provided convincing evidence that intensive diabetes treatment that improved glycemic control conferred a significant risk reduction for retinopathy, nephropathy, and neuropathy compared with conventional treatment [4,5]. Within the cohort of patients included in the DCCT, 195 were pubertal adolescents at the time of recruitment (aged 13–17 years). Compared with conventional treatment, intensive treatment of diabetes reduced the risk and progression of background retinopathy by 53% and microalbuminuria by 54% in adolescents. Clinical neuropathy was not sufficiently common for a significant treatment effect to be demonstrated (7/103 in the conventional group and 3/92 in the intensive group) [6].

After completion of the DCCT, the Epidemiology of Diabetes Interventions and Complications (EDIC) study continued to follow patients from the DCCT cohort [7–10]. During the subsequent first 4 years of EDIC there was no difference in mean Hba1c levels between the former intensive and the former conventional groups. The benefits of 7 years of randomization to intensive versus conventional diabetes treatment continued to have effect, however. Patients who previously were randomized to the intensive group were less likely to have retinopathy or microalbuminuria (Table 1). In the adolescent cohort from the DCCT, laser intervention for diabetic retinopathy was needed in 6% of the conventional group compared with 1% of the formerly treated intensive group. Although there was no significant difference in progression from normoalbuminuria to microalbuminuria between the groups, proteinuria remained less likely

Table 1

Results from the Diabetes Control and Complications Trial and Epidemiology of Diabetes Interventions and Complications trial showing the risk reduction in diabetic retinopathy and nephropathy (microalbuminuria and albuminuria) as a result of intensive compared with conventional therapy during the Diabetes Control and Complications Trial

Complication	Risk reduction in DCCT IT versus CT (%)	Risk reduction in EDIC former IT versus former CT (%)
Any retinopathy	53–70	74–78
Microalbuminuria	55	48
Albuminuria		85

Abbreviations: CT, conventional therapy; EDIC, Epidemiology of Diabetes Interventions and Complications trial; IT, intensive therapy.

Adapted from DCCT Research Group. Effect of intensive diabetes treatment on the development and progression of long-term complications in adolescents with insulin-dependent diabetes mellitus. J Pediatr 1994;125:177–88.

in patients from the former intensive group (1.3%) compared with the conventional group (9.9%).

The major adverse event associated with intensive diabetes treatment was a threefold increase in severe hypoglycemia with seizures and unconsciousness, which was more likely in the adolescent cohort [6]. No children were included in the study. Because severe hypoglycemia can have effects on the developing brain, intensive therapy must be balanced against the risk of hypoglycemia, especially in young children.

Risk factors for the development of complications

Apart from glycemic control, other factors are relevant to the development of complications. Duration of diabetes, age, family history of complications, smoking, dyslipidemia, and hypertension are known to influence the development of complications. The presence of one microvascular complication has been shown to be associated with development of another [11].

Prepubertal children younger than 12 years of age rarely develop complications of diabetes, and prepubertal years of diabetes were believed to be relatively unimportant in the development of complications [12]. More recent studies that examined prepubertal diabetes duration have shown its significance. In this center, 193 adolescents who developed prepubertal diabetes were followed through to early adulthood [13]. There was a nonuniform effect of diabetes duration for microvascular complications. Although the survival-free period of retinopathy and microalbuminuria was significantly longer (2–4 years) for persons diagnosed before 5 years of age compared with persons diagnosed after 5 years of age (Fig. 1), the risk of clinical retinopathy increased by 28% for every prepubertal year of duration and by 36% for every postpubertal year of duration [13].

Associations were observed among high cholesterol, triglyceride, and retinopathy incidence [14]. High cholesterol has been correlated with hard exudate and macular edema [15], and lower HDL-cholesterol is associated with development of retinal lesion [16]. Serum triglyceride and high level of low density cholesterol are associated with progression of retinopathy [17].

Smoking is associated with an increased risk of developing persistent microalbuminuria or macroalbuminuria [11,18–20]. The incidence rates for microalbuminuria were higher in smokers compared with non-smokers (7.9 versus 2.2 per 100 person-years) and smoking resulted in an even greater incidence rate if combined with poor glycemic control [21]. The evidence for the effect of smoking on retinopathy is less clear [22–24].

Diabetic retinopathy

Retinopathy is a leading cause of blindness among young adults in western countries [5,25]. An orderly progression of increasing severity occurs from

A

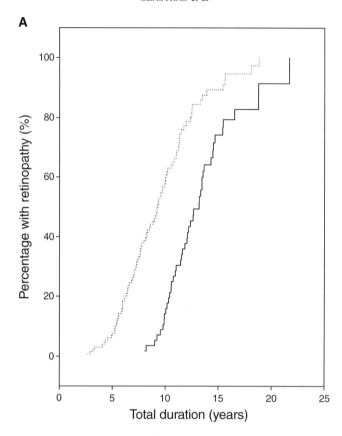

Fig. 1. (*A, B*) Cumulative percentage of retinopathy and microalbuminuria in prepubertal onset patients at Children's Hospital at Westmead according to age at diagnosis. Broken line indicates patients aged younger than 5 years. Unbroken line indicates patients aged 5 years or older.

background to proliferative retinopathy. The earliest features of background retinopathy are microaneurysms and pre- and intraretinal hemorrhages. Microaneurysms develop because of loss of supporting pericytes around the capillary wall. They are often transient and last from months to years [26]. Later features are hard exudates caused by protein and lipid leakage and microvascular abnormalities. Background retinopathy is not vision threatening and does not invariably progress to proliferative retinopathy.

Preproliferative retinopathy is characterized by vascular obstruction, progressive intraretinal microvascular abnormalities, and infarctions of the retinal nerve fibers that cause cotton wool spots. The characteristic feature of proliferative retinopathy is neovascularization. These vessels may rupture or bleed into the vitreoretinal space and cause loss of vision. Encasement in connective tissue results in adhesions, which can cause hemorrhage and retinal detachment. Visual loss may occur depending on the location and extent of neovascularization [27].

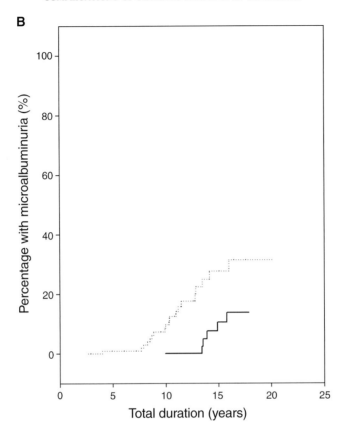

Fig. 1 (*continued*).

The Wisconsin Epidemiology Study of Diabetic Retinopathy performed baseline assessments of retinopathy from 1980 to 1982. Among patients with insulin-treated diabetes diagnosed at age younger than 30 years, retinopathy was present in 97% and proliferative retinopathy detected in 25% after 15 years of diabetes duration [28]. Our institution reported the prevalence of retinopathy to be 42% in adolescents screened between 1989 and 1992 [29] but 22% in adolescents screened between 1990 and 2002 [30]. The declining incidence in proliferative retinopathy also has been reported in Sweden and is likely the result of improvements in diabetes management [31].

The natural history of diabetic retinopathy includes progression and regression. The 4-year follow-up of the Wisconsin Epidemiology Study of Diabetic Retinopathy found that retinopathy progressed in 41%, was unchanged in 55%, and had improved in 4% [25]. In our 3-year follow-up of retinopathy in adolescents, retinopathy had progressed in 15%, remained stable in 38%, and regressed in 47% [30].

Disturbingly, the Wisconsin Epidemiology Study of Diabetic Retinopathy identified adolescents aged 15 to19 years at baseline to have the highest rate of

progression to vision-threatening retinopathy after 10 years compared with pediatric and adult patients with diabetes [5,25]. Adolescence is the time when
efforts should be directed to screening for early signs of diabetic retinopathy and
modifiable risk factors.

Assessment of retinopathy

Many techniques have been used in the detection of diabetic retinopathy,
including direct and indirect ophthalmoscopy, fluorescein angiography, stereoscopic digital and color film–based fundal photography. Stereoscopic fundal
photography provides greater sensitivity for detecting background and proliferative retinopathy compared with direct ophthalmoscopy [32]. Fluorescein angiography reveals functional abnormalities (vascular permeability) and structural
abnormalities in the blood vessels, whereas fundal photography reveals only
structural abnormalities. Fluorescein angiography requires an intravenous injection of fluorescein, however, which commonly causes nausea and may cause
anaphylactic reactions. Both methods produce a recording (hard copy or elec-
tronic) that can be referred to in subsequent assessments and can be shown to
the adolescents.

Interventions

Optimizing glycemic control is the most established therapy for preventing the development and progression of early retinopathy [6]. Improved metabolic control initially may worsen diabetic retinopathy. Within 1.5 to 3 years,
however, definite advantage of intensive treatment in the patients is evident
[33,34]. In the DCCT, the long-term benefits of intensive insulin treatment
greatly outweighed the risk of early worsening. The DCCT recommended ophthalmologic monitoring before initiation of intensive treatment and at 3-month
intervals for 6 to 12 months thereafter for patients with long-standing poor
glycemic control.

Angiotensin-converting enzyme (ACE) inhibitors have been used in clinical
trials and have been shown to reduce progression of diabetic retinopathy in normotensive subjects [35] but are not recommended yet for patients with retinopathy alone.

When vision-threatening diabetic retinopathy develops, the treatment options
are limited. The earliest possible detection of diabetic retinopathy is advisable
[36]. Panretinal photocoagulation, commonly known as laser therapy, consists of
multiple discrete outer retinal burns that are delivered to the peripheral retina
but spare the central macula. Its early use can prevent vision loss. In a study of
1758 patients with varying level of proliferative retinopathy, panretinal photocoagulation reduced the progression of visual loss by more than 50% [27].
Photocoagulation is not recommended for eyes with mild or moderate-to-severe
nonproliferative retinopathy, however [37]. Side effects of treatment are decreased night and peripheral vision and subtle changes in color perception.

Complications of laser therapy are vitrial and choroidal hemorrhages or visual sequelae of misplaced burns. In some patients treated with photocoagulation, diabetic retinopathy progresses and ongoing treatment is necessary.

Diabetic nephropathy

Diabetic renal disease characteristically follows a common clinical course. The first clinical sign is microalbuminuria. Persistent microalbuminuria predicts the development of overt diabetic nephropathy and increased cardiovascular mortality [38]. Diabetic nephropathy is characterized by frank proteinuria and often is associated with hypertension. End-stage renal failure may occur many years later and requires dialysis or kidney transplantation in some cases. It is estimated that 30% to 40% of patients with T1D develop end-stage renal failure [39]. It is responsible for most premature deaths, usually as a consequence of associated macrovascular disease [40,41].

Microalbuminuria may be detected in adolescents who have T1D but is rarely present in children who have diabetes. During adolescence, between 6% and 25% of patients who have T1D have microalbuminuria [19,42–46]. After 10 to 30 years of early-onset diabetes, approximately one third of patients have persistent microalbuminuria [47–49].

Recent evidence suggests that clinical signs of diabetic nephropathy may be present before the development of microalbuminuria. Although hypertension is rarely present at the time when microalbuminuria develops, mild increases in blood pressure, detected by 24-hour blood pressure monitoring, may precede the development of microalbuminuria in T1D [50–52]. Early rises in albumin excretion rate—although within the normal range—have been shown to predict the development of microalbuminuria and are detectable within the first few years after diagnosis in some children and adolescents [53–55]. In adolescents who have T1D, borderline albuminuria (albumin excretion rate 7.2–20 µg/min) predicted development of persistent microalbuminuria 15 to 50 months later [56].

Microalbuminuria does not always progress to overt proteinuria. Microalbuminuria and concomitant hypertension are associated with poorer prognosis than microalbuminuria alone [38]. Regression of microalbuminuria frequently has been reported [54,55,57,58]. An 8-year follow-up study of patients with microalbuminuria found that the 6-year regression rate to normoalbuminuria was 58% and progression to proteinuria only 15% [58]. Factors associated with regression have been identified and include microalbuminuria of short duration, low HbA1c, low systolic blood pressure, and low levels of cholesterol and triglycerides [54,58]. Interventions such as optimizing blood pressure control and using ACE inhibitors may increase the likelihood of regression [59,60]. New advances in interventional therapies for diabetic nephropathy may have influenced its natural history; recent data show a declining incidence of diabetic nephropathy and microalbuminuria [57,61].

Assessment of microalbuminuria

A measurement of albumin excretion rate in a timed urine collection is the gold standard for defining microalbuminuria. Microalbuminuria is defined as albumin excretion rate more than 20 μg/min but less than 200 μg/min on a minimum of two of three consecutive timed overnight urine collections [62,63]. Other estimations of microalbuminuria using a spot urine sample include albumin/creatinine ratio of 2.5 to 25 mg/μmol, albumin/creatinine ratio of 30 to 300 mg/g, or albumin concentration of 30 to 300 mg/L from an early morning urine sample [64]. The spot albumin/creatinine ratios, although easier to obtain, may be influenced by orthostatic or postexercise proteinuria. They are less sensitive for detecting rises within the normal range of albumin excretion. Regardless of the procedure used, at least two of three samples over a 3- to 6-month period should confirm microalbuminuria [63].

Interventions

Good glycemic control achieved by intensive insulin therapy and the use of ACE inhibitors may prevent or delay progression from microalbuminuria to overt diabetic nephropathy [7,39,65]. Controlling blood pressure in the normotensive range is essential in all diabetes management. ACE inhibitors seem to have renoprotective effects that are independent of lowering blood pressure, which makes them superior to other antihypertensive agents, such as calcium channel blockers [63,66]. ACE inhibitors may reduce frank proteinuria and delay the onset of end-stage renal failure in adults who have T1D and overt diabetic nephropathy [67]. They are also effective in delaying the development of proteinuria in patients who have T1D and microalbuminuria with or without hypertension [68–72]. Although currently widely used in adults who have diabetes, the data on whether ACE inhibitors preserve renal function in normotensive microalbuminuric patients are less substantive. Cessation of therapy may result in rapid progression of albumin excretion to the level of untreated patients.

The use of ACE inhibitors in children and adolescents is more contentious. Because of the small number of children and adolescents who develop microalbuminuria, few studies have investigated the use of antihypertensive agents in this age group. One study examined the effects of an ACE inhibitor, captopril, in a group of adolescents who have T1D and microalbuminuria over 3 months [65]. They found that patients treated with captopril had a significant reduction in albuminuria compared with the control group. Another study found that treatment with either an ACE inhibitor or beta blocker in young adults resulted in regression of microalbuminuria compared with placebo [73]. Given the lack of evidence for the long-term protective benefit of ACE inhibitors in children and adolescents, initial treatment should include nonpharmacologic interventions. In particular, improvements in glycemic control, the cessation of smoking, and restriction of excessive protein consumption should be actively encouraged [74].

Diabetic neuropathy

Diabetic neuropathy should be considered in a child with recurrent vomiting or persistent pain syndromes, which may be caused by autonomic and peripheral neuropathy, respectively. Prepubertal children are not necessarily protected from diabetic neuropathy [75]. A longitudinal Flemish study that followed patients who had T1D from 1947 to 1973 reported that neuropathy had developed in 45% of individuals after 20 to 25 years and that it was less common in patients with better diabetes control [76]. Despite major changes in diabetes management, electrophysiologic abnormalities are common in adolescents [77].

Assessment of neuropathy

The American Diabetes Association has generated consensus statements for the diagnosis of neuropathy. Measurement from each of the following categories is recommended: clinical symptoms, clinical examination, electrodiagnostic studies, quantitative sensory testing, and autonomic function testing [78]. The place for these tests in children and adolescents is unclear.

Autonomic neuropathy

Clinical presentations of autonomic neuropathy include postural hypotension, vomiting, diarrhea, bladder paresis, impotence, sweating abnormalities, and gastric fullness. In adults, symptomatic and subclinical autonomic neuropathy has been associated with an increased risk of sudden death and increased mortality [79,80]. Prolonged QT intervals also may predispose to arrhythmias and sudden death [81].

The most frequently used tests to evaluate the autonomic nervous system are cardiovascular and pupillary function tests. Diabetes can cause a reduction in heart rate variation and in pupillary size with attenuation of the phasic light reflex. Loss of normal diurnal variation in blood pressure and nocturnal hypertension may be the first indications of hypertension and possibly renal disease. Longitudinal studies are needed to determine the true value of autonomic nerve testing in adolescents.

Peripheral neuropathy

Peripheral neuropathy most commonly presents in a chronic insidious fashion and affects sensory modalities in a symmetrical distribution. The most commonly reported symptoms are altered pain sensations (ie, dys-, para-, hypo- or hyperesthesia), burning, and either superficial or deep pain. Pain is usually worse at night. Painful peripheral neuropathy can be disabling in young adults with childhood-onset diabetes [82]. Hyperglycemia and rapid fluxes in plasma glucose may be important in perpetuating this symptom [83]. The mechanism of pain may result from regenerating small nerve fibers. The small unmyelinated C fibers are probably first affected. Sural nerve biopsies show fiber loss and atrophy of myelinated and unmyelinated fibers and regeneration of fibers.

Physical examination typically shows sensory loss in a glove and stocking distribution and loss of deep tendon reflexes. Muscle weakness occurs later in the disease and usually involves the intrinsic foot muscles and ankle dorsiflexors. Nerve conduction studies primarily reflect the function of large myelinated motor and sensory nerves. Improvement in velocity and amplitude has been shown with reduction in blood glucose levels with intensive treatment [84,85].

Quantitative sensory tests are noninvasive and less aversive and so have potential advantages in adolescents and for repeated studies. Large myelinated fibers are tested by vibration discrimination, and small unmyelinated and thinly myelinated fibers are tested by temperature discrimination. Abnormal biothesiometry in children who have diabetes has been found to have high specificity and sensitivity for nerve conduction abnormalities [86]. In our institution, we found that heat discrimination was more frequently abnormal than vibration in the foot (12% versus 5%) and that abnormalities of heat discrimination increased over 10 years [87].

Peripheral neuropathy, measured by vibration or thermal discrimination, predisposes to foot ulceration and amputation. Poor vibration discrimination was a predictor for foot ulceration 4 years later [88] and for ulceration and amputation over a 12-year period in patients [89]. Not all patients with neuropathy develop plantar ulceration, however. Other contributors include limited joint mobility, callus formation, and high plantar pressure [90]. At our center, we found that 35% of adolescents had reduced range of motion at the subtalar joint [91] and 10% had elevated plantar pressure using pedar analysis of gait [92]. More longitudinal studies are required in adolescents and young adults to determine the significance of abnormalities and the natural history of neuropathy.

Acute presentations of neuropathy, including proximal motor neuropathies (eg, amyotrophy), ophthalmoplegias, and painful sensory neuropathies, are much less common. Acute painful neuropathy can occur at any stage of diabetes and can be located in a stocking distribution, in the thighs (ie, femoral neuropathy), or in the trunk as a radiculopathy. Correlation with physical examination and electrophysiologic abnormalities may be poor. The pain is protracted and unremitting and lasts on average 10 months, until complete recovery, when return of lost tendon reflexes may occur. Exquisite contact discomfort is characteristic. It is unrelated to other complications of diabetes and can be precipitated by a period of improved glycemic control. It has been associated with eating disorders in young women [93].

Interventions

Symptomatic improvement of diabetic neuropathy has been shown with administration of tricyclic antidepressants, serotonin reuptake inhibitors, carbamazepine, and topical capsaicin. Mexiletine, the oral analog of lignocaine, recently has been been shown to be effective in reducing pain and dysesthesia, presumably because of its capacity to block sodium channels. Aldose reductase inhibitors have been used successfully in rodents as primary prevention of neuropathy and in patients who have type 2 diabetes and subclinical or mild peripheral neuropathy [94].

Macrovascular complications

Although macrovascular disease is rare in children and adolescents who have diabetes, risk factors are frequently present and should be addressed, including hypertension, smoking, and dyslipidemia. Although higher levels of total and low density lipoprotein (LDL) cholesterol, high density lipoprotein (HDL) cholesterol, and apoproteins have been reported in children who have diabetes [95,96], the more important factor for atherosclerosis is likely the greater proportion of smaller, more atherogenic LDL particles [97,98]. Statins have been recognized as safe for use in adolescents [99].

Subclinical macrovascular disease can be detected by using specialized tools. A recent study using quantitative coronary angiography demonstrated a high prevalence of silent coronary artery disease in young adults, which is associated with long-term glycemic control [100]. Endothelial dysfunction, fundamental to the development of vascular disease, can be detected by using ultrasound in children and adolescents who have T1D of short duration [62,101]. Similarly, an increase in carotid intima-media thickness, a structural marker of early atherosclerosis, has been detected by ultra-sensitive ultrasound in children and adolescents T1D [102].

Associated autoimmune diseases

Hypothyroidism and celiac disease are the most common autoimmune diseases associated with T1D. Thyroid and celiac disease are rarely detected by overt clinical signs but rather are identified by screening tests for relevant autoantibodies [103]. Several screening tests have been used for their detection. Measurements of thyroproxidase antibody may detect autoimmune thyroiditis, but it is more clinically relevant to measure thyroid-stimulating hormone as a screening test for hypo- or hyperthyroidism. Endomysial antibody has been the most commonly used screening test for celiac disease. Celiac disease may be confirmed by small bowel biopsy. Recent study from this center has found that thyroproxidase antibody and endomysial antibody measured at diagnosis of diabetes are strong predictors for development of thyroid and celiac disease, respectively. If thyroproxidase antibody and endomysial antibody are absent at diagnosis, such autoimmune complications are much less likely and warrant screening at 2- to 3-year intervals [104]. Treatment for hypothyroidism involves thyroid replacement with thyroxine, whereas celiac disease is managed by strict avoidance of gluten-containing foods.

Screening recommendations

The current recommendation is to screen for retinopathy annually after 2 years of diabetes in adolescents and after 5 years of diabetes in prepubertal children (Table 2). At a minimum, screening should include ophthalmoscopy through dilated pupils by an observer with special expertise in diabetic eye disease [105]. Immediate expert ophthalmologic management is recommended if there is progression of retinopathy to more than 10 microaneurysms, moderate nonproliferative or preproliferative retinopathy, or visual change or deterioration, macular edema, or proliferative changes [106].

Whenever possible, screening should be undertaken by mydriatic stereoscopic fundal photography. If it is available, biennial screening is appropriate for individuals with minimal background retinopathy, diabetes duration of less than 10 years, and a HbA1c level within the target range [30]. These findings should be interpreted with caution outside the settings of health care standards in Australia, however, and other developed countries and have not yet been incorporated into standard screening guidelines.

Annual screening for nephropathy is recommended after 2 years of diabetes in adolescents and after 5 years of diabetes in prepubertal children. Screening should include spot urinary albumin/creatinine ratio or preferably timed urine collection. If test results are abnormal, then tests should be repeated within 3 months. If the condition is persistent, then screening should be undertaken at more frequent intervals and other renal investigations sought. Other causes of increased protein excretion should be excluded, including glomerulonephritis, urinary tract infections, intercurrent infections, menstrual bleeding, vaginal discharge, orthostatic proteinuria, and strenuous exercise.

The American Diabetes Association recommends screening for lipids on an annual basis for adults and every 5 years in children older than 2 years of age if initial screen at diagnosis is normal [107]. In most Australian tertiary pediatric centers, screening for lipid disorders is undertaken at the time of microvascular screening. Screening for thyroid and celiac disease is recommended every 2 to 3 years [108,109].

Discussing complications

Educating families and adolescents about diabetes and its complications is an important aspect of care. Although the threat of complications should not be made, accurate and timely information about potential complications and the importance of good glycemic control may prevent or delay their development. The information provided should be appropriate to the young person's age and level of maturity. It is convenient and timely to provide education about complications during their assessment and screening. The importance of good glycemic control should be reinforced to all persons involved in the care of a young person who has diabetes.

Table 2
Screening guidelines

	When to commence screening?	Frequency	Preferred method of screening	Other screening methods	Potential intervention
Retinopathy	After 5 years duration in prepubertal children, after 2 years in pubertal children [105]	1–2 yearly [30,105]	Fundal photography	Fluorescein angiography, mydriatic ophthalmoscopy	Improved glycemic control, laser therapy
Nephropathy	After 5 years duration in prepubertal children, after 2 years in pubertal children [105]	Annually [105]	Overnight timed urine excretion of albumin	24-h excretion of albumin, Urinary albumin/creatinine ratio	Improved glycemic control, blood pressure control, ACE inhibitors
Neuropathy	Unclear	Unclear	Physical examination	Nerve conduction, thermal and vibration threshold, Pupillometry, cardiovascular reflexes	Improved glycemic control
Macrovascular disease	After age 2 [107]	Every 5 years [106]	Lipids	Blood pressure	Statins for hyperlipidemia Blood pressure control
Thyroid disease	At diagnosis	Every 2–3 years [108,109]	TSH	Thyroid peroxidase antibody	Thyroxine
Celiac disease	At diagnosis	Every 2–3 years [108,109]	Tissue transglutaminase, endomysial antibody	Antigliadin antibodies	Gluten-free diet

References

[1] Nishikawa T, Edelstein D, Brownlee M. The missing link: a single unifying mechanism for diabetic complications. Kidney Int 2000;77:S26–30.
[2] Gabbay KH. Hyperglycemia, polyol metabolism, and complications of diabetes mellitus. Annu Rev Med 1975;26:521–36.
[3] Giugliano D, Ceriello A, Paolisso G. Oxidative stress and diabetic vascular complications. Diabetes Care 1996;19:257–67.
[4] DCCT Research Group. The effect of intensive treatment of diabetes on the development and progression of long-term complications in insulin-dependent diabetes mellitus. N Engl J Med 1993;329:977–86.
[5] Klein R, Klein BE, Moss SE, et al. The Wisconsin Epidemiologic Study of Diabetic Retinopathy: XVII. The 14-year incidence and progression of diabetic retinopathy and associated risk factors in type 1 diabetes. Ophthalmology 1998;105:1801–15.
[6] DCCT Research Group. Effect of intensive diabetes treatment on the development and progression of long-term complications in adolescents with insulin-dependent diabetes mellitus: Diabetes Control and Complications Trial. J Pediatr 1994;125:177–88.
[7] White NH, Cleary PA, Dahms W, et al. Beneficial effects of intensive therapy of diabetes during adolescence: outcomes after the conclusion of the Diabetes Control and Complications Trial (DCCT). J Pediatr 2001;139:804–12.
[8] Epidemiology of Diabetes Interventions and Complications (EDIC) Research Group. Effect of intensive therapy on the microvascular complications of type 1 diabetes mellitus. JAMA 2002; 287:2563–9.
[9] Epidemiology of Diabetes Interventions and Complications (EDIC) Research Group. Sustained effect of intensive treatment of type 1 diabetes mellitus on development and progression of diabetic nephropathy: the Epidemiology of Diabetes Interventions and Complications (EDIC) study. JAMA 2003;290:2159–67.
[10] DCCT/Epidemiology of Diabetes Interventions and Complications Research Group. Retinopathy and nephropathy in patients with type 1 diabetes four years after a trial of intensive therapy. N Engl J Med 2000;342:381–9.
[11] Rossing P, Hougaard P, Parving HH. Risk factors for development of incipient and overt diabetic nephropathy in type 1 diabetic patients: a 10-year prospective observational study. Diabetes Care 2002;25:859–64.
[12] Kostraba JN, Dorman JS, Orchard TJ, et al. Contribution of diabetes duration before puberty to development of microvascular complications in IDDM subjects. Diabetes Care 1989;12: 686–93.
[13] Donaghue KC, Fairchild JM, Craig ME, et al. Do all prepubertal years of diabetes duration contribute equally to diabetes complications? Diabetes Care 2003;26:1224–9.
[14] Chaturvedi N, Sjoelie AK, Porta M, et al. Markers of insulin resistance are strong risk factors for retinopathy incidence in type 1 diabetes. Diabetes Care 2001;24:284–9.
[15] Chew EY, Klein ML, Ferris III FL, et al. Association of elevated serum lipid levels with retinal hard exudate in diabetic retinopathy: Early Treatment Diabetic Retinopathy Study (ETDRS) Report 22. Arch Ophthalmol 1996;114:1079–84.
[16] Kordonouri O, Danne T, Hopfenmuller W, et al. Lipid profiles and blood pressure: are they risk factors for the development of early background retinopathy and incipient nephropathy in children with insulin-dependent diabetes mellitus? Acta Paediatr 1996;85:43–8.
[17] Lloyd CE, Klein R, Maser RE, et al. The progression of retinopathy over 2 years: the Pittsburgh Epidemiology of Diabetes Complications (EDC) Study. J Diabetes Complications 1995; 9:140–8.
[18] Rossing P, Rossing K, Jacobsen P, et al. Unchanged incidence of diabetic nephropathy in IDDM patients. Diabetes 1995;44:739–43.
[19] Couper JJ, Staples AJ, Cocciolone R, et al. Relationship of smoking and albuminuria in children with insulin-dependent diabetes. Diabet Med 1994;11:666–9.

[20] Chase HP, Garg SK, Marshall G, et al. Cigarette smoking increases the risk of albuminuria among subjects with type I diabetes. JAMA 1991;265:614–7.

[21] Scott LJ, Warram JH, Hanna LS, et al. A nonlinear effect of hyperglycemia and current cigarette smoking are major determinants of the onset of microalbuminuria in type 1 diabetes. Diabetes 2001;50:2842–9.

[22] Diabetes Drafting Group. Prevalence of small vessel and large vessel disease in diabetic patients from 14 centres: the World Health Organisation multinational study of vascular disease in diabetics. Diabetologia 1985;28:615–40.

[23] West KM, Ahuja MM, Bennett PH, et al. Interrelationships of microangiopathy, plasma glucose and other risk factors in 3583 diabetic patients: a multinational study. Diabetologia 1982;22: 412–20.

[24] Moss SE, Klein R, Klein BE. Cigarette smoking and ten-year progression of diabetic retinopathy. Ophthalmology 1996;103:1438–42.

[25] Klein R, Klein BE, Moss SE, et al. The Wisconsin Epidemiologic Study of Diabetic Retinopathy. IX. Four-year incidence and progression of diabetic retinopathy when age at diagnosis is less than 30 years. Arch Ophthalmol 1989;107:237–43.

[26] Kohner EM, Dollery CT. The rate of formation and disappearance of microaneurysms in diabetic retinopathy. Trans Ophthalmol Soc U K 1970;90:369–74.

[27] Diabetic Retinopathy Study. Photocoagulation treatment of proliferative diabetic retinopathy: the second report of diabetic retinopathy study findings. Ophthalmology 1978;85:82–106.

[28] Klein R, Klein BE, Moss SE, et al. The Wisconsin epidemiologic study of diabetic retinopathy. II. Prevalence and risk of diabetic retinopathy when age at diagnosis is less than 30 years. Arch Ophthalmol 1984;102:520–6.

[29] Fairchild JM, Hing SJ, Donaghue KC, et al. Prevalence and risk factors for retinopathy in adolescents with type 1 diabetes. Med J Aust 1994;160:757–62.

[30] Maguire A, Chan A, Cusumano J, et al. The case for biennial retinopathy screening in children and adolescents. Diabetes Care 2005;28:509–13.

[31] Nordwall M, Bojestig M, Arnqvist HJ, et al. Declining incidence of severe retinopathy and persisting decrease of nephropathy in an unselected population of type 1 diabetes: -the Linkoping Diabetes Complications Study. Diabetologia 2004;47:1266–72.

[32] Moss SE, Klein R, Kessler SD, et al. Comparison between ophthalmoscopy and fundus photography in determining severity of diabetic retinopathy. Ophthalmology 1985;92:62–7.

[33] The Kroc Collaborative Study Group. Blood glucose control and the evolution of diabetic retinopathy and albuminuria: a preliminary multicenter trial. N Engl J Med 1984; 311:365–72.

[34] Group DR. Early worsening of diabetic retinopathy in the Diabetes Control and Complications Trial. Arch Ophthalmol 1998;116:874–86.

[35] Chaturvedi N, Sjolie AK, Stephenson JM, et al. Effect of lisinopril on progression of retinopathy in normotensive people with type 1 diabetes: the EUCLID study group. EURODIAB controlled trial of lisinopril in insulin-dependent diabetes mellitus. Lancet 1998;351:28–31.

[36] Bailey CC, Sparrow JM, Grey RH, et al. The National Diabetic Retinopathy Laser Treatment Audit. III. Clinical outcomes. Eye 1999;13:151–9.

[37] Ferris F. Early photocoagulation in patients with either type I or type II diabetes. Trans Am Ophthalmol Soc 1996;94:505–37.

[38] Mogensen CE, Poulsen PL. Microalbuminuria, glycemic control, and blood pressure predicting outcome in diabetes type 1 and type 2. Kidney Int Suppl 2004;66:S40–1.

[39] Brink SJ. Complications of pediatric and adolescent type 1 diabetes mellitus. Curr Diab Rep 2001;1:47–55.

[40] Borch-Johnsen K, Kreiner S. Proteinuria: value as predictor of cardiovascular mortality in insulin dependent diabetes mellitus. Br Med J (Clin Res Ed) 1987;294:1651–4.

[41] Valdorf-Hansen F, Jensen T, Borch-Johnsen K, et al. Cardiovascular risk factors in type I (insulin-dependent) diabetic patients with and without proteinuria. Acta Med Scand 1987;222: 439–44.

[42] Bognetti E, Calori G, Meschi F, et al. Prevalence and correlations of early microvascular complications in young type I diabetic patients: role of puberty. J Pediatr Endocrinol 1997;10: 587–92.

[43] Olsen BS, Johannesen J, Sjolie AK, et al. Metabolic control and prevalence of microvascular complications in young Danish patients with type 1 diabetes mellitus: Danish Study Group of Diabetes in Childhood. Diabet Med 1999;16:79–85.

[44] Roe TF, Costin G, Kaufman FR, et al. Blood glucose control and albuminuria in type 1 diabetes mellitus. J Pediatr 1991;119:178–82.

[45] Mortensen HB, Marinelli K, Norgaard K, et al. A nation-wide cross-sectional study of urinary albumin excretion rate, arterial blood pressure and blood glucose control in Danish children with type 1 diabetes mellitus: Danish Study Group of Diabetes in Childhood. Diabet Med 1990;7:887–97.

[46] Dahlquist G, Rudberg S. The prevalence of microalbuminuria in diabetic children and adolescents and its relation to puberty. Acta Paediatr Scand 1987;76:795–800.

[47] Svensson M, Sundkvist G, Arnqvist HJ, et al. Signs of nephropathy may occur early in young adults with diabetes despite modern diabetes management: results from the nationwide population-based Diabetes Incidence Study in Sweden (DISS). Diabetes Care 2003;26: 2903–9.

[48] Bryden KS, Dunger DB, Mayou RA, et al. Poor prognosis of young adults with type 1 diabetes: a longitudinal study. Diabetes Care 2003;26:1052–7.

[49] Harvey JN, Allagoa B. The long-term renal and retinal outcome of childhood-onset type 1 diabetes. Diabet Med 2004;21:26–31.

[50] Lurbe E, Redon J, Kesani A, et al. Increase in nocturnal blood pressure and progression to microalbuminuria in type 1 diabetes. N Engl J Med 2002;347:797–805.

[51] Lafferty AR, Werther GA, Clarke CF. Ambulatory blood pressure, microalbuminuria, and autonomic neuropathy in adolescents with type 1 diabetes. Diabetes Care 2000;23:533–8.

[52] Poulsen PL, Hansen KW, Mogensen CE. Ambulatory blood pressure in the transition from normo- to microalbuminuria: a longitudinal study in IDDM patients. Diabetes 1994;43: 1248–53.

[53] Schultz CJ, Neil HA, Dalton RN, et al. Oxforn Regional Prospective Study G: risk of nephropathy can be detected before the onset of microalbuminuria during the early years after diagnosis of type 1 diabetes. Diabetes Care 2000;23:1811–5.

[54] Hovind P, Tarnow L, Rossing P, et al. Predictors for the development of microalbuminuria and macroalbuminuria in patients with type 1 diabetes: inception cohort study. BMJ 2004; 328:1105–9.

[55] Rudberg S, Dahlquist G. Determinants of progression of microalbuminuria in adolescents with IDDM. Diabetes Care 1996;19:369–71.

[56] Couper JJ, Clarke CF, Byrne GC, et al. Progression of borderline increases in albuminuria in adolescents with insulin-dependent diabetes mellitus. Diabet Med 1997;14:766–71.

[57] Bojestig M, Arnqvist HJ, Karlberg BE, et al. Glycemic control and prognosis in type I diabetic patients with microalbuminuria. Diabetes Care 1996;19:313–7.

[58] Perkins BA, Ficociello LH, Silva KH, et al. Regression of microalbuminuria in type 1 diabetes. N Engl J Med 2003;348:2285–93.

[59] ACE Inhibitors in Diabetic Nephropathy Trialist Group. Should all patients with type 1 diabetes mellitus and microalbuminuria receive angiotensin-converting enzyme inhibitors? A meta-analysis of individual patient data. Ann Intern Med 2001;134:370–9.

[60] Makino H, Nakamura Y, Wada J. Remission and regression of diabetic nephropathy. Hypertens Res 2003;26:515–9.

[61] Kofoed-Enevoldsen A, Borch-Johnsen K, Kreiner S, et al. Declining incidence of persistent proteinuria in type I (insulin-dependent) diabetic patients in Denmark. Diabetes 1987;36: 205–9.

[62] Donaghue KC, Fairchild JM, Chan A, et al. Diabetes complication screening in 937 children and adolescents. J Pediatr Endocrinol Metab 1999;12:185–92.

[63] Mogensen CE. Microalbuminuria and hypertension with focus on type 1 and type 2 diabetes. J Intern Med 2003;254:45−66.

[64] Meinhardt U, Ammann RA, Fluck C, et al. Microalbuminuria in diabetes mellitus: efficacy of a new screening method in comparison with timed overnight urine collection. J Diabetes Complications 2003;17:254−7.

[65] Cook J, Daneman D, Spino M, et al. Angiotensin converting enzyme inhibitor therapy to decrease microalbuminuria in normotensive children with insulin-dependent diabetes mellitus. J Pediatr 1990;117:39−45.

[66] Kasiske BL, Kalil RS, Ma JZ, et al. Effect of antihypertensive therapy on the kidney in patients with diabetes: a meta-regression analysis. Ann Intern Med 1993;118:129−38.

[67] Lewis EJ, Hunsicker LG, et al. The effect of angiotensin-converting-enzyme inhibition on diabetic nephropathy: the Collaborative Study Group. N Engl J Med 1993;329:1456−62.

[68] The EUCLID Study Group. Randomised placebo-controlled trial of lisinopril in normotensive patients with insulin-dependent diabetes and normoalbuminuria or microalbuminuria. Lancet 1997;349:1787−92.

[69] Mathiesen ER, Hommel E, Hansen HP, et al. Randomised controlled trial of long term efficacy of captopril on preservation of kidney function in normotensive patients with insulin dependent diabetes and microalbuminuria. BMJ 1999;319:24−5.

[70] The Microalbuminuria Captopril Study Group. Captopril reduces the risk of nephropathy in IDDM patients with microalbuminuria. Diabetologia 1996;39:587−93.

[71] Viberti G, Mogensen CE, Groop LC, et al. Effect of captopril on progression to clinical proteinuria in patients with insulin-dependent diabetes mellitus and microalbuminuria: European Microalbuminuria Captopril Study Group. JAMA 1994;271:275−9.

[72] O'Hare P, Bilbous R, Mitchell T, et al. Low-dose ramipril reduces microalbuminuria in type 1 diabetic patients without hypertension: results of a randomized controlled trial. ACE-Inhibitor Trial to Lower Albuminuria in Normotensive Insulin-Dependent Subjects Study Group. Diabetes Care 2000;23:1823−9.

[73] Rudberg S, Osterby R, Bangstad HJ, et al. Effect of angiotensin converting enzyme inhibitor or beta blocker on glomerular structural changes in young microalbuminuric patients with type I (insulin-dependent) diabetes mellitus. Diabetologia 1999;42:589−95.

[74] Chiarelli F, Casani A, Verrotti A, et al. Diabetic nephropathy in children and adolescents: a critical review with particular reference to angiotensin-converting enzyme inhibitors. Acta Paediatr Suppl 1998;425:42−5.

[75] White NH, Waltman SR, Krupin T, et al. Reversal of neuropathic and gastrointestinal complications related to diabetes mellitus in adolescents with improved metabolic control. J Pediatr 1981;99:41−5.

[76] Pirart J. Diabetes mellitus and its degenerative complications: a prospective study of 4,400 patients observed between 1947 and 1973. Diabet Metab 1977;3:173−82.

[77] Hyllienmark L, Brismar T, Ludvigsson J. Subclinical nerve dysfunction in children and adolescents with IDDM. Diabetologia 1995;38:685−92.

[78] Maser RE, Becker DJ, Drash AL, et al. Pittsburgh Epidemiology of Diabetes Complications Study: measuring diabetic neuropathy follow-up study results. Diabetes Care 1992;15:525−7.

[79] Ewing DJ. The natural history of diabetic autonomic neuropathy. Q J Med 1980;49:95−108.

[80] Maser RE, Mitchell BD, Vinik AI, et al. The association between cardiovascular autonomic neuropathy and mortality in individuals with diabetes: a meta-analysis. Diabetes Care 2003;26: 1895−901.

[81] Ewing DJ, Boland O, Neilson JM, et al. Autonomic neuropathy, QT interval lengthening, and unexpected deaths in male diabetic patients. Diabetologia 1991;34:182−5.

[82] Watkins PJ, Campbell IW, Clarke BF, et al. Clinical observations and experiments in diabetic neuropathy. Diabetologia 1992;35:2−11.

[83] Sindrup SH, Ejlertsen B, Gjessing H, et al. Peripheral nerve function during hyperglycemic clamping in healthy subjects. Acta Neurol Scand 1988;78:141−5.

[84] DCCT Research Group. Effect of intensive diabetes treatment on nerve conduction in the Diabetes Control and Complications Trial. Ann Neurol 1995;38:869−80.

[85] DCCT Research Group. The effect of intensive diabetes therapy on the development and progression of neuropathy. Ann Intern Med 1995;122:561–8.

[86] Davis EA, Jones TW, Walsh P, et al. The use of biothesiometry to detect neuropathy in children and adolescents with IDDM. Diabetes Care 1997;20:1448–53.

[87] Donaghue KC, Bonney M, Simpson JM, et al. Autonomic and peripheral nerve function in adolescents with and without diabetes. Diabet Med 1993;10:664–71.

[88] Sosenko JM, Kato M, Soto R, et al. Comparison of quantitative sensory-threshold measures for their association with foot ulceration in diabetic patients. Diabetes Care 1990;13:1057–61.

[89] Coppini DV, Young PJ, Weng C, et al. Outcome on diabetic foot complications in relation to clinical examination and quantitative sensory testing: a case-control study. Diabet Med 1998; 15:765–71.

[90] Veves A, Murray HJ, Young MJ, et al. The risk of foot ulceration in diabetic patients with high foot pressure: a prospective study. Diabetologia 1992;35:660–3.

[91] Duffin AC, Donaghue KC, Potter M, et al. Limited joint mobility in the hands and feet of adolescents with type 1 diabetes mellitus. Diabet Med 1999;16:125–30.

[92] Duffin AC, Kidd R, Chan A, et al. High plantar pressure and callus in diabetic adolescents: incidence and treatment. J Am Podiatr Med Assoc 2003;93:214–20.

[93] Steel JM, Young RJ, Lloyd GG, et al. Clinically apparent eating disorders in young diabetic women: associations with painful neuropathy and other complications. Br Med J (Clin Res Ed) 1987;294:859–62.

[94] Nakayama M, Nakamura J, Hamada Y, et al. Aldose reductase inhibition ameliorates pupillary light reflex and F-wave latency in patients with mild diabetic neuropathy. Diabetes Care 2001; 24:1093–8.

[95] Sosenko JM, Breslow JL, Miettinen OS, et al. Hyperglycemia and plasma lipid levels: a prospective study of young insulin-dependent diabetic patients. N Engl J Med 1980;302: 650–4.

[96] Lopes-Virella MF, Wohltmann HJ, Loadholt CB, et al. Plasma lipids and lipoproteins in young insulin-dependent diabetic patients: relationship with control. Diabetologia 1981;21: 216–23.

[97] Lyons TJ, Jenkins AJ. Lipoprotein glycation and its metabolic consequences. Curr Opin Lipidol 1997;8:174–80.

[98] Jenkins AJ, Best JD, Klein RL, et al. Lipoproteins, glycoxidation and diabetic angiopathy. Diabetes Metab Res Rev 2004;20:349–68.

[99] de Jongh S, Ose L, Szamosi T, et al. Efficacy and safety of statin therapy in children with familial hypercholesterolemia: a randomized, double-blind, placebo-controlled trial with simvastatin. Circulation 2002;106:2231–7.

[100] Larsen J, Brekke M, Sandvik L, et al. Silent coronary atheromatosis in type 1 diabetic patients and its relation to long-term glycemic control. Diabetes 2002;51:2637–41.

[101] Wiltshire EJ, Gent R, Hirte C, et al. Endothelial dysfunction relates to folate status in children and adolescents with type 1 diabetes. Diabetes 2002;51:2282–6.

[102] Jarvisalo MJ, Raitakari M, Toikka JO, et al. Endothelial dysfunction and increased arterial intima-media thickness in children with type 1 diabetes. Circulation 2004;109:1750–5.

[103] Hanukoglu A, Mizrachi A, Dalal I, et al. Extrapancreatic autoimmune manifestations in type 1 diabetes patients and their first-degree relatives: a multicenter study. Diabetes Care 2003;26: 1235–40.

[104] Glastras SJ, Craig ME, Verge CF, et al. The role of autoimmunity at diagnosis of type 1 diabetes in the development of thyroid and celiac disease and microvascular complications. Diabetes Care 2005.

[105] International Society for Pediatric and Adolescent Diabetes. Consensus guidelines for the management of type 1 diabetes mellitus in children and adolescents. Zeist, The Netherlands: Medical Forum International; 2000.

[106] Dorman JS, Laporte RE, Kuller LH, et al. The Pittsburgh insulin-dependent diabetes mellitus (IDDM) morbidity and mortality study: mortality results. Diabetes 1984;33:271–6.

[107] American Diabetes Association. Management of dyslipidemia in children and adolescents with diabetes. Diabetes Care 2003;26:2194–7.

[108] Australasian Paediatric Endocrine Group. Clinical practice guidelines: type 1 diabetes in children and adolescents, 2005. Available at: http://www.nhmrc.gov.au/publications/pdf/cp102.pdf. Accessed March 15, 2005.

[109] National Institute for Clinical Excellence. Type 1 diabetes (childhood): diagnosis and management of type 1 diabetes in children and young people. London: RCOG Press; 2005.

PEDIATRIC CLINICS

OF NORTH AMERICA

Pediatr Clin N Am 52 (2005) 1755–1778

The Psychologic Context of Pediatric Diabetes

Tim Wysocki, PhD*, Lisa M. Buckloh, PhD,
Amanda Sobel Lochrie, PhD, Holly Antal, PhD

*Nemours Children's Clinic, Division of Psychology and Psychiatry, 807 Children's Way,
Jacksonville, FL 32207, USA*

During the past few decades, there has been an explosion of behavioral science research on family management of pediatric diabetes. This article distills the major conclusions from that literature, emphasizing how primary care providers (PCPs) can apply these findings in clinical practice.

Interactions between psychologic adjustment and family management of type 1 diabetes in children and adolescents

Behavioral science research on type 1 diabetes mellitus (DM1) has shown clearly that this is best considered a family disease rather than a medical condition affecting only the child or adolescent [1]. The effectiveness of family diabetes management is influenced by such variables as family communication [2], problem solving [3], conflict resolution [4], and responsibility sharing [5]. Favorable status in these domains promotes better psychologic adjustment and quality of life [6], treatment adherence [7], glycemic control, and health care use [8]. Although DM1 poses significant psychologic threats, most families manage these challenges adequately without suffering serious psychologic problems, whereas a minority exhibit significant difficulties that compound the stress associated with

Support was provided to one or more of the authors by the following grants awarded to the first author: National Institutes of Health grants RO1-DK43802, U10-HD/DK 41918, and K24-DK67128, and National Institutes of Health research contract N01-HD-3361; and by a subcontract to American Diabetes Association Clinical Research grant 1-04-CR-18 awarded to Michael A. Harris, PhD, of Washington University in St. Louis.

* Corresponding author.

E-mail address: twysocki@nemours.org (T. Wysocki).

doi:10.1016/j.pcl.2005.07.003   ***pediatric.theclinics.com***

DM1 and its management. Research on the psychosocial aspects of DM1 management including interactions with the family environment, quality of life, emotional and behavioral problems, peer relationships, effects of diabetes on cognition and learning, and school issues is summarized next.

Family environment and parental involvement

Although youths with DM1 are understandably held accountable for regimen adherence, it is more appropriate to consider diabetes management as a family enterprise rather than an individual responsibility. Youth, especially younger children, require significant parental involvement with daily regimen tasks. Similar to other aspects of their daily care, children and adolescents cannot be expected to function independently. Given that DM1 management must be integrated into the family's lifestyle, it is likely to affect every family member. Recent research supports this perspective and further indicates that a family-centered orientation to DM1 care focused on increasing cohesion and decreasing family conflict may facilitate metabolic control [1]. A focus on achieving and maintaining parent-child teamwork in managing diabetes is indicated and the nature of this relationship must evolve as the child grows and matures.

The onset of adolescence carries many psychosocial challenges for youths and parents. Also, glycemic control becomes more difficult in adolescence because of hormonal changes that decrease insulin sensitivity [9]; changes in physical activity (eg, participation in sports); and changes in nutritional intake (eg, more eating away from home). These factors may complicate DM1 care, causing some adolescents to experience frustration, guilt, and avoidance of diabetes care activities. Parents may be frustrated with their inability to maintain control over their adolescent's behavior and vacillate between overly harsh, critical parenting versus being overly discouraged about family management of DM1. When parents withdraw prematurely from involvement in care, adult supervision and guidance of the youth's DM1 management tend to be inadequate. Because many teenagers are not able to cope independently with such responsibility, they may make errors of commission (eg, overtreating hypoglycemia) or omission (eg, less glucose monitoring, haphazard insulin administration). Research on adolescent psychology shows that more parental involvement in, and knowledge of, their adolescents' friendships, school performance, and leisure activities lower the risks of substance abuse [10], teenage pregnancy [11], and school achievement [12] and it is likely that DM1 outcomes are similar.

Many families adapt to raising adolescents with DM1 without excessive turmoil. Common factors in these families include approaching problems with warmth and empathy rather than with hostility and anger, clearly defining goals and expectations, anticipating imperfection in self-management, encouraging appropriate autonomy, using social supports, and communicating effectively to solve problems together [13]. Many parents may ask PCPs for advice on specific parenting techniques to use to improve adherence or glycemic control. Parents of younger children should be advised to maintain more direct involvement, while expressing warmth, support, confidence, and affection [14]. Parents of older youths should be advised to provide some independence to the child, yet retain consultative and supportive involvement in care because this is associated with better adherence and metabolic control [15,16]. PCPs should encourage parents to solve diabetes problems with, rather than for, older youths. Systematically negotiating parent and child responsibility for diabetes care is also valuable [5].

Quality of life

Quality of life is obviously a vitally important DM1 outcome [17]. Maintaining acceptable quality of life impacts the youth's confidence toward DM1 management, psychosocial functioning, and relationships with caregivers. Parents of children with DM1 rate their children's quality of life as significantly worse than that of children without diabetes [18], but children with DM1 do not report diminished quality of life [6,19,20]. Because diabetes poses threats to quality of life and psychologic adjustment among patients, parents, and siblings, the use of positive coping skills is critical. This includes effective problem solving, communication, and reinforcement strategies; effective stress management; and adequate social support.

Although quality of life measures are often unrelated to glycemic control [6,20], PCPs are advised routinely to ask patients and parents about their psychologic well-being, use of coping strategies, and disease management [19]. This information can guide decisions about referrals for psychologic or psychiatric services or for additional diabetes education.

Psychologic and behavioral problems

Some youths with DM1 who face significant psychologic stress or who have inadequate coping skills or family supports may be susceptible to psychologic problems, particularly depression, anxiety disorders, and eating disorders. In the first 10 years after diagnosis of DM1, 27% of youths experienced major depression and 13% experienced anxiety disorders [21]. Females with DM1 may face higher risks than males for depression, anxiety, and low self-esteem [22]. Psychologic adjustment in adolescence has been linked to glycemic control in early adulthood [23,24].

Some findings indicate that youths with DM1 may not differ from the general population in terms of general psychologic adjustment [25,26]. Nonetheless, the subsets of youths who develop these problems merit referrals for further evaluation and treatment whether or not the disorder is impeding DM1 management. Many adolescents may not present as overtly depressed or noncompliant with the regimen. Even those with very good diabetic control may perceive diabetes as having a negative influence and may suffer from depressive symptoms. PCPs should ask youths specifically about symptoms of depression and anxiety because these often are less evident to parents and teachers than are externalizing symptoms, such as anger and aggressive outbursts [19].

Disorders of eating and weight control

Disordered eating or weight control behaviors are a particular concern for patients with DM1 because of the immediate and long-term impact on glycemic control. Rates of eating disorders in preadolescent and adolescent girls with diabetes range from 8% to 30% [27,28], compared with rates of 1% to 4% in the general population [29–32]. These problems may present as insulin omission [27,28], strict dieting, excessive exercise [27], laxative use, and self-induced vomiting [31]. These behaviors are more prevalent in girls than in boys [27,32]. Eating disorders are a common finding among adolescent girls with recurrent diabetic ketoacidosis [30].

Coincidence of eating disorders and DM1 predicts increased body mass index from adolescence to adulthood for girls [27]; poor glycemic control [30,33]; and increased incidence of ketoacidosis [30], microvascular complications [30,34], neuropathy [35], and retinal lesions [36] in adulthood. Eating disorders are also associated with other psychiatric disorders (ie, depression, anxiety, substance abuse) in late adolescence to early adulthood [30]. Although many of these youths do not meet strict diagnostic criteria for an eating disorder, their behaviors may indicate serious psychologic distress. PCPs should be alert to the signs and symptoms of eating disorders in youths with DM1 (particularly girls), such as inordinate weight and body image concerns, evidence of insulin omission, and excessive exercising. Eating disorders should be included among differential diagnoses for youths, particularly girls, who experience recurrent hospitalizations for poor diabetic control [30].

Peer relationships

Peers affect youths' glycemic control, treatment adherence, and psychologic adjustment, particularly during adolescence. Adolescents spend more time with peers than with family, and often look to peers for acceptance of their behaviors. Adolescents tend to perceive more peer support than do younger children [37], who often seek support primarily from family members. Adolescents rate family members as offering more support for the diabetes regimen, but peers are more supportive emotionally [38]. Adolescents, particularly girls, are more supportive with joining in on exercising and listening to diabetes-related concerns [39]. Adolescent peer support and diabetes knowledge may be improved with participation in a group intervention [40]. The relationship between peer support and glycemic control is mixed. Although perceived peer and family support may not influence control or regimen adherence, youths with lower hemoglobin (Hb) A_{1c} had more peer-support in a recent study [38]. Girls perceive regimen-specific support as more helpful and as occurring more often than do boys [41].

Effects of diabetes on cognition and learning

Cognitive deficits and learning difficulties may occur in some children with DM1. Some studies of children with diabetes [42–44] show that impaired cognitive and learning abilities are more common among boys and children diagnosed with DM1 during infancy and the preschool years (<5 years old). Children and adolescents assessed shortly after diagnosis and at 2- and 6-year follow-ups indicated decreased ability on measures of intelligence, attention, processing speed, long-term memory, and executive skills compared with controls without diabetes [45]. Some abilities (ie, attention, processing speed, executive skills) are more vulnerable to early disease onset, whereas others may be related to severe hypoglycemia (ie, verbal and full-scale intelligence scores) [45]. Various foci of cognitive impairment have been reported, perhaps because varied assessment batteries have been used [42–44]. In addition, research has not determined if patients who develop subtle cognitive impairments have greater difficulty with diabetes management.

Identification of mechanisms causing diabetes-related cognitive deficits has been difficult because such variables as frequency of severe hypoglycemia, frequency of diabetic ketoacidosis, cumulative glycemic exposure, and duration of diabetes are intercorrelated [42]. Some studies [45] suggest that severe hypoglycemia may cause cognitive deficits, whereas other studies fail to confirm this [46]. PCPs should encourage parents to maintain good glycemic control, especially in youths diagnosed at early ages.

There are increased rates of learning disabilities among children with DM1 compared with the general population and academic difficulties are associated with poorer diabetic control [42–44,47,48]. Cognition and learning may be impaired by level of glycemic control rather than merely the presence of DM1. It is important to note that cognitive and learning deficits are found in a minority of children with diabetes, and the precise etiology has not been confirmed. PCPs should recognize these risks and consider referral for further evaluations if indicated.

School issues

Most children and adolescents with DM1 should be expected to adapt normally to school, including maintaining normal attendance, academic achievement, involvement in extracurricular activities, and social relationships. Some children with DM1, however, may experience difficulties with school adjustment. Absences caused by health concerns, teasing or mocking by peers, and lack of support from school employees are examples of barriers that may decrease the student's motivation, self-esteem, and academic progress. Although adaptation to normal school demands should be the goal for most youths with DM1, alternatives to standard educational services are discussed below.

Many common school-related problems can be remedied through provisions of Section 504 of the Rehabilitation Act of 1990, which mandates that school systems have mechanisms to prepare, implement, and monitor accommodation plans for students with defined chronic conditions, such as DM1. Accommodation plans modify school routines so that the medical condition or its management does not impede normal academic functioning. For example, a child with diabetes could be permitted to leave class early before lunch to take an insulin injection in the school clinic.

Placement in special education or exceptional student education requires documentation by a designated multidisciplinary team that the student has one of several handicapping conditions that interfere significantly with normal educational progress. Students placed in special education must receive an Individual Education Plan that meets their educational needs in the least restrictive setting that is feasible. One of the categories of special education is for children with "other health impairments," although it is unlikely that a child with DM1 qualifies on this basis unless there are other complicating conditions.

Homebound education consists of education provided by a teacher in the home several times per week. It is an alternative often presented to chronically ill children who have difficulties attending regularly because of hospitalizations or frequent illness. Disadvantages may include falling behind because of less overall instruction and a potential to extend the service beyond what is medically necessary.

Home schooling consists of educational services provided by parents with less school system oversight. This is available to all children, but may be selected by parents of chronically ill children after or in lieu of homebound education. The decision to home-school should be based on a positive rationale rather than avoidance of problems.

Summary

Whether considering the impact of DM1 on a child's emotional, familial, or educational functioning, it is important to recognize DM1 as a family issue rather than an individual concern. Although DM1 increases the risk for psychologic problems, most children and families are able to adjust to the illness, use social support, communicate effectively, and solve problems adequately. Unfortunately, those families who suffer negative psychologic side effects are more likely to report decreased quality of life and have a higher risk of complications and excess health care use. These families may benefit from psychologic interventions. The next section reviews studies that have evaluated treatments that target the key processes influencing coping with DM1 among youths and their families.

Pediatric type 1 diabetes: psychologic interventions

There are many promising psychologic interventions for youth with DM1 that have been designed to treat the barriers to effective diabetes management and control [49]. Interventions that have been investigated most thoroughly are those targeting treatment adherence, diabetes-specific coping and social skills, family communication and problem-solving, and anxiety and stress management. Interventions targeting these outcomes are reviewed next. Weight control interventions that may benefit youths with DM1 are summarized in the next section on childhood type 2 diabetes.

Treatment adherence

Few children and adolescents with diabetes demonstrate perfect adherence to their medical regimens and some demonstrate pervasive nonadherence. There have been a number of interventions that have empirical support for improving treatment adherence. For example, behavioral contracting has been shown to be an effective component in the treatment of nonadherence [49–54]. Behavioral contracting consists of helping parents and youth to negotiate an agreement by which positive reinforcement can be earned by meeting specific, short-term diabetes management goals. For example, a teenager may negotiate a later curfew for checking blood glucose at least three times daily for a week. One study [54] evaluated behavioral contracting for adherence with blood glucose monitoring using a meter with memory, and found that adherence exceeded 80% with contracting and the use of the memory meter compared with 50% and 60% for the meter alone. Others [52] found that direct reinforcement consisting of praise and a point reward system increased blood glucose monitoring in all three patients in a multiple baseline study, with maintenance of adherence and metabolic control at 4-month follow-up.

Other studies have shown that self-monitoring increases treatment adherence [51,53]. Self-monitoring involves having the youth actively record diabetes management behaviors, such as amount of exercise, blood glucose testing, insulin use, urine testing, or wearing medic alert identification. One study [51] found that two of three participants improved their diabetes management behavior during the 2-month intervention period and at 2-month follow-up.

Teaching problem-solving skills has also been found to be effective in improving treatment adherence [55,56]. Anderson and colleagues [55] taught children ages 11 to 14 five modules of problem-solving skills with a focus on using self-monitoring of blood glucose to solve diabetes management problems. Compared with standard care, youth in the treatment group performed self-monitoring of blood glucose more frequently when exercising and had lower HbA_{1c} levels. Delamater and colleagues [56] found that children and teenagers in a group receiving problem-solving skills, education, and contingent praise had lower HbA_{1c} levels and fewer dietary deviations at 2-year follow-up.

Some researchers have found family-based therapy to be an effective way to treat adherence problems [57–59]. Ellis and colleagues [59] found that a 6-month trial of multisystemic therapy with adolescents with DM1 led to improved adherence to blood glucose testing and metabolic control compared with controls, and also decreased the number of inpatient admissions 6 months postintervention. Multisystemic therapy is an intensive home-based treatment model that uses family systems and social-ecologic theories of behavior; the intervention targets several systems of the child's world, including individuals, family, peers, school, and the medical team.

Family-based treatment is particularly important for younger children with diabetes. Anderson and colleagues [58] evaluated children's participation in a "Young Children's Program," a program with a multifamily parent support group led by an endocrinologist and psychologist with regular diabetes care, additional medical appointments as needed, and a supervised activity for the young children. Families who participated regularly over a 3-year period were under better metabolic control and had fewer children with an HbA_{1c} greater than 9.9% compared with nonparticipants at 3-year follow-up. It is important to involve families early in integrated medical and psychosocial care.

Coping and social skills

Children and families must manage diabetes within a social context and youths' coping and social skills are important in doing this effectively. A number of interventions have focused on improving these skills [60–63]. Coping skills training focuses on increasing competence and mastery by replacing negative or ineffective coping styles with more constructive patterns of behavior. For example, Grey and colleagues [62] found that adolescents who received coping skills training demonstrated better diabetes self-efficacy, lower HbA_{1c} levels, better coping, and less negative impact on quality of life from DM1. Gross and colleagues [64–66] conducted a series of studies showing that social skills training improved diabetes-specific social skills, such as dealing with peer teasing. Kaplan and colleagues [67] contributed a similar evaluation of diabetes-specific social skills training.

Other studies have focused on increasing peer and family social support of diabetes care [40,68]. Anderson and colleagues [68] found that a peer group focusing on use of blood glucose data and peer support improved glycemic control and treatment adherence in adolescents. Greco and colleagues [40] conducted a four-session education and support group intervention with adolescent and peer pairs ("best friends") designed to integrate friends into diabetes management; improve social functioning and social support; and improve treatment adherence, diabetes-related family conflict, and adjustment to diabetes. The intervention significantly improved diabetes knowledge and peer support and increased the amount of peer support relative to family support. Parents also reported a significant reduction in diabetes-related conflict.

Family communication and problem solving

Family interventions with youths with DM1 have received empirical support [2,4,5]. Behaviorally oriented family therapy has shown promise in reducing general and diabetes-related family conflict [4] and in improving directly observed family communication and problem-solving skills [69]. Satin and colleagues [70] investigated a multifamily group intervention with or without parental simulation compared with a standard treatment group. Participants in the intervention groups demonstrated significantly improved glycemic control at both 3- and 6-month follow-up compared with the standard treatment group.

Wysocki and colleagues used Robin and Foster's [71] behavioral family systems therapy, 10 sessions of family therapy focusing on teaching problem solving and behavioral contracting, family communication skills, and cognitive restructuring within a family systems perspective. They found significant improvements in parent-teenager relationships and a decrease in diabetes-specific family conflicts [69] and family communication and problem-solving skills [2]. These gains persisted for 1 year [69] but there was no significant effect on glycemic control. There were delayed treatment adherence effects, with the behavioral family systems therapy group showing improved treatment adherence at 6- and 12-months follow-up, whereas control families showed deteriorated adherence [69].

Anderson and colleagues [5] developed an intervention that targeted declining parental involvement with diabetes, which has been related to decreases in glycemic control. Their four-session intervention delivered in a diabetes clinic focused on improving parent-teenager sharing of DM1 responsibilities and reducing family conflict that might affect this teamwork. The experimental group showed no significant declines in parental involvement in diabetes management and less family conflict compared with an attentional control group or standard care group.

Other interventions targeting diabetes-specific problem-solving skills have proved effective [72–74]. Cook and colleagues [73] randomized adolescents to either a 6-week problem-solving diabetes education program or a control group. Teenagers who participated in problem-solving training had better problem-solving skills, more frequent blood glucose testing, and lower HbA$_{1c}$ values. This "Choices" program focused on such problem-solving topics as "making choices and keeping records," "planning meals," and "timing your insulin."

Anxiety and stress management

Because psychologic stress can interfere with adherence and metabolic control, a number of interventions have targeted reducing anxiety and improving the management of stress with children with DM1. Fowler and colleagues [75] used biofeedback-assisted relaxation to lower blood glucose levels in the office but not at home. Rose and colleagues [76] taught progressive muscle relaxation over 6 months, which improved metabolic control in four of five girls who were treated. Boardway and colleagues [77] investigated a stress management intervention, which included identification of life stressors, self-monitoring of stress responses, and progressive muscle relaxation. This intervention reduced stress in the participants, but did not improve metabolic control or treatment adherence. Mendez and Belendez [78] designed a behavioral intervention that taught stress management, social skills, blood glucose discrimination, problem solving, and self-monitoring to adolescents and parents. This multicomponent intervention improved diabetes knowledge, blood glucose monitoring adherence, and social skills, but did not have an effect on glycemic control. Hains and colleagues [72] examined a cognitive-behavioral intervention incorporating problem-solving and cognitive restructuring on reducing anxiety, anger, and diabetes-related stress. Four of the six youths demonstrated some improvement on these variables. These interventions suggest that stress management and anxiety treatments may be useful in combination with other interventions that more directly target problem behavior, but that these interventions alone do not significantly improve metabolic control or treatment adherence.

Access to psychologic interventions

Although the preceding discussion illustrates that there are many appropriate behavioral and psychologic intervention strategies targeting problems related to DM1, access to these services by families who need them in ordinary clinical settings continues to be problematic. There are many barriers that may inhibit patients from receiving appropriate mental health services. Some communities do not have mental health professionals who have been specially trained to treat issues related to compliance and adjustment to chronic medical conditions (ie, pediatric or health psychologists). In other areas, families cannot access these services because of limited or no insurance benefits. Still other families are not familiar with the role of mental health professionals in a medical setting and may be hesitant to seek out mental health services. Coordination of medical and mental health issues can also be difficult. It is important for a mental health professional to be part of the diabetes treatment team so that families have increased access to these services. Another barrier to care is the cost to families, hospitals, and communities for the treatment of diabetes. The cost-effectiveness of psychosocial interventions needs to be evaluated so that programs can be developed that reduce costs while still maintaining high-quality care.

Future research

More intervention research is needed in a number of key areas. A recent meta-analysis suggests that interventions with this population are more likely to be effective if they address the interrelatedness of various aspects of diabetes management and assess outcomes that are explicit targets for change [49]. Future research should be driven by explicit theoretical principles with specific inclusion and exclusion criteria; clearly defined outcome variables; and valid, reliable assessment tools. In addition, research focusing on new technologies, such as telemedicine, text messaging, continuous glucose monitors, and insulin pumps, may be fruitful. Studies should address a range of outcomes, such as glycemic control, treatment adherence, quality of life, parent-child interactions, and psychosocial functioning [79]. Multisite trials including larger populations of children and adolescents could evaluate the cost-effectiveness of these interventions.

Summary of interventions

There are a number of empirically validated interventions that target specific areas of concern for children and adolescents with DM1. These interventions work best within the context of a team approach to care, involving the family, PCP, endocrinologist, diabetes educator, nurses, and mental health professionals. PCPs are in a position to promote access to and continuity of services with these professionals for the family. In addition, the integration of basic psychologic and behavioral principles into routine diabetes care may serve to prevent problems in children and adolescents with diabetes.

Childhood type 2 diabetes in a psychologic context

Type 2 diabetes mellitus (DM2) and obesity in children and adolescents is increasing dramatically in the United States and worldwide; obesity is now considered to be the most prevalent nutritional disease of children and adolescents [80]. DM2 is considered to be the new morbidity in children and adolescents [81–83]. Before 1990, it was rare for pediatric centers to report the incidence of DM2 in their pediatric population, but by 1994 DM2 pediatric patients represented up to 16% of new cases of diabetes in children in urban areas [84]. Children and adolescents who are overweight, sedentary, and at risk for DM2 or who have been diagnosed with the disease also face elevated risks of cardiovascular disease, retinopathy, nephropathy, neuropathy, impaired quality of life, and premature death, along with psychologic and social consequences [85]. The social and psychologic sequelae are often the most salient and enduring problems related to obesity and DM2 for children and adolescents and are often just as damaging as the medical morbidities [86]. Some studies have found children who are overweight or obese to be at increased risk for psychiatric disorders, such as depression, anxiety, and behavioral problems [84,87]. Other comorbid psychologic problems include eating disorders, such as binge-eating problems; behavioral problems; poor coping and problem-solving skills; low motivation; and poor self-control, many of which are also seen in children with DM1, particularly during adolescence [84,87]. Although this article summarizes the extensive behavioral science research that has been done on pediatric DM1, there are important considerations that should be taken into account when generalizing these findings to the DM2 population.

Differences in the psychologic contexts of type 1 versus type 2 diabetes mellitus

There are important differences between the psychologic contexts of DM1 and DM2. In DM1 socioeconomic status is broadly distributed, whereas DM2 disproportionately affects individuals with fewer resources (single parents, less educated, less well insured). Second, DM1 is typically diagnosed throughout childhood, whereas DM2 emerges more commonly during adolescence, when peer influence dominates, adolescents have more independence, parental control declines, and there are more adherence difficulties. Third, about 5% of families with a child diagnosed with DM1 have had previous experience with the disease compared with over 90% of families of a child with DM2 [88]. This experience has been linked to families feeling a sense of failure and futility related to weight loss and glycemic control. Finally, in DM1 major lifestyle modification beyond insulin and glucose monitoring are only needed in overweight and inactive children, whereas this is the foundation of treatment in DM2. These differences alone make DM2 more challenging and difficult to treat.

Risk factors for developing type 2 diabetes mellitus

The increasing incidence of DM2 in children and adolescents is strongly associated with increases in sedentary lifestyle and overeating. There are several additional risk factors associated with developing DM2, however, such as being in a particular racial or ethnic group, having a family history of DM2, being overweight, going through puberty, having insulin resistance, and being born too small or too large. The multiple risk factors related to obesity and DM2 in children affect physical and psychologic factors, and population-wide economic burdens related to the disease. The economic burden of childhood obesity, as reported for obesity-related hospital costs, has increased dramatically over the last 20 years, reaching $127 million per year in 2001 [89].

In addition to the changing lifestyles and composition of families, certain ethnic and racial groups are disproportionately affected by DM2 in the pediatric population. For example, American Indian and Alaska Native children in North America have a higher rate of DM2 in their pediatric population than in any other ethnic group [80]. Hispanic and African American children are also at increased risk for developing DM2 as children. In addition, in 1994, it was estimated that the odds-ratio of developing DM2 was 6.1 in African American girls and 3.5 in African American boys compared with whites [84]. A family history of DM2 is also an important risk factor associated with developing the disease. If a parent or close relative has been diagnosed with DM2, the risk increases significantly. In addition to possible genetic causation, physical, behavioral, and environmental characteristics are also important contributors to family management of the disease.

Another critical risk factor for the development of DM2 is obesity; the link between obesity and DM2 is well-established. Parallel to the increase in incidence of DM2 in children, studies have also shown that the prevalence of childhood obesity has increased from approximately 5% in the 1960s to 10% to 18% currently in children and adolescents, with some studies reporting higher prevalence rates [88]. Including adults, around 90% of people with diabetes have DM2 and most of them are overweight or obese. Worldwide, it is estimated that more than 22 million children under 5 years old are obese or overweight, and more than 17 million of them are in developing countries [84]. Obesity has also been identified as a risk factor for much of adult morbidity and mortality [85]. In addition, the likelihood that childhood obesity persists into adulthood is 20% for obese preschoolers and 80% for obese adolescents [85].

Overweight status in children and adolescents is generally caused by some combination of overeating, insufficient physical activity, and genetic predisposition [90]. A recent American Academy of Pediatrics Policy Statement [85] states that because of the increasing incidence of DM2 among obese adolescents and because diabetes-related morbidities may worsen if diagnosis is delayed, clinicians should be alert to the possibility of DM2 in all obese adolescents, especially those with a family history of early onset (younger than 40 years) DM2. Prevention of DM2 is a key public health goal for children and adolescents.

Behavioral intervention and prevention efforts

There are no published studies that have evaluated a psychologic or behavioral treatment for children with type 2 diabetes, although there are such studies under way with this population. A number of intervention studies have focused on prevention of overweight and obesity and treatment of overweight status. This discussion is limited to those studies completed with children and adolescents at risk for DM2 and to pertinent adult studies to report what has been done so far in terms of prevention and intervention. Research on behavioral interventions for treating obesity has now spanned more than 20 years. Most studies have been conducted with adults and have shown that lifestyle interventions improve glucose tolerance in individuals at high risk of developing DM2, at least over the short-term. In adults, studies have shown that long-term weight loss has so far lagged behind improvements in short-term weight loss [91].

In a recent review of empirically supported treatments in pediatric obesity, Jelalian and Saelens [92] found that there are well-established treatments for intervening in pediatric obesity in children between the ages of 8 and 12 years who do not have comorbid medical conditions or psychologic disorders. Specifically, a series of studies documented that comprehensive behavioral treatment targeting eating and physical activity was superior to wait-list control or nutrition education alone in achieving short-term weight loss in children. In addition, Epstein and colleagues [91,93] documented maintenance of treatment efficacy at long-term follow-up of up to 10 years. There is currently little research available documenting treatment efficacy for children with comorbid psychopathology, medical conditions, or who are more than 100% overweight. In adolescents there is less literature on weight loss interventions than in children. Some studies, however, have shown short-term efficacy when using behavior modification of dietary intake [94].

Studies targeting children who are overweight have shown that children, especially preadolescents, are more likely to maintain improvements in weight control than are adults [9]. For example, Epstein and colleagues [93] reported that sustained reductions in age-adjusted percentage overweight in the 10% to 15% range are achievable over follow-ups as long as 10 years. Pediatric weight control programs with long-term effectiveness tend to target both dietary intake and physical activity, to engage parents and children in the intervention, and to maintain the intervention over longer periods of time [95]. More studies are needed to assess further critical treatment components and maintenance issues and to demonstrate that effective weight control programs can be implemented with similar outcome among youths from racial and ethnic minorities with low socioeconomic status.

Studies have also evaluated preventing or delaying the onset of obesity in children who are at high risk of DM2. There are many reasons why intervening early is critical in the delay or prevention of obesity and DM2. First, there are direct and indirect health care costs associated with obesity and DM2 [96]. Treatment of diabetes and its complications currently accounts for 12% to 14% of national health care expenditures. Because children will have diabetes for longer than adults, prevention of pediatric DM2 could be offset by major savings in health care costs. Obesity also has a direct educational and financial impact on schools. Studies have shown that children who consume high levels of sugar and fat tend not to do as well academically. Poor performance and absenteeism cost money. Youths who do poorly in school tend to need more special services. Second, obesity has also been associated with diminished school performance because of sleep apnea, lack of physical exercise, social stigmatization, and peer problems. Intervening with children presents additional systemic challenges, such as encouraging healthy nutritional alternatives in schools and communities, maintaining adequate physical education programs in school, and addressing safety concerns in many communities and neighborhoods [88]. Programs designed for children have primarily targeted the schools, communities, and family and individual intervention.

School-based overweight prevention programs offer substantial promise [97]. Recent school-based randomized controlled trials have demonstrated success in reducing the prevalence and incidence of childhood obesity by decreasing children's television viewing [98,99], by improving their dietary behaviors, and by increasing their physical activity [100]. One example of such a program is Planet Health, an interdisciplinary curriculum focused on improving the heath and well-being of sixth- through eighth-grade students by increasing physical activity, improving dietary quality, and decreasing inactivity [100]. Girls in Planet Health schools, compared with those in control schools, realized reduced obesity, increased fruit and vegetable consumption, and reduced caloric intake [100]. Among girls and boys, it was effective in reducing sedentary behavior and increasing curriculum-based knowledge [98]. A similar program, Child and Adolescent Trial for Cardiovascular Health, which targets third through fifth graders, has achieved a 50% increase in moderate-to-vigorous physical activity [101]. Bienestar Health Program, a school-based program to reduce DM2 risks targeting fourth-grade Mexican American children, significantly decreased fat intake, increased fruit and vegetable intake, and increased diabetes knowledge [102].

The Zuni Diabetes Prevention Program [103] is a community-based intervention targeting Zuni high school students, using supportive social networks, development of a wellness facility, integrated diabetes education, and modification of the food supply. Results after 2 years of the implementation of this study have shown a reduction in body mass index, decreased consumption of sugar-containing beverages, increased dietary fiber, and increased insulin sensitivity.

Currently, a multisite consortium, funded primarily by the National Institute of Diabetes, Digestive and Kidney Diseases, National Institutes of Health, with additional support from the American Diabetes Association, is developing trials related to type 2 diabetes in children and adolescents. Two trials are currently being supported under this Stop Type 2 Diabetes (STOPP-T2D) consortium: the TODAY study and STOPP-T2D Prevention Trial. The purpose of the TODAY trial is to examine the safety and effectiveness of three different treatments for DM2 in the pediatric population (medication, medication plus lifestyle intervention, and control group). The TODAY trial is in progress at 12 medical centers across the United States. The STOPP-T2D Prevention Trial is a school-based trial to prevent the onset of DM2 in middle school children. The study, currently in the pilot phase, is being conducted at eight medical centers and numerous school districts around the United States.

Summary: keys to intervention

DM2 has a different risk profile and psychologic context from DM1, but there are many parallels. Several pertinent intervention points each require different kinds and levels of activities. Studies have confirmed efficacy of psychologic and behavioral treatment targeting many of these intervention points in non-DM2 samples. First and foremost, the goal of any medical treatment for children with DM2 is to normalize glycemia and HbA_{1c}. There are many other critical goals of diabetes management, however, for this population. Although not well researched yet, it is important to apply what has been learned from studies with children with chronic illnesses, particularly DM1, and adults with DM2 when choosing an intervention. Current and future research will help to clarify many of the treatment recommendations and options. Additional behavioral targets that should be included are adherence, decreasing or maintaining weight, increasing exercise, improving dietary choices, and promoting healthy emotional adjustment and quality of life.

Intervention should begin early, particularly in preadolescence, and efforts should be made to identify those children at risk by family history of DM2 and having an overweight parent. It is important for physicians and health care providers to screen for depression and anxiety in this population given the impact it has on children with chronic illnesses and children who are suffering from overweight; these may represent critical barriers to intervention and prevention and should be explored. In an optimal intervention and prevention design, the family should be the focus of treatment. It is very difficult to treat only the child, because families play key roles in both etiology and remediation of these problems. Interventions with families should focus on teaching them effective problem-solving skills and giving them practical solutions and ideas for intervention to decrease the sense of hopelessness. Lifestyle and small gradual changes should always be the goal. For example, targeting only decreasing consumption of sweetened beverages is a reasonable start for some families. It is extremely important to be flexible and allow for open communication with the family. Positive reinforcement and praise from PCPs can be very powerful influences in encouraging patients and families to initiate and maintain lifestyle changes. It is especially important for PCPs to praise families' initial behavior change efforts, however small, and to guide them in goal setting for future lifestyle changes. Although these can be sensitive issues for many families, failure to intervene almost guarantees the progression toward diabetes for high-risk youths or the acceleration of complications among those who have been diagnosed.

Psychologic aspects of pediatric diabetes: roles for primary care providers

Having reviewed research on the psychologic aspects of pediatric diabetes, six important contributions that PCPs can make to manage these issues are now presented.

Prevent adjustment problems and promote family teamwork

Several factors influence coping with the challenges of diabetes among youths and their families. PCPs can promote healthy adaptation to diabetes by helping families to anticipate and cope with imperfection, by guiding families in negotiating realistic goals for diabetes management, and by assisting families in maintaining parental support for diabetes management well into adolescence.

Striving for excellent diabetic control must be balanced with the capacity to cope with falling short of tight control. Families who can manage these dual priorities effectively tend to have an easier time coping with diabetes during adolescence. Rigid perfectionism may lead to conflict, discouragement, and problems with adherence, parent-adolescent relationships, and psychologic adjustment. Imperfection, inconsistency, and frustration are natural parts of living with diabetes and these experiences should be anticipated so that youths and family members maintain healthy self-efficacy regarding diabetes care.

Many families do not have clear goals for diabetes care or metabolic control. PCPs can help families in clarifying who will do what, when, and how often and in achieving a consensus on acceptable glucose targets. Achieving blood glucose in the normal range in 50% of tests equates to an HbA_{1c} of about 7% [104]. Stating a goal in those terms decreases the emotional significance of isolated glucose results and keeps attention appropriately on the broader profile.

Families also must prepare their children to increase their responsibility for diabetes care gradually. Historically, youths were encouraged toward independence in diabetes care [105,106], but recent studies show that premature withdrawal of parents from diabetes care is associated with adverse outcomes [15,107–111]. Teenagers who enjoy supportive, consultative, and affirming interactions with their parents around diabetes are more likely to enjoy favorable diabetes outcomes during adolescence [15,110,111]. PCPs should encourage an evolution of parental involvement in diabetes management from an authoritative role during late childhood to a cooperative and monitoring role during early adolescence to a consultative role during later adolescence. Complete cessation of parental interest in diabetes care may never be appropriate.

Finally, how families talk about diabetes and its treatment may be as important as what they say. Cross-sectional and prospective studies show that family communication is a key factor affecting diabetes management and outcomes [3,112–114]. Healthy family communication about diabetes and its management should be direct, calm, reciprocal, open, fair, constructive, and positive. There should be a minimum of criticism, sarcasm, interruption, domination of the conversation, threats, demands, or anger. PCPs can encourage weekly family meetings about diabetes management using healthy communication habits. Behavioral interventions can improve communication skills of youths with diabetes and their parents [2,69].

Detect adjustment problems early

Like medical problems, early detection of psychologic disorders enables more treatment options and enhances outcomes. Although youths with diabetes may or may not have elevated rates of psychopathology [115,116], psychologic disorders predispose youths to problems with treatment adherence, metabolic control, and preventable hospitalizations [21,117,118]. PCPs should anticipate a more difficult course during and after the transition to adolescence. Periodic screening for depression, anxiety disorders, eating disorders, and learning disabilities is indicated because these are the most common disorders that have been reported [119]. Also, school phobia is a common etiology of chronically poor metabolic control and so this should be evaluated as a possible contributing factor in such cases [120]. PCPs can communicate with school staff and provide clear criteria for allowing school absence.

Childhood diabetes is a threat to the entire family and PCPs are well-situated to recognize adverse psychologic effects on siblings, parents, and couples. Because adjustment difficulties of any family member can impede diabetes care, PCPs should refer for appropriate services promptly and maintain timely communication with the diabetes team.

Refer for appropriate services and encourage engagement

PCPs should regularly assess the need for psychiatric or psychologic services of patients and families. The optimal arrangement is integration of these services into a comprehensive diabetes management program with active participation of one or more mental health professionals as members of the diabetes team. If that is not available, a good alternative is to refer to providers who are familiar with psychologic aspects of pediatric medical conditions [121]. Once referred, PCPs should follow-up to encourage continuity of psychiatric or psychologic services and to promote communication between those providers and the diabetes team.

Advocate for health promotion on a community level

PCPs may also be engaged in community health promotion and advocacy activities that may benefit youths with diabetes and prediabetes. These may include community advocacy for obesity prevention and treatment and enhanced opportunities for exercise, organized sports, and physical education. For teen-agers with diabetes, reproductive health concerns and the transition from pe-diatric to adult care are systemic needs that PCPs can promote. PCPs can also facilitate school management of diabetes and maintain a healthy skepticism regarding the approval of homebound instruction or special education placement based on health impairments for children with diabetes. Finally, because PCPs must often approve coverage for mental health services, another valuable role is advocating with third-party payers regarding the need for specialized psychologic and psychiatric services for this population.

Counsel patients and families regarding advances in medical care

Diabetes therapy is constantly evolving, with new types of insulin, new methods of insulin delivery, continuous glucose monitoring, and various means of islet cell transplantation all in varying stages of development [122–125]. Families may ask PCPs for guidance about these advances, many of which entail increased regimen demands. The authors recommend encouraging careful con-sideration of adding new therapy or monitoring options to the regimen, ideally including evaluation by a mental health professional to enhance the prospects of successful outcomes of these decisions. PCPs should assess the expectations of parents and patients regarding these advances and temper them as appropriate. Regarding long-term complications of diabetes, PCPs should express a realistic but optimistic perspective, while stressing maintenance of good metabolic control and early detection as the best assurances of long-term health maintenance.

Seek continuing education regarding psychologic aspects of diabetes

There are many practical resources available to PCPs that can assist them and their pediatric patients in coping with diabetes. Also, members of regional diabetes teams may be able to provide or recommend additional resources, such as those listed below:

Books
    Anderson BJ, Rubin R, editors. Practical psychology for diabetes clinicians. 2nd edition. Alexandria (VA): American Diabetes Association; 2003.

Wysocki T. The ten keys to helping your child grow up with diabetes. 2nd edition. Alexandria (VA): American Diabetes Association; 2004.
Internet websites
diabetes.org (American Diabetes Association)
jdrfi.org (Juvenile Diabetes Research Foundation)
childrenwithdiabetes.com (Children with Diabetes)
diabetes.niddk.nih.gov (National Diabetes Information Clearinghouse)
Practice guidelines
American Diabetes Association. Diabetes care in the school and daycare setting (position statement). Diab Care 2004;27(Suppl 1):S122–8.

Summary

This article reviews an extensive body of empirical research demonstrating that careful appreciation of the psychologic context of pediatric diabetes is essential to promoting adaptation to the many challenges imposed by these conditions. PCPs who are familiar with this literature should be better equipped to help patients and families deal with these challenges so that they can achieve and maintain optimal physical and psychologic health.

References

[1] Hanson CL, De Guire MJ, Schinkel AM, et al. Empirical validation for a family-centered model of care. Diabetes Care 1995;18:1347–56.
[2] Wysocki T, Miller KM, Greco P, et al. Behavior therapy for families of adolescents with diabetes: effects on directly observed family interactions. Behav Ther 1999;30:507–25.
[3] Wysocki T. Associations among parent-adolescent relationships, metabolic control and adjustment to diabetes in adolescents. J Pediatr Psychol 1993;18:443–54.
[4] Wysocki T, Harris MA, Greco P, et al. Randomized, controlled trial of behavior therapy for families of adolescents with insulin dependent diabetes mellitus. J Pediatr Psychol 2000; 25:23–33.
[5] Anderson BJ, Brackett J, Ho J, et al. An office-based intervention to maintain parent-adolescent teamwork in diabetes management. Diabetes Care 1999;22:713–21.
[6] Laffel LMB, Connell A, Vangsness L, et al. General quality of life in youth with type 1 diabetes. Diabetes Care 2003;11:3067–73.
[7] Moreland EC, Tovar A, Zuehlke JB, et al. The impact of physiological, therapeutic and psychosocial variables on glycemic control in youth with type 1 diabetes mellitus. J Pediatr Endocrinol Metab 2004;17:1533–44.
[8] Glasgow AM, Weissberg-Benchell DR, Tynan WD, et al. Re-admissions of children with diabetes mellitus to a children's hospital. Pediatrics 1991;88:98–104.
[9] Amiel SA, Sherwin RS, Simonson DC, et al. Impaired insulin action in puberty: a contributing factor to poor glycemic control in adolescents with diabetes. N Engl J Med 1986;315:215–9.
[10] Hawkins JD, Catalano RF, Miller JY. Risk and protective factors for alcohol and other drug problems in adolescence and early adulthood: implications for substance abuse and prevention. Psychol Bull 1992;112:64–105.
[11] Billy J, Udry J. Patterns of adolescents' friendship and effects on sexual behavior. Soc Psychol Q 1985;48:27–41.

[12] Stevenson DL, Baker DP. The family-school relation and the child's school performance. Child Dev 1987;58:1348–57.

[13] Wysocki T. Parents, teens, and diabetes. Diabetes Spectrum 2002;15:6–8.

[14] Davis CL, Delamater AM, Shaw KH, et al. Parenting styles, regimen adherence, and glycemic control in 4- to 10-year-old children with diabetes. J Pediatr Psychol 2001;26: 123–9.

[15] Anderson B, Ho J, Brackett J, et al. Parental involvement in diabetes management tasks: relationships to blood glucose monitoring adherence and metabolic control in young adolescents with insulin-dependent diabetes mellitus. J Pediatr 1997;130:257–65.

[16] Couper JJ, Taylor J, Fotheringham M, et al. Failure to maintain the benefits of home-based intervention in adolescents with poorly controlled type 1 diabetes. Diabetes Care 1999;22: 1933–7.

[17] Kaplan RM. Behavior as the central outcome in health care. Am Psychol 1990;45:1211–20.

[18] Hesketh KD, Wake MA, Cameron FJ. Health-related quality of life and metabolic control in children with type 1 diabetes. Diabetes Care 2004;27:415–20.

[19] Oneil KJ, Jonnalagadda SS, Hopkins BL, et al. Quality of life and diabetes knowledge of young persons with type 1 diabetes: influence of treatment modalities and demographics. J Am Diet Assoc 2005;105:85–91.

[20] Grey M, Boland EA, Yu C, et al. Personal and family factors associated with quality of life in adolescents with diabetes. Diabetes Care 1998;21:909–14.

[21] Kovacs M, Goldston D, Obrosky DS, et al. Psychiatric disorders in youths with IDDM: rates and risk factors. Diabetes Care 1997;20:36–44.

[22] Kovacs M, Goldston D, Obrosky DS, et al. Major depressive disorder in youths with IDDM. Diabetes Care 1997;20:45–51.

[23] Bryden KS, Peveler RC, Stein A, et al. Clinical and psychological course of diabetes from adolescence to young adulthood. Diabetes Care 2001;24:1536–40.

[24] Wysocki T, Hough BS, Ward KM, et al. Diabetes mellitus in the transition to adulthood: adjustment, self-care, and health status. J Dev Behav Pediatr 1992;13:194–201.

[25] Cohen DM, Lumley MA, Naar-King S, et al. Child behavior problems and family functioning as predictors of adherence and glycemic control in economically disadvantaged children with type 1 diabetes: a prospective study. J Pediatr Psychol 2004;29:171–84.

[26] Davis WB, Coon H, Whitehead P, et al. Predicting diabetic control from competence, adherence, adjustment, and psychopathology. J Am Acad Child Adolesc Psychiatry 1995;34: 1629–36.

[27] Bryden KS, Neil A, Mayou RA, et al. Eating habits, body weight, and insulin misuse. Diabetes Care 1999;22:1956–60.

[28] Pollock M, Kovacs M, Charron-Prochownik D. Eating disorders and maladaptive dietary/ insulin management among youths with childhood-onset insulin-dependent diabetes mellitus. J Am Acad Child Adolesc Psychiatry 1995;34:291–6.

[29] Colton P, Olmsted M, Daneman D, et al. Disturbed eating behavior and eating disorders in preteen and early teenage girls with type 1 diabetes. Diabetes Care 2004;27:1654–9.

[30] Peveler RC, Bryden KS, Neil HAW, et al. The relationship of disordered eating habits and attitudes to clinical outcomes in young adult females with type 1 diabetes. Diabetes Care 2005;28:84–8.

[31] Jones JM, Lawson ML, Daneman D, et al. Eating disorders in adolescent females with and without type 1 diabetes: cross sectional study. BMJ 2000;320:1563–6.

[32] Grylli V, Hafferl-Gattermayer A, Wagner G, et al. Eating disorders and eating problems among adolescents with type 1 diabetes: exploring relationships with temperament and character. J Pediatr Psychol 2005;30:197–206.

[33] Peveler RC, Fairburn CG, Boller I, et al. Eating disorders in adolescents with IDDM. Diabetes Care 1992;15:1356–60.

[34] Rydall AC, Rodin GM, Olmsted MP, et al. Disordered eating behavior and microvascular complications in young women with insulin-dependent diabetes mellitus. N Engl J Med 1997;26:1849–54.

[35] Steel JM, Young RJ, Lloyd GG, et al. Clinically apparent eating disorders in young diabetic women: associations with painful neuropathy and other complications. BMJ 1987;294: 859–62.

[36] Colas C, Mathieu P, Techobroutsky G. Eating disorders and retinal lesions in type 1 (insulin-dependent) diabetic women. Diabetologia 1991;34:288.

[37] Shroff-Pendley J, Kasmen LJ, Miller DL, et al. Peer and family support in children and adolescents with type 1 diabetes. J Pediatr Psychol 2002;27:429–38.

[38] La Greca AM, Auslander WF, Greco P, et al. I get by with a little help from my family and friends: adolescents' support for diabetes care. J Pediatr Psychol 1995;26:279–82.

[39] La Greca AM, Bearman KJ. The diabetes social support questionnaire-family version: evaluating adolescents' diabetes-specific support from family members. J Pediatr Psychol 2002; 27:665–76.

[40] Greco P, Shroff Pendley J, McDonell K, et al. A peer group intervention for adolescents with type 1 diabetes and their best friends. J Pediatr Psychol 2001;26:485–90.

[41] Bearman KJ, La Greca AM. Assessing friend support of adolescents' diabetes care: the diabetes social support questionnaire-friends version. J Pediatr Psychol 2002;27:417–28.

[42] Ryan CM. Effects of diabetes mellitus on neuropsychological function: a lifespan perspective. Semin Clin Neuropsychiatry 1997;2:4–14.

[43] Rovet J, Ehrlich RM, Czuchta D, et al. Psychoeducational characteristics of children and adolescents with insulin-dependent diabetes mellitus. J Learn Disabil 1993;26:7–22.

[44] Holmes CS, Cant M, Fox MA, et al. Disease and demographic risk factors for disrupted cognitive functioning in children with insulin-dependent diabetes mellitus (IDDM). Sch Psychol Rev 1999;28:215–27.

[45] Northam EA, Anderson PJ, Jacobs R, et al. Neuropsychological profiles of children with type 1 diabetes 6 years after disease onset. Diabetes Care 2001;24:1541–6.

[46] Wysocki T, Harris M, Mauras N, et al. Absence of adverse effects of severe hypoglycemia on cognitive function in school-aged children with diabetes over 18 months. Diabetes Care 2003;26:1100–5.

[47] Holmes CS, Dunlap WP, Chen RS, et al. Gender differences in the learning status of diabetic children. J Consult Clin Psychol 1992;60:698–704.

[48] McCarthy AM, Lindgren S, Mengeling MA, et al. Effects of diabetes on learning in children. Pediatrics 2002;109:E9.

[49] Hampson SE, Skinner TC, Hart J, et al. Effects of educational and psychosocial interventions for adolescents with diabetes mellitus: a systematic review. Health Technol Assess 2001; 5:1–79.

[50] Epstein LH, Beck S, Figueroa J, et al. The effects of targeting improvement in urine glucose on metabolic control in children with insulin-dependent diabetes mellitus. J App Behav Anal 1981;14:365–75.

[51] Schafer LC, Glasgow RE, McCaul KD. Increasing the adherence of diabetic adolescents. J Behav Med 1982;5:353–62.

[52] Carney RM, Schechter K, Davis T. Improving adherence to blood glucose monitoring in insulin-dependent diabetic children. Behav Ther 1983;14:247–54.

[53] Snyder J. Behavioral analysis and treatment of poor diabetic self-care and antisocial behavior: a single-subject experimental study. Behav Ther 1987;18:251–63.

[54] Wysocki T, Green LB, Huxtable K. Blood glucose monitoring by diabetic adolescents: compliance and metabolic control. Health Psychol 1989;8:267–84.

[55] Anderson BJ, Wolf FM, Burkhart MT, et al. Effects of a peer group intervention on metabolic control of adolescents with IDDM: randomized outpatient study. Diabetes Care 1989; 12:184–8.

[56] Delamater AM, Bubb J, Davis SG, et al. Randomized prospective study of self-management training with newly diagnosed diabetic children. Diabetes Care 1990;13:492–8.

[57] Delamater AM, Smith JA, Bubb J, et al. Family-based behavior therapy for diabetic adolescents. In: Johnson JH, Johnson SB, editors. Advances in child health psychology. Gainesville (FL): University of Florida Press; 1991. p. 293–306.

[58] Anderson BJ, Loughlin C, Goldberg E, et al. Comprehensive, family-focused outpatient care for very young children living with chronic disease: lessons from a program in pediatric diabetes. Child Serv Soc Policy Res Pract 2001;4:235–50.

[59] Ellis DA, Naar-King S, Frey M, et al. Use of multisystemic therapy to improve regimen adherence among adolescents with type 1 diabetes in poor metabolic control: a pilot investigation. J Clin Psychol Med Settings 2004;11:315–24.

[60] Grey M, Boland EA, Davidson M, et al. Short-term effects of coping skills training as adjunct to intensive therapy in adolescents. Diabetes Care 1998;21:902–8.

[61] Grey M, Boland E, Davidson M, et al. Coping skills training for youth with diabetes on intensive therapy. Appl Nurs Res 1999;12:3–12.

[62] Grey M, Boland E, Davidson M, et al. Coping skills training for youth on intensive therapy has long-lasting effects on metabolic control and quality of life. J Pediatr 2000;137:107–13.

[63] Knight KM, Bundy C, Morris R, et al. The effects of group motivational interviewing and externalizing conversations for adolescents with type-1 diabetes. Psychol Health Med 2003;8:149–57.

[64] Gross AM, Johnson WG, Wildman H, et al. Coping skills training with insulin-dependent preadolescent diabetics. Child Behav Ther 1981;3:141–55.

[65] Gross AM, Heimann L, Shapiro R, et al. Children with diabetes: social skills training and HbA1c levels. Behav Modif 1983;7:151–63.

[66] Gross AM, Magalnick LJ, Richardson P. Self management training with families of insulin-dependent diabetic children: a long term controlled investigation. Child Fam Behav Ther 1985;3:141–53.

[67] Kaplan RM, Chadwick MW, Schimmel LE. Social learning intervention to promote metabolic control in type 1 diabetes mellitus: pilot experiment results. Diabetes Care 1985;8:152–5.

[68] Anderson BJ, Wolf FM, Burkhart MT, et al. Effects of a peer group intervention on metabolic control of adolescents with IDDM: randomize outpatient study. Diabetes Care 1989;12:184–8.

[69] Wysocki T, Greco P, Harris MA, et al. Behavior therapy for families of adolescents with diabetes: maintenance of treatment effects. Diabetes Care 2001;24:441–6.

[70] Satin W, La Greca AM, Zigo S, et al. Diabetes in adolescence: effects of multifamily group intervention and parent simulation of diabetes. J Pediatr Psychol 1989;14:259–76.

[71] Robin AL, Foster SL. Negotiating parent-adolescent conflict: a behavioral family systems approach. New York: Guilford Press; 1989.

[72] Hains AA, Davies WH, Parton E, et al. Brief report: a cognitive behavioral intervention for distressed adolescents with type 1 diabetes. J Pediatr Psychol 2001;26:61–6.

[73] Cook S, Herold K, Edidin DV, et al. Increasing problem solving in adolescents with type 1 diabetes: the Choices diabetes program. Diabetes Educ 2002;28:115–23.

[74] Silverman AH, Haines AA, Davies WH, et al. A cognitive behavioral adherence intervention for adolescents with type 1 diabetes. J Clin Psychol Med Settings 2003;10:119–27.

[75] Fowler J, Budzynski T, Vandebergh R. Effects of an EMG biofeedback relaxation program on control of diabetes: a case study. Biofeedback Self Regul 1976;1:105–12.

[76] Rose MI, Firestone P, Heick HMC, et al. The effect of anxiety management training on the control of juvenile diabetes. J Behav Med 1983;6:381–95.

[77] Boardway RH, Delamater AM, Tomakowsky J, et al. Stress management training for adolescents with diabetes. J Pediatr Psychol 1993;18:29–45.

[78] Mendez FJ, Belendez M. Effects of a behavioral intervention on treatment adherence and stress management in adolescents with IDDM. Diabetes Care 1997;20:1370–5.

[79] Delamater AM, Jacobson AM, Anderson B, et al. Psychosocial therapies in diabetes: report of the psychosocial therapies working group. Diabetes Care 2001;24:1286–92.

[80] Gahagan S, Silverstein J. Prevention and treatment of type 2 diabetes mellitus in children, with special emphasis on American Indian and Alaska Native Children. Pediatrics 2003;112: e328–38.

[81] Rosenbloom AL, Joe JR, Winter WE. Emerging epidemic of type 2 diabetes in youth. Diabetes Care 1999;22:345–54.

[82] American Diabetes Association. Type 2 diabetes in children and adolescents. Pediatrics 2000;105:671–80.

[83] Ludwig DS, Ebbeling CB. Type 2 diabetes mellitus in children-primary care and public health considerations. JAMA 2001;286:1427–30.

[84] Kaufman FR. Type 2 diabetes in children and youth. Rev Endocr Metab Disord 2003;4:33–42.

[85] American Academy of Pediatrics. Prevention of pediatric overweight and obesity. Pediatrics 2003;112:424–30.

[86] Mustillo S, Worthman C, Erkanli A, et al. Obesity and psychiatric disorder: developmental trajectories. Pediatrics 2003;111:851–9.

[87] Krahnstoever Davison K, Lipps Birch L. Weight status, parent reaction, and self-concept in five-year-old girls. Pediatrics 2001;107:46–52.

[88] Rosenbloom AL, Silverstein JH. Type 2 diabetes in children and adolescents: a guide to diagnosis, epidemiology, pathogenesis, prevention, and treatment. Alexandria (VA): American Diabetes Association; 2003.

[89] Wang G, Dietz WH. Economic burden of obesity in youths aged 6 to 7 years: 1979–1999. Pediatrics 2002;109:E81.

[90] Freedman D, Khan L, Serdula M, et al. Interrelationships among childhood BMI, childhood height, and adult obesity: the Bogalusa Heart Study. Int J Obes Relat Metab Disord 2003;28:10–6.

[91] Jeffrey RW, Epstein LH, Wilson GT, et al. Long-term maintenance of weight loss: current status. Health Psychol 2000;19:5–16.

[92] Jelalian E, Saelens B. Empirically supported treatments in pediatric psychology: pediatric obesity. J Pediatr Psychol 1999;24:223–48.

[93] Epstein LH, Valoski A, Wing RR, et al. Ten-year outcomes of behavioral family-based treatment for childhood obesity. Health Psychol 1994;13:373–83.

[94] Brownell KD, Kelman JH, Stunkard AJ. Treatment of obese children with and without their mothers: changes in weight and blood pressure. An Pediatr (Barc) 1983;71:515–23.

[95] Wysocki T, Buckloh LM. Endocrine, metabolic, nutritional and immune disorders. In: Boll TJ, editor. Handbook of health psychology, vol 1. Washington: American Psychological Association; 2002. p. 65–99.

[96] Silverstein JH, Rosenbloom AL. Treatment of type 2 diabetes in children and adolescents. J Pediatr Endocrinol Metab 2003;13:1403–9.

[97] Kann L, Warren CW, Harris WA, et al. Youth risk behavior surveillance-United States, 1993. J Sch Health 1995;65:163–71.

[98] Gortmaker SL, Peterson K, Wiecha J, et al. Reducing obesity via school-based interdisciplinary intervention among youth: Planet Health. Arch Pediatr Adolesc Med 1999;153: 409–18.

[99] Robinson TN. Reducing children's television viewing to prevent obesity: a randomized controlled trial. JAMA 1999;282:1561–7.

[100] Wiecha JL, Alison ME, Fuemmeler BF, et al. Diffusion of an integrated health education program in an urban school system: Planet Health. J Pediatr Psychol 2004;29:467–74.

[101] Holescher DM, Kelder SH, Murray N, et al. Dissemination and adoption of the Child and Adolescents Trial for Cardiovascular Health (CATCH): a case study in Texas. J Public Health Manag Pract 2001;7:90–100.

[102] Trevino RP, Pugh JA, Hernandez AE, et al. Bienestar: a diabetes risk factor prevention program. J Sch Health 1998;68:62–7.

[103] Teufel NI, Ritenbaugh CK. Development of a primary prevention program: insight gained in the Zuni Diabetes Prevention Program. Clin Pediatr (Phila) 1998;37:131–41.

[104] Brewer KW, Chase HP, Owen S, et al. Slicing the pie: correlating HbA1c values with average blood glucose values in a pie chart form. Diabetes Care 1998;21:209–12.

[105] American Diabetes Association. Curriculum for youth education. Alexandria (VA): American Diabetes Association; 1983.

[106] Baker L, Lyen K. Laying the foundation for juvenile diabetes management. Drug Ther 1981;10:63–73.

[107] Wysocki T, Taylor A, Hough BS, et al. Deviation from developmentally appropriate self care autonomy: association with diabetes outcomes. Diabetes Care 1996;19:119–25.

[108] Allen DA, Tennen H, McGrade BJ, et al. Parent and child perceptions of the management of juvenile diabetes. J Pediatr Psychol 1983;8:129–41.

[109] Ingersoll G, Orr DP, Herrold AJ, et al. Cognitive maturity and self- management among adolescents with insulin-dependent diabetes mellitus. J Pediatr 1986;108:620–3.

[110] Palmer D, Berg CA, Wiebe DJ, et al. The role of autonomy and pubertal status in understanding age differences in maternal involvement in diabetes responsibility across adolescence. J Pediatr Psychol 2004;29:35–46.

[111] Weibe DJ, Berg CA, Korbel C, et al. Children's appraisals of maternal involvement in coping with diabetes: enhancing our understanding of adherence, metabolic control, and quality of life across adolescence. J Pediatr Psychol 2005;30:167–78.

[112] Anderson BJ, Coyne JC. Miscarried helping in the families of children and adolescents with chronic diseases. In: Johnson JH, Johnson SB, editors. Advances in child health psychology. Gainesville (FL): University of Florida Press; 1991. p. 167–77.

[113] Bobrow ES, AvRuskin TW, Siller I. Mother-daughter interactions and adherence to diabetes regimens. Diabetes Care 1985;8:146–51.

[114] Miller-Johnson S, Emery RE, Marvin RS, et al. Parent-child relationships and the management of insulin-dependent diabetes mellitus. J Consult Clin Psychol 1994;62:603–10.

[115] Hanson CL, Rodrigue J, Henggeler SW, et al. The perceived self-competence of adolescents with insulin-dependent diabetes mellitus: deficit or strength? J Pediatr Psychol 1990;15: 605–18.

[116] Hauser ST, Jacobson AM, Wertlieb DM, et al. The contribution of family environment to perceived competence and illness adjustment in diabetic and acutely ill adolescents. Fam Relat 1985;34:99–108.

[117] Kovacs M, Mukerji P, Iyengar S, et al. Psychiatric disorder and metabolic control among youths with IDDM: a longitudinal study. Diabetes Care 1996;19:318–23.

[118] White K, Kolman ML, Wexler P, et al. Unstable diabetes and unstable families: a psychosocial evaluation of children with recurrent diabetic ketoacidosis. Pediatrics 1984;73:749–55.

[119] Wysocki T, Greco P, Buckloh LM. Childhood diabetes in psychological context. In: Roberts MC, editor. Handbook of pediatric psychology. 3rd edition. New York: Guilford Press; 2003. p. 304–20.

[120] Glaab LA, Brown R, Daneman D. School attendance in children with type 1 diabetes. Diabet Med 2005;22:421–6.

[121] Wysocki T. For parents: mental health resources for kids. Diabetes Self Manag 2000;18: 96–101.

[122] Weissberg-Benchell J, Antisdel-Lomaglio J, Seshadri R. Insulin pump therapy: a meta-analysis. Diabetes Care 2003;26:1079–87.

[123] Johnson SB. Screening programs to identify children at risk for diabetes mellitus: psychological impact on children and parents. J Pediatr Endocrinol Metab 2001;14(Suppl 1):653–9.

[124] Kruger D, Marcus AO. Psychological motivation and patient education: a role for continuous glucose monitoring. Diabetes Technol Ther 2000;2:S93–7.

[125] Saab PG, McCalla JR, Coons HL, et al. Technological and medical advances: implications for health psychology. Health Psychol 2004;23:142–6.

ELSEVIER
SAUNDERS

Pediatr Clin N Am 52 (2005) 1779–1804

PEDIATRIC CLINICS
OF NORTH AMERICA

A Look to the Future: Prediction, Prevention, and Cure Including Islet Transplantation and Stem Cell Therapy

Anna Casu, MD, Massimo Trucco, MD,
Massimo Pietropaolo, MD*

*Division of Immunogenetics, Department of Pediatrics, Rangos Research Center,
Children's Hospital of Pittsburgh, University of Pittsburgh School of Medicine, 3460 Fifth Avenue,
Pittsburgh, PA 15213, USA*

Critical to the success of intervention strategies is the identification of individuals at risk of developing the disease in an effort to delay or prevent the clinical onset of type 1 diabetes mellitus (T1DM). The ability to predict T1DM progression with 50% to 80% accuracy is the sine qua non for the accomplishment of successful intervention strategies in relatives of T1DM probands. Even with this high degree of predictability, the current comfort level with intervention therapies is such that there are still very few clinical trials in the preclinical phase of T1DM, with most of these trials being conducted in newly diagnosed T1DM patients.

Prediction of type 1 diabetes

Islet autoantibodies

T1DM is caused by autoimmune destruction or dysfunction of the insulin-secreting cells within the islets of Langerhans and represents the end point of a

This work was supported by NIH grants R01 DK53456 and R01 DK56200 (M. Pietropaolo), by NIH R01 DK24021 (M. Trucco), and by an American Diabetes Association Career Development Award (M. Pietropaolo).

* Corresponding author.

E-mail address: pietroma@pitt.edu (M. Pietropaolo).

progressive decline in β-cell function [1,2]. This long prodromic period before overt T1DM development offers a large window of opportunity not only to predict the disease onset but also to intervene with safe therapeutic agents [2]. Similar to many autoimmune diseases, T1DM is characterized by humoral and cellular autoimmune responses directed against multiple target antigens of pancreatic islet cells. The immunologic diagnosis of autoimmune diseases relies mainly on the detection of autoantibodies in the serum of T1DM patients. Although their pathogenic significance still remains unclear, they serve as surrogate markers for specific autoimmune responses. Multiple antibodies are present in most newly diagnosed T1DM patients and their presence is highly predictive of disease progression in otherwise healthy first-degree relatives. The currently used markers for prediction studies are islet cell antibodies (ICA), glutamic acid decarboxylase autoantibodies (GAD65 AA), tyrosine-phosphatase–like protein IA-2 autoantibodies (IA-2/ICA512 AA), and insulin autoantibodies (IAA).

During the past decade, the use of islet-related autoantibodies has allowed major advances in prediction studies. All of these studies have suggested that a combination of humoral immunologic markers detecting autoantibodies to these islet antigens, rather than any single test, gives a high predictive value for T1DM in first-degree relatives, and great sensitivity without significant loss of specificity [3–7]. The detection of GAD65 AA, IA-2/ICA512 AA, and IAA is now a clear prerequisite for identifying individuals at risk of developing insulin-requiring diabetes. In particular, the presence of two or more of these auto-antibodies to islet antigens is now used as entry criteria for intervention trials aiming at mitigating the deterioration in insulin secretion after T1DM onset or at preventing the disease process in first-degree relatives of T1DM probands.

ICA were the first disease-specific antibodies identified in patients affected by T1DM. These antibodies are detected by indirect immunofluorescence using human pancreatic sections [8]. The Immunology of Diabetes Society has repeatedly demonstrated a marked variability between laboratories and even within the same laboratory performing ICA assays. Nonetheless, the authors provided evidence suggesting that ICA predict a more rapid progression to insulin-requiring diabetes in GAD65 AA– and IA-2 AA–positive relatives. Despite marked variability of the ICA assay formats, the authors strongly support the conclusion that cytoplasmic ICA should remain part of the assessment of T1DM risk for future intervention trials [9]. Their data also provided indirect evidence for the presence of an important subset of ICA that apparently reacts with unidentified islet autoantigens. The general view is that cytoplasmic ICA represents a heterogeneous group of immunoglobulins that specifically react with a family of autoantigens on frozen pancreatic sections. Thus far, the best-characterized subsets of ICA react with GAD and IA-2 [10–13].

The availability of molecularly characterized islet autoantigens represents an unlimited source of reagents that are readily used for experimental and diagnostic purposes. Some of these molecules include GAD65 and IA-2, and they have been used to optimize fluid-phase radioimmunoassays with much higher reproducibility as compared with immunofluorescence assays used for ICA detection [14,15].

The presence of GAD65 and IA-2/ICA512 AA is now a prerequisite to enroll subjects in prevention trials.

Insulin was the first identified T1DM-related autoantigen [16] and IAA are detected using a radiobinding immunoassay [17–19]. They have a specificity almost as high as 100%, but the sensitivity seems to be rather low (compared with the sensitivity of GAD65 AA), as suggested by the results of proficiency workshops organized by the Diabetes Autoantibodies Standardization Program [20]. Nonetheless, IAA are detected in as much as 90% of newly diagnosed patients below 5 years of age, in 71% between 5 and 10 years, and in 50% of T1DM patients 10 to 15 years old [21,22].

GAD autoantibodies were identified in 1990 [23] and they are mainly directed against the 65- kDa isoform of this enzyme. They are detected using a semiquantitative fluid-phase radiobinding assay, using in vitro transcribed and translated ^{35}S-labeled human recombinant GAD65. The Diabetes Autoantibodies Standardization Program reported a median specificity of 94% and median sensitivity of 77% [20]. GAD autoantibodies in T1DM seem to be mainly directed toward disease-specific epitopes, which are localized within the middle region and the COOH-terminus of the molecule. These epitopes have been identified by competition assays between GAD65-positive sera and cloned GAD65-specific recombinant Fab, and the results seem to be useful to improve T1DM prediction. Some crucial residues for autoantibodies binding to GAD65 have been demonstrated in the same area as a result of homolog-scanning mutagenesis experiments. These studies suggested that GAD65 epitopes are conformational and that the native molecule is recognized by GAD65-specific antibody responses [24,25].

The neuroendocrine antigens ICA512 and IA-2β (phogrin) are both targets of T1DM-related autoantibody responses. A radioligand-binding assay format similar to that used to detect GAD65 AA is currently applied to detect autoantibodies to IA-2 and IA-2β. The specificity of this assay approaches 100% with a sensitivity of nearly 60% [20]. All antigenic constructs used include the intracellular portion of the molecule (IA-2ic aa. 601-979), which contains most of the immunoreactive epitopes as demonstrated by binding and competition analysis with multiple chimeric ICA512-phogrin constructs [26]. One of the immunodominant IA-2 epitopes, termed "Fragment 1" (aa 761-964), has been proposed to be one of the most significant IA-2 epitopes. Of note, autoantibodies against IA-2/Fragment 1 can be detected in 16% of patients that test negative for IA-2 AA measured by the conventional radioassay [27]. Recent results showed that the presence of autoantibodies against the IA-2 intracellular domain epitopes conferred a cumulative risk of diabetes progression significantly higher than the one in relatives with no detectable AA against Fragment 1 and IA-2ic. Because the group of relatives with detectable autoantibodies against Fragment 1 and IA-2ic did not have different titer or prevalence of GAD65, IAA, and ICA when compared with negative subjects, this means that only the presence of antibodies against one of the two IA-2 epitopes conferred the increased risk [28]. These data suggest that biochemical assays detecting autoantibodies against

IA-2 intracellular domain epitopes enhance not only sensitivity but also identify rapid progressors of T1DM onset as compared with conventional markers alone. First-degree relatives carrying IA-2ic and Fragment 1 AA should be included in the highest T1DM risk category and in the inclusion criteria for enrollment in intervention trials aimed at preventing T1DM.

Autoantibodies against more than 20 putative targets of islet autoimmunity have been identified in T1DM patients, but they are less well characterized. Those include ICA69, carboxypeptidase H, CD38, glima 38, the glucose transporter 2 the islet ganglioside GM2-1, heat shock protein 60 kd, ICA12/SOX13 [12,29–31], and a number of other molecules.

Many well-defined epidemiologic studies are currently ongoing in the United States and around the world, such as the Bart's Windsor, Joslin, Denver, Pittsburgh, Seattle, Gainesville, BabyDiab in Germany, and other studies [32–36]. These studies provide the groundwork to understand the natural history of the disease process and to improve prediction of T1DM in first-degree relatives of T1DM probands and ultimately in the general population [21,37–40]. There is a high degree of concordance among these groups that multiple autoantibodies to islet autoantigens confer a cumulative risk of developing diabetes of 75% to 90% during 5 to 10 years of prospective follow-up in first-degree relatives (Fig. 1) [3,5,41–43]. The antibody titer also seems to be an important predictive risk factor, in that higher autoantibody titers are associated with a higher risk of de-

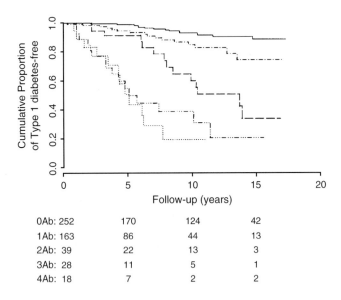

Fig. 1. Progression to insulin-requiring diabetes among first-degree relatives (N = 500) in relation to the number of autoantibodies (Ab) to insulin, GAD65, IA-2, and ICA. Relatives who are positive for three or four Ab are at much greater risk of developing diabetes compared with relatives with two Ab alone. Log rank: $P = .0096$ and .001, respectively. (*From* Pietropaolo M, Becker DJ, LaPorte RE, et al. Progression to insulin-requiring diabetes in seronegative prediabetic subjects: the role of two HLA-DQ high-risk haplotypes. Diabetologia 2002;45:66–76; with permission.)

veloping the disease [4,44–46]. T1DM risk can be further stratified by taking into consideration a high titer of IA-2 AA and IAA [46]. In particular, first-degree relatives with titers of IA-2 AA in the upper three quartiles have significantly higher diabetes risk than relatives with their IA-2 AA titer in the lowest quartile. Similar results were obtained for IAA but not for GAD65 AA. High titer of IA-2 AA and IAA seems to be a strong predictor of T1DM development [46].

To assess the predictive role of the islet-related AA, a number of studies have been undertaken in the general population, particularly in schoolchildren [21,37–40]. These studies concluded that ICA or other islet AA in subjects with no family history of disease conferred an increased risk of T1DM development. It must be emphasized that the predictive value of islet-related AA is lower in the general population compared with that in first-degree relatives [21,37–39]. This is because of a low prevalence of the disease in the general population. For uncommon diseases like T1DM (eg, prevalence of 1.2–1.5 per 1000 in the United States) [47,48], a large proportion of individuals with positive screening test results, including multiple autoantibodies to islet antigens, will inevitably be found not to develop the disease. According to Bayes' theorem, the positive predictive value of screening tests varies dramatically based on the prevalence of the disease in a given population [49,50]. For example, because the prevalence of T1DM is quite low, the positive predictive value of GAD AA and IA-2 AA alone or in combination is also likely to be quite low, even when using assays with high sensitivity and specificity. Until proved otherwise, the only intervention strategy for T1DM that should be proposed in the general population is an innocuous nutritional or vaccination program, because the presence of positive markers, such as ICA, does not guarantee progression to clinical disease. By contrast, with a disease such as polio, it is not necessary to identify individuals at risk for the development of the disease, because the benefits of a safe massive vaccination program outweigh by far the devastating risk of poliomyelitis for the society [49].

The role of major histocompatibility complex in type 1 diabetes mellitus prediction studies

The role of HLA in T1DM susceptibility remains unquestionable, because there is convincing evidence that inherited susceptibility to T1DM is primarily associated and linked with genes within the major histocompatibility complex [51–53]. The HLA locus is termed *IDDM1* according to a more recent nomenclature [54]. Genome-wide scans in T1DM have identified over 18 putative loci of statistical significance but only linkage to HLA seems incontestable.

Early studies found that HLA-DR3 and -DR4 alleles were strongly associated with T1DM susceptibility [51,55]. Approximately 95% of patients with T1DM were heterozygous for DR3/4 or expressed at least one of these alleles, and heterozygous individuals seemed to be more susceptible to the disease than the homozygous ones. Restriction fragment length polymorphism analysis of DNA from T1DM patients and nondiabetic controls showed an even stronger association between the HLA-DQ locus and disease susceptibility. Analysis of the DQβ chain showed that a negatively charged aspartic acid at position 57 correlated with resistance, whereas non–aspartic acid at position 57 correlated with susceptibility [56,57]. Also, it was shown that arginine at position 52 of the DQα chain correlated with disease susceptibility. The ability of HLA-DQ molecules to influence susceptibility or resistance to the disease is explained by the different interactions between DQ molecules, antigens, and T-cell receptors. The presence of susceptible HLA alleles also correlates with the presence of islet autoantibodies.

The addition of HLA-DQ genotypes to screening strategies does not increase sensitivity of combined autoantibody assays. Unidentified autoimmune phenomena may well be present in seronegative relatives who eventually develop insulin-requiring diabetes if they possess two HLA-DQ high-risk haplotypes (Fig. 2) [58,59].

Although HLA is not the optimal primary screening tool for T1DM and it is not sufficient alone to predict the disease onset, the evaluation of HLA genotyping in relatives with ICA positivity can significantly improve the ability to predict T1DM progressors versus nonprogressors [60–62]. In seronegative relatives who developed insulin-requiring diabetes, the presence of two HLA-DQ high-risk haplotypes conferred an increased cumulative risk of developing insulin requirement (see Fig. 2) [58].

The prevalence of HLA-DR2 is decreased in patients with T1DM, and in many populations the DQB1*0602 allele is rarely found among patients with T1DM. This suggests that this allele may play a protective role in the disease

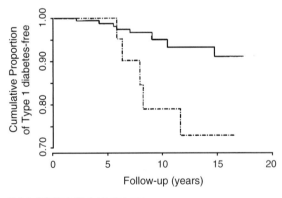

Number of HLA-DQ High Risk Haplotypes			
0 or 1: 221	149	110	36
2 : 31	21	14	6

Fig. 2. Progression to insulin-requiring diabetes for seronegative relatives (N = 252) who carry two compared with zero or one *HLA-DQ* high-risk haplotypes. Two *HLA-DQ* high-risk haplotypes conferred a cumulative risk of insulin-requiring diabetes of 27% after a follow-up of 12.5 years, compared with a risk of 6% for relatives who had zero or one *HLA-DQ* high-risk haplotypes (log rank $P = .01$) or two *HLA-DQ* high-risk haplotypes. (*From* Pietropaolo M, Becker DJ, LaPorte RE, et al. Progression to insulin-requiring diabetes in seronegative prediabetic subjects: the role of two HLA-DQ high-risk haplotypes. Diabetologia 2002;45:66–76; with permission.)

process. At present, carrying a protective DQB*0602 allele is considered a criterion of exclusion for enrolling first-degree relatives of diabetic patients in clinical trials, such as the Diabetes Prevention Trial 1 (DPT-1) or the TrialNet, which is being performed in the United States. These trials have been designed to use any effective therapeutic regimen that could delay and ultimately prevent the clinical onset of T1DM in individuals considered at high risk of developing the disease.

Other genes

Several studies revealed an association between the disease and 18 chromosomal regions other than major histocompatibility complex that may contain susceptibility loci. Some of those associations were not confirmed in subsequent studies. The main non–major histocompatibility complex loci related to T1DM are the insulin gene region (INS) known as *IDDM2*, the immunoglobulin heavy chain genes (*IDDM11*), and CTLA-4 (*IDDM12*). To date, none of them has been shown to have any role in the prediction of T1DM [51].

Pancreatic β-cell function

In individuals with islet antibodies, the first-phase insulin response (FPIR) after an intravenous glucose tolerance test predicts time to diabetes onset [50,63–68]. The FPIR is determined as the first plus third minute plasma insulin concentration (mU/L) after the midpoint of intravenous injection of 0.5 g of glucose per kilogram body weight with a maximum of 35 g. Oral glucose tolerance is not impaired until the FPIR is less than the first percentile (<50 mU/L in prepubertal children and <100 mU/L in older individuals) on two occasions 3 to 6 months apart, which corresponds to a very late stage of the natural history of the disease [50].

A low FPIR underlies an advanced autoimmune process and is the outcome of a profound reduction in β-cell function. A FPIR less than the first percentile is associated with an estimated risk of diabetes of 100% within a 4-year follow-up, regardless of the presence of one or more islet autoantibodies [5].

Proposed guidelines for screening

The Immunology of Diabetes Society has proposed a number of guidelines for screening and assessing diabetes risk in unaffected first-degree relatives of T1DM probands. According to these guidelines, testing for GAD65 AA, IA-2/ICA512 AA, and IAA can identify approximately 85% of either newly diagnosed or future T1DM cases. To maximize sensitivity, IAA testing should be included as primary screening strategy for children <10 years of age. Cytoplasmic ICA should be included as a secondary screening methodology, because it increases the predictive value of combined biochemical autoantibody markers. As a general rule, subjects that are positive for one or more islet autoantibodies should be further evaluated by using other markers (genetic and metabolic) to define the risk more precisely. Participation of laboratories in workshop or proficiency programs is strongly advised. HLA class II typing may be useful in identifying infants who would be subsequently followed to document closely the occurrence of islet autoantibodies and ultimately to recruit them into intervention trials. The FPIR assessment is generally used to identify a subgroup of individuals with the highest risk of developing diabetes within a short period of time. Findings from studies in first-degree relatives should not be assumed to apply to the general population [21,37–39,69] because the predictive value obtained in this population is lower than those obtained for first-degree relatives. At this stage, all prediction should be considered as investigational but not yet applicable to the general population or general physician.

Prevention strategies

The rationale for undertaking prevention studies in humans stems from the evidence that in animal models of autoimmune diabetes, such as the nonobese diabetic (NOD) mouse and the biobreeding rat, the disease process can be prevented using many different therapeutic approaches.

Prevention strategies can be classified into three categories based on the timing of intervention: (1) primary prevention, aimed at preventing the disease in high-risk populations before any serologic evidence of islet autoimmunity; (2) secondary prevention, aimed at delaying and, possibly, suppressing β-cell damage in euglycemic subjects with evidence of islet autoimmunity; and (3) tertiary prevention, initiated after diabetes onset, aimed at inducing prolonged remission or β-cell regeneration. This also seems to be useful in preserving the remaining β-cell function, which has been correlated with a reduced incidence of chronic complications [70–72]. First-degree relatives of patients with T1DM represent an accessible and highly motivated population, for the most part, to be screened and included in primary and secondary prevention trials, whereas newly diagnosed diabetic patients are included in tertiary prevention strategy.

Several drugs, such as cyclosporine [73,74] and azathioprine [75–77], have been used to preserve β-cell function after T1DM onset. These immunosuppressive therapies were administered in newly diagnosed T1DM and yielded a transient beneficial effect in terms of maintaining higher C-peptide levels over time compared with the placebo-treated patients. Because of the development of serious side effects, these therapeutic regimens are no longer considered appropriate treatments for T1DM. Other approaches have also been proposed in humans (Table 1).

Primary prevention

Only one primary prevention trial is ongoing and it is based on the possible role of cow's milk proteins in inducing diabetes. Cow's milk protein have been

Table 1
Prevention trials in type 1 diabetes

Name of the study	Strategy	Type of study	Agent	Population	Result
TRIGR	Primary prevention	Randomized, placebo-controlled, double-blind	Hydrolyzed cow's milk formula	FDR at high genetic risk	Ongoing
ENDIT	Secondary prevention	Randomized, placebo-controlled, double-blind	Nicotinamide	High-risk FDR: ICA+	No prevention
DPT-1 parenteral	Secondary prevention	Randomized, no placebo	Parenteral insulin	High-risk relatives	No prevention
DPT-1 oral	Secondary prevention	Randomized, placebo-controlled, double-blind	Oral insulin	Moderate-risk relatives	Reduced incidence of T1DM in relatives with IAA $\geq$ 80 U
Cyclosporine	Tertiary prevention	Randomized, placebo-controlled, double-blind	Cyclosporine	New-onset T1DM patients	Temporary remission of T1DM
Azathioprine	Tertiary prevention	Randomized, placebo-controlled, double-blind	Azathioprine	New-onset T1DM patients	No effect
Azathioprine, prednisone	Tertiary prevention	Randomized, unblind	Azathioprine, prednisone	New-onset T1DM patients	Partial, temporary remission of T1DM
Anti-CD3 treatment	Tertiary prevention	Randomized, placebo-controlled	hOKT3γ(Ala-Ala)	New-onset T1DM patients	Prevention of loss of C peptide
Anti-CD20	Tertiary prevention	Randomized, placebo-controlled	Anti-CD20 monoclonal antibodies	New-onset T1DM patients	To be started
Thymoglobulin	Tertiary prevention	Randomized, placebo-controlled	Antithymocyte polyclonal antibodies	New-onset T1DM patients	To be started
DIPP	Secondary prevention	Randomized, placebo-controlled, double-blind	Nasal insulin	High-risk subjects	Ongoing
NBI-6024 Neurocrine	Tertiary prevention	Randomized, placebo-controlled, double-blind	Altered peptide ligand insulin B:9-23	New-onset T1DM patients	Ongoing
Peptor HSP60	Tertiary prevention	Randomized, placebo-controlled, double-blind	Heat shock protein 60	New-onset T1DM adult patients	Ongoing; prevention of loss of C peptide
BCG vaccination	Tertiary prevention	Randomized, placebo-controlled, double-blind	BCG vaccine	New-onset T1DM adult patients	No effect

Abbreviations: BCG, bacillus Calmette-Guerin; FDR, first degree relatives; IAA, insulin antibodies; ICA, islet cell antibodies; T1DM, type 1 diabetes mellitus.

suggested to play a role in T1DM pathogenesis following prospective studies, which showed that breastfeeding was associated with a somewhat lower incidence of children developing T1DM [78–80] as compared with children who were exposed to cow's milk. A role for cow's milk proteins in diabetes has also been reported in animal models of T1DM [80–82]. A decreased incidence of T1DM was found in animals weaned to hydrolyzed proteins instead of intact foreign proteins. Some evidence now suggests that a similar relationship may exist in humans [83]. The Trial to Reduce Insulin-dependent Diabetes in Genetically at Risk (TRIGR) is an ongoing randomized controlled trial aimed at determining whether the absence of cow's milk proteins in the diet protects from T1DM progression in first-degree relatives of T1DM patients carrying high-risk HLA alleles. This is a primary prevention trial in subjects with no evidence of autoimmunity. This study will also determine whether or not breastfeeding is associated with a reduced T1DM risk during a 10-year follow-up. All families whose offspring are included in the study receive the recommendation to breastfeed for at least the first 6 months of life in accordance with the World Health Organization recommendations. If a mother is unable exclusively to breastfeed before the baby is 8 months of age, her child is randomly assigned to one of two groups. One group receives breastfeeding supplements of a trial formula based on extensively hydrolyzed protein whose fragments do not stimulate the immune system; the other group receives a trial formula containing intact proteins. This study is designed not to interfere with infant feeding practices, except to emphasize and encourage breastfeeding. What makes this intervention attractive is its safety, because hydrolyzed formulas have been used for decades to treat cow's milk protein allergies with no occurrence of serious adverse effects. Theoretically, this intervention may be applied to the general population as a form of primary intervention.

The results of the pilot study for TRIGR performed in Finland, Estonia, and Sweden have recently been published [83]. At the end of the 2-year observation period, the proportion of subjects positive for at least one autoantibody was lower in the hydrolyzed group compared with the control group. In addition, during a follow-up of up to 4 years (only for the Finnish subjects), the number of children who developed overt diabetes was higher in the control group, although this difference was not statistically significant. The completion of the larger TRIGR study is needed to confirm the trends shown by the pilot study.

Secondary prevention

Most prevention trials have been conducted in first-degree relatives of T1DM patients when many of these subjects have already developed signs of islet autoimmunity documented by the presence of both humoral immunologic and metabolic abnormalities. The most important secondary prevention studies are the European Nicotinamide Diabetes Intervention Trial (ENDIT) and DPT-1. Their results have been recently reported [84,85].

Nicotinamide (European Nicotinamide Diabetes Intervention Trial)

Initial observations indicated that high doses of nicotinamide could prevent the development of T1DM in streptozotocin-treated rats. This drug also seems to prevent or delay the onset of diabetes in NOD mice, possibly preserving β-cell function [86]. Initial pilot studies suggested that nicotinamide might prevent diabetes development in ICA-positive schoolchildren [87]. Following these initial observations, a double-blind placebo trial was undertaken in first-degree relatives of T1DM patients carrying ICA autoantibodies [84,85]. More than 30,000 first-degree relatives were screened for cytoplasmic ICA and 552 of them with ICA titer >20 Juvenile Diabetes Foundation units were randomized and then nicotinamide or placebo were administered. The sample size was sufficiently large and powered to estimate a reduction in progression to overt diabetes from 35% to 21% assuming a 20% drop out rate. These subjects were followed for 5 years with regular clinical and metabolic assessment, such as intravenous glucose tolerance test, FPIR, and oral glucose tolerance test. The results of this study indicated that nicotinamide treatment, at the dose used in this trial (1.2 g/m^2 daily up to a maximum of 3 g/d in two doses), did not decrease the incidence of T1DM. The mean FPIR was not different between the two groups, so nicotinamide did not stop the decrease of β-cell function. Body weight and height were monitored to ascertain any possible effect of the drug on growth. No differences were seen with respect to growth and no adverse events were reported between the two groups [84,85].

Parenteral and oral insulin: Diabetes Prevention Trial Type 1

Thus far, both insulin and proinsulin are considered the only candidate pancreatic β-cell–specific autoantigens. There is evidence in both NOD mice and biobreeding rats that the administration of insulin can modify the natural history of autoimmune diabetes in these animals [88–90]. Although a pilot study performed in relatives at risk of developing T1DM showed that parenteral insulin administration delayed the onset of the disease, this conclusion was not confirmed by a more robust recent trial conducted by the DPT-1 diabetes study group [91,92]. A number of research groups have reported the expression of islet autoantigens within cells of the thymus and lymphoid organs [93–96] and in peripheral lymphoid organs [97], two tissues thought to be vital to the maintenance of immunologic self-tolerance. One may postulate that disruption of genetic elements regulating transcript and protein expression (eg, insulin) in the thymus and lymphoid tissues could short circuit mechanisms necessary for maintaining immune self-tolerance to endogenous antigens, such as insulin. This hypothesis was corroborated by the demonstration that diabetes development is accelerated in NOD mice deficient for proinsulin-2 expression within both the thymus and the β-cells [98].

The hypothesis was further strengthened by reports that the insulin epitope has experimentally blocked the development of T1DM in NOD mice and that oligoclonally expanded T-cells from pancreatic lymph nodes of type 1 diabetic mice recognized the insulin A:1-15 epitope.

In the DPT-1 trial, relatives with a risk of developing diabetes ≥ 50% in 5 years were enrolled in the parenteral insulin trial and randomized to receive subcutaneous insulin twice daily (0.125 U/kg of body weight) and intravenous insulin once a month or observation (a placebo was not administered) [92]. Relatives with projected 5-year risk of 26% to 50% were assigned to an oral insulin trial, to assess the effect of oral insulin therapy in preventing T1DM (7.5 mg of insulin crystals per day) [99]. Starting from 1996, more than 84,000 relatives were screened and 339 with a risk of developing diabetes ≥ 50% in 5 years underwent randomization. After a median follow-up of 3.7 years, the cumulative incidence of diabetes was similar in the two groups as was the mean C-peptide levels. Similarly, insulin taken orally did not delay or prevent T1DM in 372 relatives at moderate risk of developing the disease. Compared with the placebo group, however, a small effect of oral insulin administration in preventing T1DM was seen in relatives with confirmed high levels of IAA (≥ 80 nU/mL) (Fig. 3) [99]. It is possible that a more potent beneficial effect of oral insulin may be present in relatives enrolled in the trial with higher IAA levels (ie, ≥ 200 nU/mL).

Finally, a trial conducted by a company called Neurocrine, using an altered insulin peptide ligand of insulin B:9-23, is currently underway in humans in which the peptide is delivered without the use of an adjuvant or other immuno-modulation [100].

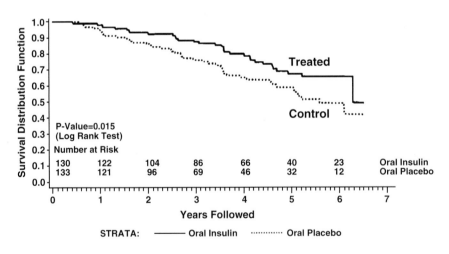

Fig. 3. Kaplan-Meier curves showing the proportion of subjects without diabetes during the trial by treatment assignment for subjects with baseline confirmed IAA ≥ 80 nU/mL. The number of subjects at risk in each group at each year of follow-up is enumerated at the bottom of the figure. The log-rank test was used for comparison between the groups, with the *P* values as indicated. (*From* Effects of oral insulin in relatives of patients with type 1 diabetes: the Diabetes Prevention Trial-Type 1. Diabetes Care 2005;28:1068–76; with permission from the American Diabetes Association).

Lessons from secondary prevention trials

Both the DPT-1 and ENDIT trials have been instrumental in paving the way for designing new intervention trials. First, it was learned that large preventive trials of T1DM are feasible in first-degree relatives. This major commitment has also contributed in creating a large network of investigators working cooperatively and collegially. Both trials re-emphasized that diabetes can be predicted and the natural history of T1DM has been further elucidated. It is to be noticed that both trials identified high-risk relatives on the basis of ICA titer and competitive IAA assays, whereas now a better prediction is achieved by using IA-2/ICA512 AA and GAD AA. A rigorous follow-up of subjects to be enrolled in these trials permits an earlier diagnosis of the disease with less frequency of ketoacidosis and implementation of insulin therapy when higher C-peptide levels still are present. The outcome of these initial trials raised questions regarding the most appropriate dose of antigen that may be effective to prevent diabetes.

Tertiary prevention

A different preventive approach can be undertaken in newly diagnosed diabetic patients. The aims of tertiary prevention can be summarized as follows. First, to preserve the remaining β-cell function. This is associated with better metabolic control, less hypoglycemic events, and decrease of chronic complication in diabetic patients [70,101]. Second, to test the safety and efficacy of preventive strategies in new-onset T1DM patients before moving to high-risk populations, such as first-degree relatives.

The rationale for conducting these interventions is based on the assumption that at least 10% of β-cells are still viable at the onset of the disease, but the potential for functional recovery could even be greater. Furthermore, The Diabetes Control and Complications Trial provided evidence that preservation of residual insulin production is of clinical value and that it might result in lowering hemoglobin A_{1c} levels [70,71]. To date, the quantification of the efficacy of these therapies, undertaken after the onset of insulin requirement, hinges on the assessment of baseline and stimulated C-peptide levels. Although there is concordance in interpreting the metabolic data (ie, C peptide), there is a paucity of data addressing whether the immunotherapies induce antigen-related or regulatory tolerance. In the case of insulin trials started after diabetes onset, immune responses to insulin, such as IAA (epitope, affinity, immunoglobulin subclasses) and T-cell responses using the ELISPOT, were evaluated to assess whether this therapy may induce changes in IAA and cytokine secretion patterns. It is important to develop assays to assess whether regulatory tolerance is being generated as a result of these antigen-based therapies.

For these reasons, the Immunology of Diabetes Society has recently established Guidelines for Intervention Trials in Subjects with Newly Diagnosed Type 1 Diabetes to stratify for disease risk and maximize the information gained from these studies [102]. The goal for these studies is to preserve β-cell function.

Thus far, the only reliable screening marker for β-cell function is C peptide. In fact, it is produced by cleavage of the proinsulin molecule to obtain insulin. C peptide is cosecreted along with insulin, but it is subjected to less first-pass clearance by the liver. Its long half-life is a prerequisite for its accurate and reproducible detection in the blood. Although hemoglobin A_{1c} is a valuable clinical hallmark of glycemic control, it is an insensitive marker of β-cell function. Despite some limitations, C-peptide measurement under standardized conditions provides a sensitive, well-accepted, and validated assessment of β-cell function. It represents the most suitable primary outcome for clinical trials aimed at preserving or improving endogenous insulin secretion in T1DM patients; even a modest effect on preserving C-peptide secretion seems to impart benefits in terms of prevention of chronic complications (Fig. 4) [70,71,101].

The benefits of tertiary prevention trials could be transient; also, some interventions that might be effective if used in the early phase of the disease might be ineffective in its terminal stage. Of note, nearly all of the prevention treatments in NOD mice are of no value if started after the clinical onset of the disease [86]. Treatment with anti-CD3 antibodies represents an exception to this rule [103,104]. Other possible treatments in newly diagnosed T1DM patients are under evaluation. The most promising ones seem to be the immuno-suppressant therapy with mycophenolate mofetil-daclizumab [105,106], the anti-CD20 antibody, therapy with antithymocyte globulin [107], and the antigen-based vaccination using the heat shock peptide DiaPep 277 [108]. Large, multicenter, controlled trials are required to confirm evidence for beneficial effects in initial pilot studies and to address the potential toxicity and long-term safety of the agent used.

Anti-CD3 treatment

The rationale for undertaking this approach derives from a study showing a beneficial effect before and after disease onset in NOD mice treated with anti-CD3 antibodies (OKT3) [103,104,109]. The remission seemed to be long lasting with preservation of the capacity to mount an immune response to foreign antigens. To be effective, this treatment should be started within 7 days of the clinical onset, presumably when a sufficient β-cell mass is still present [103,104]. Unfortunately, the use of OKT3 in humans was precluded because of significant side effects as a result of massive cytokine release, particularly tumor necrosis factor-α. A monoclonal antibody, termed hOKT3gl(Ala-Ala), has been developed and it contains the binding region of OKT3 in which the CH2 region has been modified by site-directed mutagenesis to alter FcR-binding activity. Apparently, this humanized hOKT3gl(Ala-Ala) monoclonal antibody treatment does not lead to major adverse effects because of release of cytokines by activated T cells, such as fever, headache, hypotension, and so forth, which are common following anti-CD3 monoclonal antibody treatment (OKT3). These antibodies have been used successfully for the treatment of acute renal allograft rejection [110] and psoriasis [111].

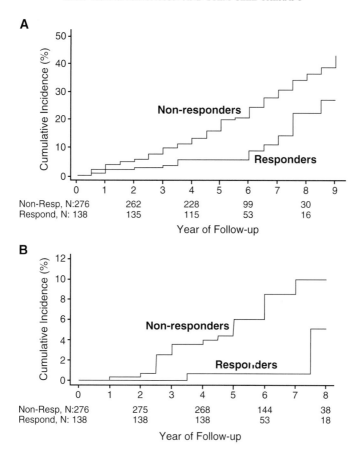

Fig. 4. (*A*) Cumulative incidence of any three or more step progression of retinopathy among base-line C peptide responders versus nonresponders in the intensive treatment group of the DCCT. (*B*) Cumulative incidence of a sustained three-step or more progression. (*From* Palmer JP, Fleming GA, Greenbaum CJ, et al. C-peptide is the appropriate outcome measure for type 1 diabetes clinical trials to preserve beta-cell function: report of an ADA workshop, 21–22 October 2001. Diabetes 2004;53:250–64; with permission.)

A randomized placebo-controlled phase I-II trial was performed in newly diagnosed T1DM patients using this drug [112]. Twelve patients were enrolled in the intervention group and 12 were enrolled in the control group. The treatment consisted of intravenous infusion of the drug for 14 days (1.42 µg per kilogram of body weight on day 1; 5.67 µg per kilogram of body weight on day 2; 11.3 µg per kilogram of body weight on day 3; 22.6 µg per kilogram of body weight on day 4; and 45.4 µg per kilogram of body weight on days 5 through 14). The monoclonal antibody treatment resulted in a reduced decline of the C-peptide response to mixed meal tolerance test in 9 out of 12 patients (Fig. 5) and it lasted for more than 1 year. This treatment also induced a significant decrease in

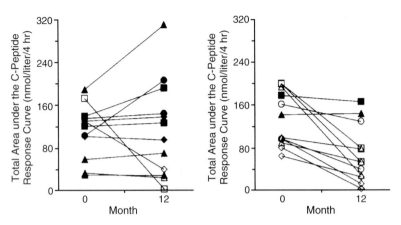

Fig. 5. Changes from study entry to 12 months in the total C peptide response to mixed-meal tolerance testing. Data from each control and antibody-treated subject are shown. Solid symbols represent patients who had a sustained or increased C peptide response, and open symbols represent patients who had a reduced response. (*From* Herold KC, Hagopian W, Auger JA, et al. Anti-CD3 monoclonal antibody in new-onset type 1 diabetes mellitus. N Engl J Med 2002;346:1692–8; with permission.)

hemoglobin A_{1c} levels along with a significant reduction in daily exogenous insulin requirement. In the treatment group, patients experienced mild side effects, such as mild or moderate anemia, nausea, vomiting, arthralgia, headache, and urticarial rash, but with no evidence of long-term toxic effects [112]. Among patients who responded to the therapy and those who did not, there was no substantial difference in terms of clinical presentation, autoantibody titers, isotype subclasses of the autoantibodies, and HLA-DQA1 and DQB1 genotypes. No difference was found between responders and nonresponders to treatment in terms of frequency of the HLA alleles that are associated with protection or susceptibility to T1DM [112]. The mechanism of action of this drug is still unknown. It has been hypothesized that hOKT3g may affect the dynamics of regulatory T-cell populations, such as selective deletion of activated Th1 cells or activation of Th2 cells and their protective cytokines. Alterations in the number and function of regulatory cells may contribute to the generation of an auto-immune state in T1DM [109,113]. Dysfunction or loss of CD1-restricted T cells, T cells with γ/δ receptors, $CD4^+$ and $CD25^+$ T cells, and natural killer T cells may all theoretically contribute to disease pathogenesis through inefficient suppression of pathogenic autoreactive T cells. For instance, in monozygotic twins who are discordant for diabetes, levels of CD1-restricted T cells seem to be diminished in the affected twin. The antigens that activate regulatory T cells are unknown, and the mechanisms in which these cells exert their effect on immune responses still remains unclear. Of note, in vitro studies have demonstrated that alloantigen tolerance induced by costimulatory blockade is maintained by $CD4^+$ and $CD25^+$ T cells [114].

Antithymocyte globulin

Antithymocyte globulin is being used in organ transplantation and little is known about its potential beneficial effects in T1DM. Preclinical studies have shown that antilymphocyte serum treatment in NOD mice with recent-onset diabetes can induce disease remission. An early study that was performed in newly diagnosed T1DM patients (using equine antithymocyte globulin) seemed to prolong the honeymoon phase of the disease. Subsequently, to evaluate both safety and efficacy of the rabbit polyclonal antithymocyte globulin, a phase II study has been undertaken in newly diagnosed T1DM patients. This randomized, placebo-controlled trial should determine whether antithymocyte globulin (6.5 mg/kg of antithymocyte globulin is administered over 4 days) induces immunologic tolerance and thereby prolongs endogenous insulin secretion in adult patients affected by newly diagnosed T1DM. The primary end point is the presence of residual endogenous insulin secretion at 12-month follow-up. Metabolic and mechanistic studies will also be conducted over 24-month intervals. The anticipated outcome is that the treated group will maintain a sustained endogenous insulin secretion and will exhibit a lower daily exogenous insulin requirement as compared with the control group. This study is supported by both the Immuno-Tolerance Network and TrialNet [107].

Anti-CD20

Rituximab, an anti-CD20 monoclonal antibody, has been used for the treatment of β-cell neoplasia and antibody-mediated autoimmune diseases. A recent study showed that rituximab is effective in rheumatoid arthritis [115] and other antibody-mediated autoimmune diseases. It has never been used in autoimmune diseases that seem to have a cell-mediated pathogenesis. For this reason TrialNet is evaluating the possibility of starting a trial to determine its safety and efficacy in preserving C-peptide levels in new-onset T1DM.

Pancreas and islet transplantation

A major goal of clinical investigation in T1DM is to restore a physiologic insulin secretion after engrafting the pancreas or the pancreatic islets into T1DM diabetic recipients. Although ectopancreatic transplantation of donor pancreas has proved fairly effective in normalizing blood glucose levels with partial to complete restoration of C-peptide production in selected groups of patients, islet transplantation gave less promising results [116]. It should be noted that pancreas and islet transplantation cannot be considered as life-saving procedures, and the benefit and risk of these procedures must be thoroughly weighed, particularly if one is dealing with pediatric patients that need long-lasting chronic immunosuppressant therapy to prevent allorejection of the graft. The improvement of new immunosuppressive regimens is an important objective to achieve before considering pancreas and islet transplantation as the standard of care for T1DM [117].

Over the past few years, Shapiro and coworkers [118] have been able to reverse T1DM following islet implantation and the success of the Edmonton protocol has again sparked interest for islet transplantation. Shapiro and co-workers [118] administered a steroid-free immunosuppression regimen along with a larger number of transplanted islets compared with previous islet trans-plantation protocols; sirolimus (0.2 mg/kg/d orally, followed by 0.1 mg/kg/d); low-dose tacrolimus (<2 mg/d orally); and daclizumab (1 mg/kg intravenously every 14 days), an anti interleukin-2 receptor antibody [118]. Side effects were those related to transhepatic puncture and intrahepatic infusion and those related to immunosuppression, such as ulceration of the buccal mucosa, nausea and vomiting, arthralgias, diarrhea, and anemia. Some of the patients had low white blood cell count and a rise in serum creatinine. After a median follow-up of 20 months, 11 transplanted patients were off insulin. According to the American Diabetes Association criteria for diagnosis of diabetes after oral glucose toler-ance test, however, only two subjects met the criteria for normal glucose tol-erance and the remainder had diabetes [119]. The Edmonton protocol has been widely adopted; however, data on long-term follow-up are not yet available.

Stem cell therapy, gene therapy, and other therapies

With the initial success of the Edmonton protocol and increased interest for islet transplantation [118], a number of concerns have arisen, including the insufficient number of donors to yield a sufficient number of implantable islets and the need for a life-long immunosuppressive therapy to prevent both allograft rejection and autoimmunity recurrence. These major obstacles have shifted the interest to alternative approaches to create less immunoreactive and potentially endless alternative sources of islet cells, or to regenerate pancreatic β-cells (reviewed in [120]). The shortage of implantable islets could be overcome by a number of new approaches, including transformed insulin-producing cell lines, transfection of different cell types enabled to produce insulin, in vivo trans-differentiation of liver cells, and isolation of xenogeneic porcine islets [117, 120,121].

It has been hypothesized that newly formed islets derive from the duct epithelium [122], or alternatively from the islet cells themselves [123] or from islet neogenesis, a precursor that may be able to compensate for islet loss. Islet neogenesis may be the end result of a dedifferentiation of pancreatic epithe-lial cells, or newly formed islets might originate from common endocrine, multipotent progenitors. These islet progenitors seem also to be present within the pancreatic islet microenvironment [124]. It might be easier to derive precur-sor cells from stem cells, adult or embryonic, and use them to regenerate the damaged endocrine pancreas. Embryonic stem cell lines might give rise to a potentially unlimited source of insulin-producing cells. Even if embryonic stem cells were soon made available for the scientific community, however, their differentiation toward insulin-producing cells would still remain very difficult to direct. In contrast, achieving transdifferentiation into β-cells from adult stem cells obtained from tissues that belong to other lineages might be a more feasible task. The latter could be an attractive approach to avoid the serious problems related to allorejection because adult tissues can be obtained from an autologous living donor. Nevertheless, this approach is not likely to prevent the recurrence of autoimmunity if it is not combined with immunotherapy.

A similar strategy is based on converting the patient's nonislet cells of different lineages into insulin-producing cells. This has been accomplished using gene-engineered hepatocytes that were able to produce insulin after transfecting them with *pdx1* under the control of the rat insulin 1 promoter [125]. Although not yet confirmed, this observation suggests that engineered surrogate β-cells or insulin-producing cells obtained from cells of different lineages could be exploited to restore insulin secretion.

Other alternative sources of insulin-producing cells include xenogeneic donor manipulated cells that could provide an indefinite supply of β-cells for transplantation. In an elegant set of experiments, the generation of a transgenic pig that was deficient for $\alpha(1,3)$-galactosyltransferase resulted in the dissipation of the hyperacute xenograft rejection response. This was a major advance that might set the stage toward the attainment of the first clinical trial in humans using xenogeneic islet donors [126–129].

Although many of these approaches seem to hold great promise as alternative strategies to cure T1DM, it is unlikely that the recurrence of islet autoimmunity can be prevented without an appropriate immunotherapeutic treatment. In T1DM patients, the autoimmune process not only damages the pancreatic β-cells, leading to the clinical onset of the disease, but also limits the regeneration of newly formed β-cells that will eventually replace those cells that are lost. The recurrence of autoimmunity in combination with allorejection is probably what differentiates transplanted patients with T1DM from patients who received islet autotransplantation and were able to maintain long-lasting glucose homeostasis [117,130]. Strategies aimed at blocking this autoimmune process, or at manipulating potentially less immunoreactive transplanted cells, should yield more encouraging results. These strategies include patient's own cells of different lineages converted into insulin-producing cells; xenogeneic donor manipulated cells; and other manipulated insulin-producing cells, which are likely less immunoreactive. Furthermore, the autoimmune process is successfully averted by blocking the autoreactive T cells with an anti–T-cell antibody (antilymphocyte serum) and by inducing a mixed allogeneic chimerism by transplanting bone marrow from a diabetes-resistant donor [131]. Hematopoietic precursors do not directly participate in islet cell regeneration, although they might be necessary to promote an effective regenerative process, which is independent of the ability to block the autoimmune process [132]. A better understanding of the autoimmune process and the ability to restrain this process not only could prevent the disease, but also help restore residual islet function following islet trans-plantation or regeneration.

Summary

There is common agreement indicating that the occurrence of multiple antibodies against islet autoantigens serves as a surrogate marker of disease in primary or secondary intervention strategies aimed at halting the disease process. To date, a number of intervention strategies are in the pipeline and some of them seem promising. These therapies include anti-CD3 humanized monoclonal antibody; antilymphocyte serum; and a number of antigen-specific therapies, such as oral insulin. The DPT-1 has recently performed a subgroup analysis suggesting potential benefit of oral insulin for relatives with high insulin auto-antibody titers. A trial conducted by Neurocrine using an altered insulin peptide ligand of insulin B:9-23 is currently underway in humans in which the peptide is delivered without the use of an adjuvant or other immunomodulation. Many of these antigen-specific therapies for T1DM and other autoimmune diseases have not been approved. There is both a growing effort and a large opportunity for exploring new specific strategies alone or in combination with immunomodu-lation. It is possible that gene-engineered cell therapeutics if combined with immunotherapy may effectively replace the pancreatic β-cell loss in T1DM. The hope to induce pancreatic islet regeneration and, ultimately, to transplant insulin-producing cells with a sustained secretagogue capacity propels confidence that the cure of T1DM is within reach.

References

[1] Atkinson MA, Maclaren NK. The pathogenesis of insulin-dependent diabetes mellitus. N Engl J Med 1994;331:1428–36.
[2] Eisenbarth GS. Type I diabetes mellitus: a chronic autoimmune disease. N Engl J Med 1986; 314:1360–8.
[3] Bingley PJ, Christie MR, Bonifacio E, et al. Combined analysis of autoantibodies improves prediction of IDDM in islet cell antibody-positive relatives. Diabetes 1994;43:1304–10.
[4] Verge CF, Gianani R, Kawasaki E, et al. Number of autoantibodies (against insulin, GAD or ICA512/IA2) rather than particular autoantibody specificities determines risk of type I diabetes. J Autoimmun 1996;9:379–83.
[5] Verge CF, Gianani R, Kawasaki E, et al. Prediction of type I diabetes in first-degree relatives using a combination of insulin, GAD, and ICA512bdc/IA-2 autoantibodies. Diabetes 1996;45: 926–33.
[6] Pietropaolo M, Peakman M, Pietropaolo SL, et al. Combined analysis of GAD65 and ICA512(IA-2) autoantibodies in organ and non-organ-specific autoimmune diseases confers high specificity for insulin-dependent diabetes mellitus. J Autoimmun 1998;11:1–10.
[7] Wiest-Ladenburger U, Hartmann R, Hartmann U, et al. Combined analysis and single-step detection of GAD65 and IA2 autoantibodies in IDDM can replace the histochemical islet cell antibody test. Diabetes 1997;46:565–71.

[8] Bottazzo GF, Florin-Christensen A, Doniach D. Islet-cell antibodies in diabetes mellitus with autoimmune polyendocrine deficiencies. Lancet 1974;2:1279–83.
[9] Pietropaolo M, Yu S, Libman I, et al. Viva ICA: cytoplasmic islet cell antibodies 30 years later [abstract]. Diabetes 2004;53(Suppl 2):A64.
[10] Genovese S, Bonifacio E, McNally JM, et al. Distinct cytoplasmic islet cell antibodies with different risks for type 1 (insulin-dependent) diabetes mellitus. Diabetologia 1992;35:385–8.
[11] Gianani R, Pugliese A, Bonner-Weir S, et al. Prognostically significant heterogeneity of cytoplasmic islet cell antibodies in relatives of patients with type I diabetes. Diabetes 1992;41:347–53.
[12] Atkinson MA, Kaufman DL, Newman D, et al. Islet cell cytoplasmic autoantibody reactivity to glutamate decarboxylase in insulin-dependent diabetes. J Clin Invest 1993;91:350–6.
[13] Myers MA, Rabin DU, Rowley MJ. Pancreatic islet cell cytoplasmic antibody in diabetes is represented by antibodies to islet cell antigen 512 and glutamic acid decarboxylase. Diabetes 1995;44:1290–5.
[14] Gianani R, Rabin DU, Verge CF, et al. ICA512 autoantibody radioassay. Diabetes 1995;44:1340–4.
[15] Grubin CE, Daniels T, Toivola B, et al. A novel radioligand binding assay to determine diagnostic accuracy of isoform-specific glutamic acid decarboxylase antibodies in childhood IDDM. Diabetologia 1994;37:344–50.
[16] Palmer JP, Asplin CM, Clemons P, et al. Insulin antibodies in insulin-dependent diabetics before insulin treatment. Science 1983;222:1337–9.
[17] Williams AJ, Bingley PJ, Bonifacio E, et al. A novel micro-assay for insulin autoantibodies. J Autoimmun 1997;10:473–8.
[18] Naserke HE, Dozio N, Ziegler AG, et al. Comparison of a novel micro-assay for insulin autoantibodies with the conventional radiobinding assay. Diabetologia 1998;41:681–3.
[19] Vardi P, Dib SA, Tuttleman M, et al. Competitive insulin autoantibody assay: prospective evaluation of subjects at high risk for development of type I diabetes mellitus. Diabetes 1987;36:1286–91.
[20] Bingley PJ, Bonifacio E, Mueller PW. Diabetes Antibody Standardization Program: first assay proficiency evaluation. Diabetes 2003;52:1128–36.
[21] Bingley PJ, Bonifacio E, Williams AJ, et al. Prediction of IDDM in the general population: strategies based on combinations of autoantibody markers. Diabetes 1997;46:1701–10.
[22] Feeney SJ, Myers MA, Mackay IR, et al. Evaluation of ICA512As in combination with other islet cell autoantibodies at the onset of IDDM. Diabetes Care 1997;20:1403–7.
[23] Baekkeskov S, Aanstoot HJ, Christgau S, et al. Identification of the 64K autoantigen in insulin-dependent diabetes as the GABA-synthesizing enzyme glutamic acid decarboxylase. Nature 1990;347:151–6.
[24] Padoa CJ, Banga JP, Madec AM, et al. Recombinant Fabs of human monoclonal antibodies specific to the middle epitope of GAD65 inhibit type 1 diabetes-specific GAD65Abs. Diabetes 2003;52:2689–95.
[25] Schwartz HL, Chandonia JM, Kash SF, et al. High-resolution autoreactive epitope mapping and structural modeling of the 65 kDa form of human glutamic acid decarboxylase. J Mol Biol 1999;287:983–99.
[26] Kawasaki E, Yu L, Rewers MJ, et al. Definition of multiple ICA512/phogrin autoantibody epitopes and detection of intramolecular epitope spreading in relatives of patients with type 1 diabetes. Diabetes 1998;47:733–42.
[27] Farilla L, Tiberti C, Luzzago A, et al. Application of phage display peptide library to autoimmune diabetes: identification of IA-2/ICA512bdc dominant autoantigenic epitopes. Eur J Immunol 2002;32:1420–7.
[28] Casu A, Becker DJ, Pietropaolo S, et al. Humoral autoimmunity to IA-2 intracellular domain epitopes increases the cumulative risk of type 1 diabetes (T1D) progression [abstract]. Diabetes 2005;OR121.
[29] Pietropaolo M, Castano L, Babu S, et al. Islet cell autoantigen 69 kD (ICA69)L: molecular cloning and characterization of a novel diabetes-associated autoantigen. J Clin Invest 1993;92:359–71.

[30] Horvath L, Cervenak L, Oroszlan M, et al. Antibodies against different epitopes of heat-shock protein 60 in children with type 1 diabetes mellitus. Immunol Lett 2002;80:155–62.

[31] Lieberman SM, DiLorenzo TP. A comprehensive guide to antibody and T-cell responses in type 1 diabetes. Tissue Antigens 2003;62:359–77.

[32] Kostraba JN, Gay EC, Cai Y, et al. Incidence of insulin-dependent diabetes mellitus in Colorado. Epidemiology 1992;3:232–8.

[33] Barmeier H, McCulloch DK, Neifing JL, et al. Risk for developing type 1 (insulin-dependent) diabetes mellitus and the presence of islet 64K antibodies. Diabetologia 1991;34:727–33.

[34] Riley WJ, Maclaren NK, Krischer J, et al. A prospective study of the development of diabetes in relatives of patients with insulin-dependent diabetes. N Engl J Med 1990;323:1167–72.

[35] Maclaren NK. How, when, and why to predict IDDM. Diabetes 1988;37:1591–4.

[36] LaPorte RE, Drash AL, Wagener D, et al. The Pittsburgh Insulin-Dependent Diabetes Mellitus (IDDM) Registries: the descriptive epidemiology of racial differences. In: Mimura G, et al, editors. Clinico-genetic genesis of diabetes mellitus. International Congress Series. Amsterdam, The Netherlands: Excerpta Medica; 1982. p. 66–77.

[37] Strebelow M, Schlosser M, Ziegler B, et al. Karlsburg type I diabetes risk study of a general population: frequencies and interactions of the four major type I diabetes-associated auto-antibodies studied in 9419 schoolchildren. Diabetologia 1999;42:661–70.

[38] LaGasse JM, Brantley MS, Leech NJ, et al. Successful prospective prediction of type 1 diabetes in schoolchildren through multiple defined autoantibodies: an 8-year follow-up of the Washington State Diabetes Prediction Study. Diabetes Care 2002;25:505–11.

[39] Kulmala P, Rahko J, Savola K, et al. Beta-cell autoimmunity, genetic susceptibility, and progression to type 1 diabetes in unaffected schoolchildren. Diabetes Care 2001;24:171–3.

[40] Schatz D, Krischer J, Horne G, et al. Islet cell antibodies predict insulin-dependent diabetes in United States school age children as powerfully as in unaffected relatives. J Clin Invest 1994; 93:2403–7.

[41] Maclaren N, Lan M, Coutant R, et al. Only multiple autoantibodies to islet cells (ICA), insulin, GAD65, IA-2 and IA-2beta predict immune-mediated (type 1) diabetes in relatives. J Auto-immun 1999;12:279–87.

[42] Hummel M, Bonifacio E, Schmid S, et al. Brief communication: early appearance of islet autoantibodies predicts childhood type 1 diabetes in offspring of diabetic parents. Ann Intern Med 2004;140:882–6.

[43] Bonifacio E, Hummel M, Walter M, et al. IDDM1 and multiple family history of type 1 diabetes combine to identify neonates at high risk for type 1 diabetes. Diabetes Care 2004;27:2695–700.

[44] Verge CF, Stenger D, Bonifacio E, et al. Combined use of autoantibodies (IA-2 autoantibody, GAD autoantibody, insulin autoantibody, cytoplasmic islet cell antibodies) in type 1 diabetes: Combinatorial Islet Autoantibody Workshop. Diabetes 1998;47:1857–66.

[45] Kulmala P, Savola K, Petersen JS, et al. Prediction of insulin-dependent diabetes mellitus in siblings of children with diabetes: a population-based study. The Childhood Diabetes in Finland Study Group. J Clin Invest 1998;101:327–36.

[46] Achenbach P, Warncke K, Reiter J, et al. Stratification of type 1 diabetes risk on the basis of islet autoantibody characteristics. Diabetes 2004;53:384–92.

[47] Dorman JS, McCarthy BJ, O'Leary AL, et al. Risk factors for insulin-dependent diabetes. NIH Publication No. 95–1468. 1995.

[48] LaPorte RE, Matsushima M, Chang Y-F. Prevalence and incidence of insulin-dependent diabetes. NIH Publication No. 95–1468. 1995.

[49] Pietropaolo M, Becker DJ. Type 1 diabetes intervention trials. Pediatr Diabetes 2001;2:2–11.

[50] Harrison LC. Risk assessment, prediction and prevention of type 1 diabetes. Pediatr Diabetes 2001;2:71–82.

[51] Pietropaolo M, Trucco M. Major histocompatibility locus and other genes that determine the risk for development of type 1 diabetes mellitus. In: Le Roith DT, Olefsky JM, editors. Diabetes mellitus. A fundamental and clinical text. 3rd edition. Philadelphia: Lippincott Williams and Wilkins; 2004.

[52] Noble JA, Valdes AM, Cook M, et al. The role of HLA class II genes in insulin-dependent diabetes mellitus: molecular analysis of 180 caucasian, multiplex families. Am J Hum Genet 1996;59:1134–48.

[53] Rewers M, Bugawan TL, Norris JM, et al. Newborn screening for HLA markers associated with IDDM: diabetes autoimmunity study in the young (DAISY). Diabetologia 1996;39:807–12.

[54] Todd JA, Farrall M. Panning for gold: genome-wide scanning for linkage in type 1 diabetes. Hum Mol Genet 1996;5(Spec No):1443–8.

[55] Wolf E, Spencer KM, Cudworth AG. The genetic susceptibility to type 1 (insulin-dependent) diabetes: analysis of the HLA-DR association. Diabetologia 1983;24:224–30.

[56] Morel PA, Dorman JS, Todd JA, et al. Aspartic acid at position 57 of the HLA-DQ beta chain protects against type I diabetes: a family study. Proc Natl Acad Sci U S A 1988;85: 8111–5.

[57] McDevitt H. Closing in on type 1 diabetes. N Engl J Med 2001;345:1060–1.

[58] Pietropaolo M, Becker DJ, LaPorte RE, et al. Progression to insulin-requiring diabetes in seronegative prediabetic subjects: the role of two HLA-DQ high-risk haplotypes. Diabetologia 2002;45:66–76.

[59] Cornell CN. Absence of islet autoantibodies at diabetes onset does not rule out type 1A diabetes. Diabetes 2000;49(Suppl 1):A69.

[60] Lipton RB, Kocova M, LaPorte RE, et al. Autoimmunity and genetics contribute to the risk of insulin-dependent diabetes mellitus in families: islet cell antibodies and HLA DQ heterodimers. Am J Epidemiol 1992;136:503–12.

[61] Hahl J, Simell T, Ilonen J, et al. Costs of predicting IDDM. Diabetologia 1998;41:79–85.

[62] Dahlquist G. Potentials and pitfalls in neonatal screening for type 1 diabetes. Acta Paediatr Suppl 1999;88:80–2.

[63] Greenbaum CJ, Sears KL, Kahn SE, et al. Relationship of beta-cell function and autoantibodies to progression and nonprogression of subclinical type 1 diabetes: follow-up of the Seattle Family Study. Diabetes 1999;48:170–5.

[64] Becker DJ, Cakan N, Laporte RE, et al. High risk DQ alleles improve IDDM prediction in ICA + ve first-degree relatives with decreased insulin secretion [abstract]. Diabetologia 1995; 38(Suppl 1):A42.

[65] Pietropaolo M, Trucco M, Cakan N, et al. Autoantibodies to GAD65 and ICA512/IA-2 improve IDDM prediction in first-degree relatives with decreased first phase insulin response and ICA positivity [abstract]. Autoimmunity 1996;24(Suppl 1):51.

[66] Eisenbarth GS, Gianani R, Yu L, et al. Dual-parameter model for prediction of type I diabetes mellitus. Proc Assoc Am Physicians 1998;110:126–35.

[67] Colman PG, McNair P, Margetts H, et al. The Melbourne Pre-Diabetes Study: prediction of type 1 diabetes mellitus using antibody and metabolic testing. Med J Aust 1998;169:81–4.

[68] Vardi P, Crisa L, Jackson RA. Predictive value of intravenous glucose tolerance test insulin secretion less than or greater than the first percentile in islet cell antibody positive relatives of type 1 (insulin-dependent) diabetic patients. Diabetologia 1991;34:93–102.

[69] Bingley PJ, Bonifacio E, Ziegler AG, et al. Proposed guidelines on screening for risk of type 1 diabetes. Diabetes Care 2001;24:398.

[70] Group TDC. Effect of intensive therapy on residual beta-cell function in patients with type 1 diabetes in the diabetes control and complications trial: a randomized, controlled trial. Ann Intern Med 1998;128:517–23.

[71] Group TDR. Effects of age, duration and treatment of insulin-dependent diabetes mellitus on residual beta-cell function: observations during eligibility testing for the Diabetes Control and Complications Trial (DCCT). J Clin Endocrinol Metab 1987;65:30–6.

[72] Rosenbloom AL, Schatz DA, Krischer JP, et al. Therapeutic controversy: prevention and treatment of diabetes in children. J Clin Endocrinol Metab 2000;85:494–522.

[73] Bougneres PF, Landais P, Boisson C, et al. Limited duration of remission of insulin dependency in children with recent overt type I diabetes treated with low-dose cyclosporin. Diabetes 1990;39:1264–72.

[74] Group TC-ERCT. Cyclosporin-induced remission of IDDM after early intervention: association of 1 yr of cyclosporin treatment with enhanced insulin secretion. Diabetes 1988;37: 1574–82.

[75] Cook JJ, Hudson I, Harrison LC, et al. Double-blind controlled trial of azathioprine in children with newly diagnosed type I diabetes. Diabetes 1989;38:779–83.

[76] Harrison LC, Colman PG, Dean B, et al. Increase in remission rate in newly diagnosed type I diabetic subjects treated with azathioprine. Diabetes 1985;34:1306–8.

[77] Silverstein J, Maclaren N, Riley W, et al. Immunosuppression with azathioprine and prednisone in recent-onset insulin-dependent diabetes mellitus. N Engl J Med 1988;319:599–604.

[78] Akerblom HK, Knip M. Putative environmental factors in type 1 diabetes. Diabetes Metab Rev 1998;14:31–67.

[79] Akerblom HK, Vaarala O, Hyoty H, et al. Environmental factors in the etiology of type 1 diabetes. Am J Med Genet 2002;115:18–29.

[80] Gerstein HC. Cow's milk exposure and type I diabetes mellitus: a critical overview of the clinical literature. Diabetes Care 1994;17:13–9.

[81] Elliott RB, Martin JM. Dietary protein: a trigger of insulin-dependent diabetes in the BB rat? Diabetologia 1984;26:297–9.

[82] Elliott RB, Reddy SN, Bibby NJ, et al. Dietary prevention of diabetes in the non-obese diabetic mouse. Diabetologia 1988;31:62–4.

[83] Akerblom HK, Virtanen SM, Ilonen J, et al. Dietary manipulation of beta cell autoimmunity in infants at increased risk of type 1 diabetes: a pilot study. Diabetologia 2005;48:829–37.

[84] Group ENDIT. Intervening before the onset of type 1 diabetes: baseline data from the European Nicotinamide Diabetes Intervention Trial (ENDIT). Diabetologia 2003;46:339–46.

[85] Gale EA, Bingley PJ, Emmett CL, et al. European Nicotinamide Diabetes Intervention Trial (ENDIT): a randomised controlled trial of intervention before the onset of type 1 diabetes. Lancet 2004;363:925–31.

[86] Atkinson MA, Leiter EH. The NOD mouse model of type 1 diabetes: as good as it gets? Nat Med 1999;5:601–4.

[87] Elliott RB, Pilcher CC, Fergusson DM, et al. A population based strategy to prevent insulin-dependent diabetes using nicotinamide. J Pediatr Endocrinol Metab 1996;9:501–9.

[88] Zhang ZJ, Davidson L, Eisenbarth G, et al. Suppression of diabetes in nonobese diabetic mice by oral administration of porcine insulin. Proc Natl Acad Sci U S A 1991;88:10252–6.

[89] Muir A, Schatz D, Maclaren N. Antigen-specific immunotherapy: oral tolerance and subcutaneous immunization in the treatment of insulin-dependent diabetes. Diabetes Metab Rev 1993;9:279–87.

[90] Gottlieb PA, Handler ES, Appel MC, et al. Insulin treatment prevents diabetes mellitus but not thyroiditis in RT6-depleted diabetes resistant BB/Wor rats. Diabetologia 1991;34:296–300.

[91] Keller RJ, Eisenbarth GS, Jackson RA. Insulin prophylaxis in individuals at high risk of type I diabetes. Lancet 1993;341:927–8.

[92] Group DPTTDS. Effects of insulin in relatives of patients with type 1 diabetes mellitus. N Engl J Med 2002;346:1685–91.

[93] Pugliese A, Zeller M, Fernandez Jr A, et al. The insulin gene is transcribed in the human thymus and transcription levels correlated with allelic variation at the INS VNTR-IDDM2 susceptibility locus for type 1 diabetes. Nat Genet 1997;15:293–7.

[94] Vafiadis P, Bennett ST, Todd JA, et al. Insulin expression in human thymus is modulated by INS VNTR alleles at the IDDM2 locus. Nat Genet 1997;15:289–92.

[95] Sospedra M, Ferrer-Francesch X, Dominguez O, et al. Transcription of a broad range of self-antigens in human thymus suggests a role for central mechanisms in tolerance toward peripheral antigens. J Immunol 1998;161:5918–29.

[96] Pietropaolo M, Giannoukakis N, Trucco M. Cellular environment and freedom of gene expression. Nat Immunol 2002;3:335 [author reply: 336].

[97] Pugliese A, Brown D, Garza D, et al. Self-antigen-presenting cells expressing diabetes-associated autoantigens exist in both thymus and peripheral lymphoid organs. J Clin Invest 2001;107:555–64.

[98] Jaeckel E, Lipes MA, von Boehmer H. Recessive tolerance to preproinsulin 2 reduces but does not abolish type 1 diabetes. Nat Immunol 2004;5:1028–35.
[99] Skyler J, Krischer J, Wolfsdorf J, et al. Effects of oral insulin in relatives of patients with type 1 diabetes: the Diabetes Prevention Trial-Type 1. Diabetes Care 2005;28:1068–76.
[100] Alleva DG, Gaur A, Jin L, et al. Immunological characterization and therapeutic activity of an altered-peptide ligand, NBI-6024, based on the immunodominant type 1 diabetes autoantigen insulin B-chain (9–23) peptide. Diabetes 2002;51:2126–34.
[101] Palmer JP, Fleming GA, Greenbaum CJ, et al. C-peptide is the appropriate outcome measure for type 1 diabetes clinical trials to preserve beta-cell function: report of an ADA workshop, 21–22 October 2001. Diabetes 2004;53:250–64.
[102] Greenbaum CJ, Harrison LC. Guidelines for intervention trials in subjects with newly diagnosed type 1 diabetes. Diabetes 2003;52:1059–65.
[103] Chatenoud L, Primo J, Bach JF. CD3 antibody-induced dominant self tolerance in overtly diabetic NOD mice. J Immunol 1997;158:2947–54.
[104] Chatenoud L, Thervet E, Primo J, et al. Anti-CD3 antibody induces long-term remission of overt autoimmunity in nonobese diabetic mice. Proc Natl Acad Sci U S A 1994;91:123–7.
[105] Hao L, Chan SM, Lafferty KJ. Mycophenolate mofetil can prevent the development of diabetes in BB rats. Ann N Y Acad Sci 1993;696:328–32.
[106] TrialNet. MMF/DZB study. Available at: http://www.diabetestrialnet.org/en/public/ommf.html. Accessed May 12, 2005.
[107] Gitelman SE. Immune Tolerance Network. Trial of Thymoglobulin for treatment of new onset type 1 diabetes mellitus. Available at: http://www.immunetolerance.org/research/autoimmune/trials/gitelman.html. Accessed May 10, 2005.
[108] Raz I, Elias D, Avron A, et al. Beta-cell function in new-onset type 1 diabetes and immuno-modulation with a heat-shock protein peptide (DiaPep277): a randomised, double-blind, phase II trial. Lancet 2001;358:1749–53.
[109] Bach JF. Immunotherapy of insulin-dependent diabetes mellitus. Curr Opin Immunol 2001;13:601–5.
[110] Woodle ES, Xu D, Zivin RA, et al. Phase I trial of a humanized, Fc receptor nonbinding OKT3 antibody, huOKT3gamma1(Ala-Ala) in the treatment of acute renal allograft rejection. Transplantation 1999;68:608–16.
[111] Utset TO, Auger JA, Peace D, et al. Modified anti-CD3 therapy in psoriatic arthritis: a phase I/II clinical trial. J Rheumatol 2002;29:1907–13.
[112] Herold KC, Hagopian W, Auger JA, et al. Anti-CD3 monoclonal antibody in new-onset type 1 diabetes mellitus. N Engl J Med 2002;346:1692–8.
[113] Kukreja A, Cost G, Marker J, et al. Multiple immuno-regulatory defects in type-1 diabetes. J Clin Invest 2002;109:131–40.
[114] Taylor PA, Noelle RJ, Blazar BR. CD4(+)CD25(+) immune regulatory cells are required for induction of tolerance to alloantigen via costimulatory blockade. J Exp Med 2001;193:1311–8.
[115] Edwards JC, Szczepanski L, Szechinski J, et al. Efficacy of B-cell-targeted therapy with rituximab in patients with rheumatoid arthritis. N Engl J Med 2004;350:2572–81.
[116] Bottino R, Trucco M, Balamurugan AN, et al. Pancreas and islet cell transplantation. Best Pract Res Clin Gastroenterol 2002;16:457–74.
[117] Bottino R, Balamurugan AN, Giannoukakis N, et al. Islet/pancreas transplantation: challenges for pediatrics. Pediatr Diabetes 2002;3:210–23.
[118] Shapiro AM, Lakey JR, Ryan EA, et al. Islet transplantation in seven patients with type 1 diabetes mellitus using a glucocorticoid-free immunosuppressive regimen. N Engl J Med 2000;343:230–8.
[119] Ryan EA, Lakey JR, Paty BW, et al. Successful islet transplantation: continued insulin reserve provides long-term glycemic control. Diabetes 2002;51:2148–57.
[120] Trucco M. Regeneration of the pancreatic beta cell. J Clin Invest 2005;115:5–12.
[121] Trucco M. Stem cells and diabetes. Pediatr Diabetes 2004;5(Suppl 2):2–4.
[122] Bonner-Weir S, Sharma A. Pancreatic stem cells. J Pathol 2002;197:519–26.

[123] Dor Y, Brown J, Martinez OI, et al. Adult pancreatic beta-cells are formed by self-duplication rather than stem-cell differentiation. Nature 2004;429:41–6.

[124] Seaberg RM, Smukler SR, Kieffer TJ, et al. Clonal identification of multipotent precursors from adult mouse pancreas that generate neural and pancreatic lineages. Nat Biotechnol 2004;22: 1115–24.

[125] Ferber S, Halkin A, Cohen H, et al. Pancreatic and duodenal homeobox gene 1 induces expression of insulin genes in liver and ameliorates streptozotocin-induced hyperglycemia. Nat Med 2000;6:568–72.

[126] Dai Y, Vaught TD, Boone J, et al. Targeted disruption of the alpha1,3-galactosyltransferase gene in cloned pigs. Nat Biotechnol 2002;20:251–5.

[127] Koike C, Friday RP, Nakashima I, et al. Isolation of the regulatory regions and genomic organization of the porcine alpha1,3-galactosyltransferase gene. Transplantation 2000;70: 1275–83.

[128] Koike C, Fung JJ, Geller DA, et al. Molecular basis of evolutionary loss of the alpha 1,3-galactosyltransferase gene in higher primates. J Biol Chem 2002;277:10114–20.

[129] Phelps CJ, Koike C, Vaught TD, et al. Production of alpha 1,3-galactosyltransferase-deficient pigs. Science 2003;299:411–4.

[130] Tzakis AG, Ricordi C, Alejandro R, et al. Pancreatic islet transplantation after upper abdominal exenteration and liver replacement. Lancet 1990;336:402–5.

[131] Zorina TD, Subbotin VM, Bertera S, et al. Distinct characteristics and features of allogeneic chimerism in the NOD mouse model of autoimmune diabetes. Cell Transplant 2002;11: 113–23.

[132] Zorina TD, Subbotin VM, Bertera S, et al. Recovery of the endogenous beta cell function in the NOD model of autoimmune diabetes. Stem Cells 2003;21:377–88.

ELSEVIER
SAUNDERS

PEDIATRIC CLINICS
OF NORTH AMERICA

Pediatr Clin N Am 52 (2005) 1805–1872

Cumulative Index 2005

Note: Page numbers of article titles are in **boldface** type.

Anorexia nervosa. *See* Eating disorders
(anorexia nervosa and bulimia nervosa).

Anovulation
bleeding in, 182
in polycystic ovary syndrome, 184–186

Anterior cruciate ligament, injury of, in college
athletes, 45–46

Anterior drawer test, for ankle injury, 42

Antiarrhythmic drugs, sudden cardiac death
due to, 1381, 1385

Antibiotics. *See also specific drugs.*
autistic symptoms attributed to,
1471–1472
selection of, **869–894**
adverse reactions and, 892
for arthritis, 879
for central nervous system
infections, 889–890
for endocarditis, 885–886
for gastrointestinal infections,
886–888
for oropharyngeal infections,
881–882
for osteomyelitis, 878–879
for otitis media, 880–881
for respiratory infections, 882–885
for sinusitis, 881
for skin and soft tissue infections,
876–878
for urinary tract infections,
888–889
host factors in, 892
microbiology and, 870–872
Monte Carlo simulation in,
875, 892
pharmacodynamics and, 872–873
pharmacokinetics and, 873–875

Anticardiolipin antibodies
in antiphospholipid antibody syndrome,
469, 471–472, 485
in juvenile localized scleroderma, 536
in systemic lupus erythematosus,
462–463

Anticholinergic effects, of tricyclic antidepressants, 120

Anticoagulants, for antiphospholipid antibody
syndrome, 486–488

Anticonvulsants, for neuropathic pain, 1018

Antidepressants
for attention-deficit/hyperactivity
disorder, 75–77
for depression
discontinuation of, 127–128
indications for, 115–117

monoamine oxidase inhibitors, 116,
118, 121, 125–127
selection of, 117
selective serotonin reuptake
inhibitors, 116–118,
121–124
tricyclic, 115, 118–121
types of, 115–117
for eating disorders, 94
for fibromyalgia, 625–626
for juvenile idiopathic arthritis, 631
for neuropathic pain, 1018
for obsessive-compulsive disorder, 108
for panic disorder, 107

Antifungal agents, **895–915**
azoles, 897, 900–905
doses for, 897
echinocandins, 897, 906–908
polyenes, 896–899
pyrimidine analogues, 897, 899–900
spectrum of activity of, 896

Antigenic drift and antigenic shift, in influenza
virus, 699

Antigen-presenting cells, in juvenile idiopathic
arthritis, 343

Antihistamines, for pruritus, 1009

Antihypertensive drugs, amenorrhea due
to, 191

Antimonial drugs, for leishmaniasis, 922–923,
926–927

Anti-neutrophil cytoplasmic antibodies
in Churg–Strauss syndrome, 568–569
in microscopic polyangiitis, 568
in Wegener's granulomatosis, 566–568

Antinuclear antibodies
in juvenile localized scleroderma, 536
in juvenile systemic sclerosis, 528
in systemic lupus erythematosus,
462–463

Antiparasitic therapy, **917–948**
for *Acanthamoeba* infections, 936
for amebiasis, 923, 927–928
for babesiosis, 931, 933–934
for blood and tissue nematodes, 938,
940–941
for cestodes, 938, 941–942
for cryptosporidiosis, 929–930, 933
for *Cyclospora* infections, 930, 933
for giardiasis, 928–930
for intestinal nematodes, 937–938, 940
for isosporosis, 930, 933
for leishmaniasis, 922–923, 926–927
for malaria, 918–921, 924
for microsporidiosis, 936
for *Naegleria fowleri* infections, 932, 936

Blood culture
in central venous catheter infections,
1193–1195
in osteomyelitis, 1086
in pneumonia, 1064
in septic arthritis, 1093–1094

Blood glucose monitoring.
See Glucose monitoring.

Blood group incompatibility, diabetes mellitus
and, 1562

Blood-brain barrier, encephalitis and, 1107–1108

Blood-doping, in college athletes, 38

Body maps, in pain assessment, 614, 616

Body outline figures, in pain assessment, 614

Bohan and Peter criteria, for inflammatory
myopathies, 500–501

Bone
culture of, in osteomyelitis, 783–784
infections of. See Osteomyelitis.
postoperative healing of, analgesics
and, 1000

Bone marrow transplantation, mucositis in, 1014

Bone scan
in osteomyelitis, 784, 1087
in septic arthritis, 1094

Borreliosis
pyogenic arthritis in, 788
scleroderma in, 532
treatment of, 891
versus juvenile idiopathic arthritis,
429–430

Brachydactyly, in juvenile idiopathic
arthritis, 424

Bradykinin, in juvenile idiopathic arthritis,
340–341

Brain
abscess of, 804, 889
aneurysms of, in polyarteritis nodosa,
399–400
edema of, in diabetic ketoacidosis,
1158–1160, 1625–1627
hypoglycemia effects on, 1710,
1713–1720
injury of, in college athletes, 32–37
lesions of
in inflammatory myopathies,
508–509
in NOMID/CINCA syndrome,
599–600
in systemic lupus erythematosus,
392–393, 450–455
in Wegener's granulomatosis, 401

primary angiitis of, 566
thrombosis in, in antiphospholipid
antibody syndrome, 476–477

Brainstem, inflammation of, 1110

Breastfeeding, for diabetes mellitus protection,
1561–1562, 1788

Brodie abscess, 1090

Bronchiolitis, **1047–1057**
clinical presentation of, 1050–1051
complications of, 1052–1053
definition of, 1047
differential diagnosis of, 1051
epidemiology of, 1047–1048
etiology of, 1048
hospitalization rate in, 1048
human metapneumovirus, 704–705
mortality in, 1052
parainfluenza virus, 705–706
pathogenesis of, 1048–1050
prevention of, 1053–1054
respiratory syncytial virus, 696–698
treatment of, 1051–1052

Bronchoconstriction, in asthma, 14

Bronchodilators
for asthma, 15–16
for bronchiolitis, 1051

Bronchoscopy, in pneumonia, 1068

Brudzinski sign, in meningitis, 797

Brugada syndrome, 1290–1291
arrhythmogenic right ventricular
dysplasia/cardiomyopathy and,
1240–1241
clinical features of, 1297–1298
electrocardiography in,
1358–1359, 1363
electrophysiology studies in,
1368–1370
genetics of, 1298
heart rate variability measurement
in, 1365
implantable cardioverter-defibrillator
for, 1299
in college students, 258
sudden cardiac death in, 1226, 1383
T-wave alternans in, 1367

Brugia malayi infections, 939–941

Brugia timori infections, 939–941

Bulimia nervosa. See Eating disorders
(anorexia nervosa and bulimia nervosa).

Bullous morphea, 533

Bundle branch block, in Brugada
syndrome, 1237

for antiphospholipid antibody
syndrome, 486
for asthma, 15–16
for bronchiolitis, 1051–1052
for infectious mononucleosis, 12
for inflammatory myopathies, 512–513
for juvenile idiopathic arthritis, 421,
424–425, 432, 631
for juvenile systemic sclerosis, 528
for Kawasaki disease, 561
for PFAPA syndrome, 591–592
for systemic lupus erythematosus,
458–459

Cortisol, elevated, in diabetic
ketoacidosis, 1613

Corynebacterium diphtheriae infections,
pharyngitis in, 730, 734

Cough
in asthma, 14
in bronchiolitis, 1050

Counseling, in diabetes mellitus, 1772

Cow's milk, early exposure to, diabetes
mellitus and, 1561–1562, 1786, 1788

Coxsackievirus infections, arrhythmogenic
right ventricular dysplasia in, 1240

Cranberry juice, for urinary tract infection
prevention, 22

Cranial neuropathy
in juvenile systemic sclerosis, 527
in systemic lupus erythematosus, 454
in viral encephalitis, 1110

Craniosacral therapy, for international
adoptees, 1473

C-reactive protein
in osteomyelitis, 783, 1086
in pneumonia, 1064

Creatine supplements, college athletes using, 40

Croup, parainfluenza virus, 705–706

Cruciate ligaments, anterior, injury of, in
college athletes, 45–46

Cryopyrin proteins, defects of
in CIAS1 (cold-induced autoinflamma-
tory syndrome), 598–599
in periodic fever syndromes, 578–579

Cryotherapy, for anogenital warts, 201

Cryptosporidiosis, 929–930, 933

Cultural issues
in eating disorders, 88
in international adoption, 1232–1235,
1435, 1496–1501

Culture
blood
in central venous catheter
infections, 1193–1195
in osteomyelitis, 1086
in pneumonia, 1064
in septic arthritis, 1093–1094
bone, in osteomyelitis, 783–784
cerebrospinal fluid, in meningitis, 798
sputum, in pneumonia, 1064–1065
stool, in *Campylobacter* infections,
766–767
synovial fluid, in septic arthritis,
790, 1093
throat, in pharyngitis, 735–736, 744

Cutaneous larva migrans (hookworms),
937–938

Cyanosis, in apnea, 1129, 1132

Cyclic neutropenia, fever in, 824–825,
827–829

Cyclooxygenase 2 inhibitors
for juvenile idiopathic arthritis, 431–432
for pain, 997, 1000–1001

Cyclophosphamide
for antiphospholipid antibody syndrome,
486–487
for Henoch-Schönlein purpura, 555
for inflammatory myopathies, 514
for juvenile systemic sclerosis, 529
for polyarteritis nodosa, 565
for systemic lupus erythematosus,
458–459

Cyclospora infections, 930, 933

Cyclosporine
for diabetes mellitus prevention,
1786–1787
for inflammatory myopathies, 514

Cystic fibrosis, diabetes mellitus in, 1548,
1645–1646

Cystic fibrosis transmembrane conductance
regulator, in *Escherichia coli* infections,
755–756

Cysticercosis, 939, 941–942

Cystitis, 20–22, 888

Cytokines. *See also specific cytokines.*
in diabetic ketoacidosis, 1619
in juvenile systemic sclerosis, 523–524
in meningitis, 797

Cytolethal distending toxin, in *Campylobacter*
infections, 766

Cytomegalovirus infections, 838–848
in international adoptees, 1281, 1304

meningococcal *(Neisseria meningitidis),*
    230–232, 235, 680–681, 805
pertussis, 681–682
pneumococcal, 294, 679, 711–713, 805
policy for, 671–674
program for, challenges to, 674–677
public health impact of, 669–670
respiratory syncytial virus, 1053–1054
rotavirus, 683–684
safety of, 675–677
schedule for, 670–671
shortages of, 674–675
Streptococcus pneumoniae, 294, 679,
    711–713, 805
subsidization of, 673–674
varicella, 236, 684
websites on, 671

Immunodeficiency, pneumonia in, 1073–1074

Immunodysregulation, polyendocrinopathy,
    enteropathy, and X-linked disorders,
    diabetes mellitus in, 1643

Immunoglobulin, intravenous
    for acute disseminated
        encephalomyelitis, 1122
    for inflammatory myopathies, 513–514
    for Kawasaki disease, 560–562

Immunoglobulin D, elevated, in hyper-IgD
    syndrome, 596–598

Immunotherapy, for respiratory syncytial virus
    infections, 697–698

Impetigo, 876

Implantable cardioverter-defibrillators,
    1289–1303
    complications of, 1295–1298
    components of, 1292
    development of, 1291–1293
    experience with, 1293–1295
    for channelopathies, 1299–1301
    for hypertrophic cardiomyopathy,
        1332–1334, 1391–1392
    growth considerations in, 1390–1391
    implantation of, 1390–1391
    indications for, 1293, 1299, 1390–1392
    psychological impact of, 1299–1300
    pulse generator replacement in,
        1292–1293

Incretins, in insulin regulation, 1537

Indinavir, for HIV infection, 857

Individual with Disabilities Act, applied to
    international adoptees, 1428

Individualized education plan, for international
    adoptees, 1430–1431, 1456–1457

Indomethacin, for juvenile idiopathic
    arthritis, 431

Infanticide, apparent life-threatening event
    and, 1136

Infection(s). *See also specific infections.*
    bacterial, antibiotics for. *See* Antibiotics.
    bone and joint, **779–794,** 879
    central nervous system, 889–890
    central venous catheter, 1177
        in medically complex children,
            1189–1199
    control of, for pneumonia
        prevention, 1075
    fungal, antifungal agents for, **895–915**
    gastrointestinal, **749–777,** 886–888
    heart (endocarditis), 816, 885–886
    Henoch-Schönlein purpura in, 553
    immunizations for. *See* Immunizations.
    in diabetes mellitus development, 1560
    in international adoption
        cytomegalovirus, 1281, 1304
        gastrointestinal, 1301–1302
        hepatitis B, 1296, 1298–1300
        hepatitis C, 1296, 1303–1304
        human immunodeficiency virus
            infection, 1296, 1303
        in family, **1271–1286**
        immunizations for,
            1273–1275,
            1280–1281
        malaria, 1275–1276
        travel preparation in,
            1272–1273
        traveler's diarrhea, 1276–1277
    parasitic, 1296, 1300–1301
    screening for, 1295–1305
    syphilis, 1296, 1302–1303
    tuberculosis, 1295–1298
    inflammatory myopathies in, 498–499
    Kawasaki disease and, 556–557
    meningitis, **795–810**
    oropharyngeal, 881–882
    otitis media, **711–728**
    parasitic, **917–948**
    periodic fever syndromes in, **811–835**
    pharyngitis, **729–747,** 882
    respiratory. *See* Respiratory infections.
    skin and soft tissue, 876–878
    urinary tract, 20–22, 888–889, 1053
    vasculitis in, 569–570
    viral. *See* Antiviral agents; Viral infections.

Infectious mononucleosis
    in college students, 9–13
    pharyngitis in, 734

Infective endocarditis, in college students,
    263–264

Infertility
    in juvenile idiopathic arthritis, 348–349
    in polycystic ovary syndrome, 184–186

Tetralogy of Fallot
corrected
electrocardiography in, 1360–1361
electrophysiology studies in, 1370
sudden cardiac death after, 1395,
1397, 1411–1412
exercise recommendations in,
1411–1412
in college students, 255
sudden cardiac death in, 1266–1267

Thermography, in juvenile localized
scleroderma, 537

Thiabendazole, for intestinal nematodes,
937–938

Thiazolidinediones, for diabetes mellitus,
1597, 1692–1694

Throat, infections of. See Pharyngitis.

Throat culture, in pharyngitis, 735–736, 744

Thrombocytopenia
in antiphospholipid antibody syndrome,
479, 488
in systemic lupus erythematosus,
459–460

Thrombophilia. See also Antiphospholipid
antibody syndrome.
differential diagnosis of, 480

Thrombosis
from oral contraceptives, 144
in antiphospholipid antibody syndrome,
469–470, 476–480, 486–487
in diabetic ketoacidosis, 1625
in systemic lupus erythematosus,
452–453, 460
of central venous catheters,
1176–1177

Thyroid disorders
in systemic lupus erythematosus, 462
menstrual disorders in, 187

Ticarcillin
for osteomyelitis, 879
for skin and soft tissue infections, 876

Ticarcillin-clavulanate, for skin and soft tissue
infections, 876

Tinidazole, for giardiasis, 928–930

TNFRSF1A gene mutations, in tumor necrosis
factor receptor–associated periodic
syndrome, 593, 595

TNN3 gene mutations, in hypertrophic
cardiomyopathy, 1244

TNNT2 gene mutations, in hypertrophic
cardiomyopathy, 1244–1245

Tobacco
college student use of, 37, 293–294,
310–313
prenatal exposure to, 1380–1382

Tobramycin
for meningitis, 801
for osteomyelitis, 879

Today contraceptive sponge, 151

TODAY (Treatment Options for T2DM
in Adolescents and Youth) study,
1700, 1769

Todd's paralysis, in hypoglycemia, 1713

Toilet training, of international adoptees, 1319,
1339–1340

Tolbutamide, for diabetes mellitus, 1692, 1695

Tolmetin, for juvenile idiopathic arthritis, 431

Tongue, strawberry, in Kawasaki disease, 557

Tonsillectomy
analgesia after, 999–1000
for periodic fever, aphthous stomatitis,
pharyngitis and cervical
adenopathy, 592, 827

Toxins
in Campylobacter infections, 765–766
in Escherichia coli infections,
754–755

Toxocara cani infections, 939, 941

Toxocariasis, in international adoptees, 1301

Toxoplasmosis, 931, 934

TPM1 gene mutations, in hypertrophic
cardiomyopathy, 1244

Tracheitis, 882

Tracheostomy, in medically complex children,
1175–1176

Transdermal hormonal contraception,
145–146

Transdisciplinary coordination, in care of
medically complex children, 1169–1171

Transient ischemic attack, in antiphospholipid
antibody syndrome, 476–477

Transient synovitis, radiology in, 386

Transition programs, for college-bound
students with learning disabilities,
62–64, 66

Translators, for international adoptees, 1333,
1458–1459

Vaginal ring, for contraception, 148–149

Valacyclovir
for herpes simplex virus infections, 223–224
for herpesvirus infections, 842–843

Valganciclovir, for herpesvirus infections, 845–846

Valgus stress test, for medial collateral ligament sprain, 47

Valproate, for migraine, 20

Valvular heart disease, in antiphospholipid antibody syndrome, 478

Vancomycin
for central nervous system infections, 890
for endocarditis, 885
for gastrointestinal infections, 886, 888
for meningitis, 800–801
for osteomyelitis, 878, 1088
for otitis media, 722
for pneumonia, 1067
for pyogenic arthritis, 792, 879
for pyomyositis, 1098
for respiratory infections, 882–884
for septic arthritis, 1095
for skin and soft tissue infections, 876–878

Vancouver model, for transition to adult care of rheumatic diseases, 647–649

Varicella
immunization for, 684
in college students, 236
in international adoptees, 1293
necrotizing fasciitis in, 1101
treatment of, 838–848

Varicella-autoantibody syndrome, 481

Varicocele, in college students, 204–206

Varni-Thompson Pediatric Pain Questionnaire (PPQ), 613–616

Vascular cell adhesion molecule-1, in inflammatory myopathies, 499

Vasculitis, **547–575**
Churg–Strauss syndrome, 568–569
classification of, 549–551
diagnosis of, 547–549
epidemiology of, 551
Henoch-Schönlein purpura, 430, 552–555
hypersensitivity, 554–555
in familial Mediterranean fever, 584
in inflammatory myopathies, 508
in systemic lupus erythematosus, 449–450

Kawasaki disease, 398–399, 430, 555–563
laboratory tests in, 548–549
microscopic polyangiitis, 568
pathogenesis of, 551–552
polyarteritis nodosa, 399–400, 563–565
primary, 550
primary angiitis of central nervous system, 566
radiology in, 398–402
secondary, 550, 569–570
Takayasu's arteritis, 401–402, 565–566
treatment of, transition to adult care. See Rheumatic diseases, transition to adult care.
Wegener's granulomatosis, 400–401, 566–568

Vasopressin, for ventricular fibrillation, 1219

Venlafaxine, for depression, 118

Venous thrombosis
from oral contraceptives, 144
in antiphospholipid antibody syndrome, 476

Ventilation, mechanical. See Mechanical ventilation.

Ventricle(s)
left
hypertrophy of, in cardiomyopathy, 1320
outflow obstruction of, in cardiomyopathy, 1324–1325
right, in arrhythmogenic right ventricular dysplasia, 1238–1239

Ventricular fibrillation, **1211–1221**
as re-entry, 1211–1213
cellular metabolic factors in, 1216–1218
clinical implications of, 1219–1220
defibrillation in, 1214–1216. See also Automated external defibrillators.
definition of, 1211
epidemiology of, 1445–1446
factors favoring, 1213–1214
in commotio cordis, 1347–1350
pharmacology of, 1218–1219
sudden cardiac death in, 1206
versus atrial fibrillation, 1213

Ventricular myosin essential light chain 1 defects, in hypertrophic cardiomyopathy, 1243–1244

Ventricular myosin regulatory light chain 2 defects, in hypertrophic cardiomyopathy, 1243–1244

Ventricular septal defect
in college students, 256
sudden cardiac death in, in athletes, 1411

United States Postal Service
Statement of Ownership, Management, and Circulation

1. Publication Title	2. Publication Number	3. Filing Date
Pediatric Clinics of North America	0 0 3 1 - 3 9 5 5	9/15/05

4. Issue Frequency	5. Number of Issues Published Annually	6. Annual Subscription Price
Feb, Apr, Jun, Aug, Oct, Dec	6	$135.00

7. Complete Mailing Address of Known Office of Publication *(Not printer)* *(Street, city, county, state, and ZIP+4)*

Elsevier Inc.
6277 Sea Harbor Drive
Orlando, FL 32887-4800

Contact Person
Gwen C. Campbell
Telephone
215-239-3685

8. Complete Mailing Address of Headquarters or General Business Office of Publisher *(Not printer)*

Elsevier Inc., 360 Park Avenue South, New York, NY 10010-1710

9. Full Names and Complete Mailing Addresses of Publisher, Editor, and Managing Editor *(Do not leave blank)*

Publisher *(Name and complete mailing address)*

Tim Griswold, Elsevier Inc., 1600 John F. Kennedy Blvd., Suite 1800, Philadelphia, PA 19103-2899

Editor *(Name and complete mailing address)*

Carin Davis, Elsevier Inc., 1600 John F. Kennedy Blvd., Suite 1800, Philadelphia, PA 19103-2899

Managing Editor *(Name and complete mailing address)*

Heather Cullen, Elsevier Inc., 1600 John F. Kennedy Blvd., Suite 1800, Philadelphia, PA 19103-2899

10. Owner *(Do not leave blank. If the publication is owned by a corporation, give the name and address of the corporation immediately followed by the names and addresses of all stockholders owning or holding 1 percent or more of the total amount of stock. If not owned by a corporation, give the names and addresses of the individual owners. If owned by a partnership or other unincorporated firm, give its name and address as well as those of each individual owner. If the publication is published by a nonprofit organization, give its name and address.)*

Full Name	Complete Mailing Address
Wholly owned subsidiary of	4520 East-West Highway
Reed/Elsevier Inc., US holdings	Bethesda, MD 20814

11. Known Bondholders, Mortgagees, and Other Security Holders Owning or Holding 1 Percent or More of Total Amount of Bonds, Mortgages, or Other Securities. If none, check box ▸ ☐ None

Full Name	Complete Mailing Address
N/A	

12. Tax Status *(For completion by nonprofit organizations authorized to mail at nonprofit rates)* *(Check one)*
The purpose, function, and nonprofit status of this organization and the exempt status for federal income tax purposes:
☐ Has Not Changed During Preceding 12 Months
☐ Has Changed During Preceding 12 Months *(Publisher must submit explanation of change with this statement)*

(See Instructions on Reverse)

PS Form 3526, October 1999

13. Publication Title	14. Issue Date for Circulation Data Below
Pediatric Clinics of North America	August 2005

15.	Extent and Nature of Circulation	Average No. Copies Each Issue During Preceding 12 Months	No. Copies of Single Issue Published Nearest to Filing Date
a.	Total Number of Copies *(Net press run)*	8450	7700
b. Paid and/or Requested Circulation	(1) Paid/Requested Outside-County Mail Subscriptions Stated on Form 3541. *(Include advertiser's proof and exchange copies)*	4677	4398
	(2) Paid In-County Subscriptions Stated on Form 3541 *(Include advertiser's proof and exchange copies)*		
	(3) Sales Through Dealers and Carriers, Street Vendors, Counter Sales, and Other Non-USPS Paid Distribution	2326	2233
	(4) Other Classes Mailed Through the USPS		
c.	Total Paid and/or Requested Circulation [Sum of 15b. (1), (2), (3), and (4)] ▸	7003	6631
d. Free Distribution by Mail (Samples, complimentary, and other free)	(1) Outside-County as Stated on Form 3541	105	109
	(2) In-County as Stated on Form 3541		
	(3) Other Classes Mailed Through the USPS		
e.	Free Distribution Outside the Mail *(Carriers or other means)*		
f.	Total Free Distribution *(Sum of 15d. and 15e.)* ▸	105	109
g.	Total Distribution *(Sum of 15c. and 15f.)* ▸	7108	6740
h.	Copies not Distributed	1342	960
i.	Total *(Sum of 15g. and h.)* ▸	8450	7700
j.	Percent Paid and/or Requested Circulation *(15c. divided by 15g. times 100)*	99%	98%

16. Publication of Statement of Ownership
☐ Publication required. Will be printed in the **December 2005** issue of this publication. ☐ Publication not required.

17. Signature and Title of Editor, Publisher, Business Manager, or Owner   Date

[signature] Jean Tamucci — Executive Director of Subscription Services   9/15/05

I certify that all information furnished on this form is true and complete. I understand that anyone who furnishes false or misleading information on this form or who omits material or information requested on the form may be subject to criminal sanctions (including fines and imprisonment) and/or civil sanctions (including civil penalties).

Instructions to Publishers

1. Complete and file one copy of this form with your postmaster annually on or before October 1. Keep a copy of the completed form for your records.

2. In cases where the stockholder or security holder is a trustee, include in items 10 and 11 the name of the person or corporation for whom the trustee is acting. Also include the names and addresses of individuals who are stockholders who own or hold 1 percent or more of the total amount of bonds, mortgages, or other securities of the publishing corporation. In item 11, if none, check the box. Use blank sheets if more space is required.

3. Be sure to furnish all circulation information called for in item 15. Free circulation must be shown in items 15d, e, and f.

4. Item 15h., Copies not Distributed, must include (1) newsstand copies originally stated on Form 3541, and returned to the publisher, (2) estimated returns from news agents, and (3), copies for office use, leftovers, spoiled, and all other copies not distributed.

5. If the publication had Periodicals authorization as a general or requester publication, this Statement of Ownership, Management, and Circulation must be published; it must be printed in any issue in October or, if the publication is not published during October, the first issue printed after October.

6. In item 16, indicate the date of the issue in which this Statement of Ownership will be published.

7. Item 17 must be signed.

Failure to file or publish a statement of ownership may lead to suspension of Periodicals authorization.

PS Form 3526, October 1999 *(Reverse)*

Changing Your Address?

Make sure your subscription changes too! When you notify us of your new address, you can help make our job easier by including an exact copy of your Clinics label number with your old address (see illustration below.) This number identifies you to our computer system and will speed the processing of your address change. Please be sure this label number accompanies your old address and your corrected address—you can send an old Clinics label with your number on it or just copy it exactly and send it to the address listed below.

We appreciate your help in our attempt to give you continuous coverage. Thank you.

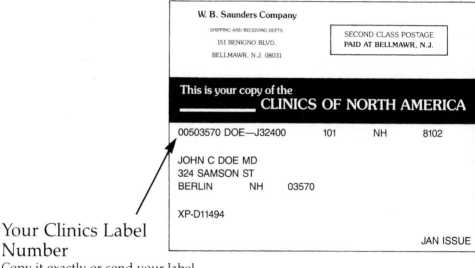

Your Clinics Label Number
Copy it exactly or send your label
along with your address to:
W.B. Saunders Company, Customer Service
Orlando, FL 32887-4800
Call Toll Free 1-800-654-2452

Please allow four to six weeks for delivery of new subscriptions and for processing address changes.